LECTURE NOTES ON

Clinical Medicine

DAVID RUBENSTEIN

MA MD FRCP
Consultant Physician
Addenbrooke's Hospital
Cambridge

DAVID WAYNE

MA BM FRCP
Consultant Physician
James Paget Hospital
Great Yarmouth

WITHDRAWN

JOHN BRADLEY

B Med Sci MA DM FRCP
Consultant Physician
Addenbrooke's Hospital
Cambridge

Sixth edition

Blackwell
Science

First published 1976
Reprinted 1977, 1978, 1979
Second edition 1980
Reprinted 1981, 1982, 1983, 1984
Third edition 1985
Reprinted 1986, 1987, 1990
Portuguese translation 1981
Spanish translation 1984
German translation 1986

Fourth edition 1991
Reprinted 1992, 1994, 1995, 1996,
1997
Four Dragons edition 1991
Reprinted 1992, 1994, 1996
Fifth edition 1997
Reprinted 1998, 2000, 2001
Sixth edition 2003
7   2009

Library of Congress Cataloging-in-Publication Data
Rubenstein, David.
   Lecture notes on clinical medicine / David Rubenstein, David Wayne, John
Bradley.—6th ed.
      p. ; cm.
   Includes index.
     ISBN 978-0-6320-6505-9
     1. Clinical medicine—Handbooks, manuals, etc.
   [DNLM: 1. Clinical Medicine—Handbooks. WB 39 R895L 2002] I. Wayne, David.
   II. Bradley, John, MRCP. III. Title.
   RC48 .R8 2002
     616—dc21

                                                          2002006193

ISBN 978-0-6320-6505-9

A catalogue record for this title is a available from the British Library

Set in 9/11.5pt Gill Sans by Graphicraft Limited, Hong Kong
Printed and bound in Malaysia by KHL Printing Co Sdn Bhd

Commissioning Editor: Vicki Noyes
Production Editor: Jessica Mautner
Production Controller: Kate Charman

For further information on Blackwell Publishing, visit our website:
www.blackwellpublishing.com

Contents

Preface to the Sixth Edition

The sixth edition follows the format of the previous editions of this book with two sections: The Clinical Approach and Essential Background Information. The chapters on haematology, dermatology and diabetes, previously divided between the two sections, have been amalgamated.

Following many helpful suggestions from our readers, we have supplied further illustrations, and added chest X-rays (PA and lateral) with explanatory line diagrams, and CT scans of the chest and abdomen, also with line diagrams.

It is rewarding to discover how many readers have found the text useful for study, for revision and for the practice of clinical medicine. Please continue to let us have your views.

David Rubenstein
David Wayne
John Bradley

Preface to the First Edition

This book is intended primarily for the junior hospital doctor in the period between qualification and the examination for Membership of the Royal Colleges of Physicians. We think that it will also be helpful to final-year medical students and to clinicians reading for higher specialist qualifications in surgery and anaesthetics.

The hospital doctor must not only acquire a large amount of factual information but also use it effectively in the clinical situation. The experienced physician has acquired some clinical perspective through practice: we hope that this book imparts some of this to the relatively inexperienced. The format and contents are designed for the examination candidate but the same approach to problems should help the hospital doctor in his everyday work.

The book as a whole is not suitable as a first reader for the undergraduate because it assumes much basic knowledge and considerable detailed information has had to be omitted. It is not intended to be a complete textbook of medicine and the information it contains must be supplemented by further reading. The contents are intended only as lecture notes and the margins of the pages are intentionally large so that the reader may easily add additional material of his own.

The book is divided into two parts: the *clinical approach* and *essential background information*. In the first part we have considered the situation which a candidate meets in the clinical part of an examination or a physician in the clinic. This part of the book thus resembles a manual on techniques of physical examination, though it is more specifically intended to help the candidate carry out an examiner's request to perform a specific examination. It has been our experience in listening to candidates' performances in examinations and hearing the examiner's subsequent assessment, that it is the failure of a candidate to examine cases systematically and his failure to behave as if he were used to doing this every day of his clinical life that leads to adverse comments.

In the second part of the book a summary of basic clinical facts is given in the conventional way. We have included most common diseases but not all, and we have tried to emphasise points which are understressed in many textbooks. Accounts are given of many conditions which are relatively rare. It is necessary for the clinician to know about these and to be on the lookout for them both in the clinic and in examinations. Supplementary reading is essential to understand their basic pathology but the information we give is probably all that need be remembered by the non-specialist reader and will provide adequate working knowledge in a clinical situation. It should not be forgotten that some rare diseases are of great importance in practice because they are treatable or preventable, e.g. infective endocarditis, hepatolenticular degeneration, attacks of acute porphyria. Some conditions are important to examination candidates because patients are ambulant and appear commonly in examinations, e.g. neurosyphilis, syringomyelia, atrial and ventricular septal defects.

We have not attempted to cover the whole of medicine but by cross-referencing between the two sections of the book and giving information in summary form we have completely omitted few subjects. Some highly specialised fields such as the treatment of leukaemia were thought unsuitable for inclusion.

A short account of psychiatry is given in the section on neurology since many patients with mental illness attend general clinics and it is hoped that readers may be warned of gaps in their knowledge of this important field. The section on dermatology is incomplete but should serve for quick revision of common skin disorders.

Wherever possible we have tried to indicate the relative frequency with which various conditions are likely to be seen in hospital practice in this country and have selected those clinical features which in our view are most commonly seen and where possible have listed them in order of importance. The frequency with which a disease is encountered by any individual physician will depend upon its prevalence in the district from which his cases are drawn and also on his known special interests. Nevertheless, rare conditions are rarely seen; at least in the clinic. Examinations, however, are a 'special case'.

We have used many generally accepted abbreviations, e.g. ECG, ESR, and have included them in the index instead of supplying a glossary.

Despite our best efforts, some errors of fact may have been included. As with every book and authority, question and check everything—and please write to us if you wish.

We should like to thank all those who helped us with producing this book and in particular, Sir Edward Wayne and Sir Graham Bull who have kindly allowed us to benefit from their extensive experience both in medicine and in examining for the Colleges of Physicians.

David Rubenstein
David Wayne
November 1975

The Clinical Approach

Nervous System

The candidate is usually asked to examine a specific area, e.g. 'Examine the cranial nerves', 'Examine the lower limbs', 'Examine the arms' or 'Examine the eyes'. The most common neurological disorders suitable for a clinical examination are multiple sclerosis and the results of cerebrovascular disease. Diabetes is a common disorder that gives rise to neurological manifestations. Carcinomatous neuropathy should always be considered when the signs are difficult to synthesize. Parkinsonism is relatively common. Motor neuron disease (MND), myopathies, myasthenia gravis and the neurological manifestations of vitamin B_{12} deficiency are all rare in practice but more frequently seen in examinations.

In terms of examination technique the practising physician must examine case after case, both normal and abnormal, in order to develop a system which is rapid, accurate and which becomes second nature. An appearance of professionalism in your neurological examination may encourage the examiner to take a kinder view of minor errors than if you appear hesitant, clumsy or imprecise. Analysis of clinical signs is improved if you can remember some anatomical diagrams such as those in this chapter.

Cranial nerves

'Examine the cranial nerves' Many abnormalities of the cranial nerves are the results of chronic disease. Such patients are commonly seen in examinations.

The most common disorders in examinations are multiple sclerosis (optic atrophy, nystagmus (often ataxic), cerebellar dysarthria), stroke and Bell's palsy. The manifestations of cerebral tumour, aneurysm, dystrophia myotonica and myasthenia gravis are seen much less frequently. It is useful to memorize diagrams of cross-sections of the brainstem and of the floor of the fourth ventricle (Figs 1.1–1.3) because these may greatly improve analysis of a cranial nerve lesion. Do not spend long on the 1st or 2nd cranial nerves unless there is good reason to suspect an abnormality. If the optic fundus is abnormal, the examiner is likely to ask you to look at it specifically. Eye movements must be carefully examined. Do not confuse ptosis (3rd nerve or sympathetic) with paresis of the orbicularis oculi (7th nerve). Make sure you can explain clearly and concisely the difference between an upper and lower motor neuron (UMN and LMN) lesion of the 7th nerve. The corneal reflex is an essential part of the complete examination of the cranial nerves.

The following approach is recommended.

Smell
'Has there been any recent change in your sense of smell?' If so, test formally with fresh 'smell bottles' (e.g. freshly ground coffee or instant coffee granules). Colds and sinusitis are the most likely cause. However, previous head trauma may have resulted in severance of the 1st cranial nerve at the cribriform plate with resultant isolated anosmia.

Eyes
Observe, and test when necessary, for the following.
• Visual acuity, either quickly with literature from the bedside locker, formally with Snellen charts or counting fingers if vision is very poor.

THE SPINAL CORD

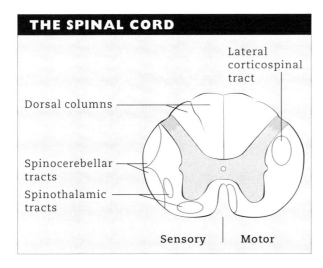

Lateral corticospinal tract

Dorsal columns

Spinocerebellar tracts

Spinothalamic tracts

Sensory | Motor

Fig. 1.1 Cross-section through the spinal cord.

THE OPEN MEDULLA

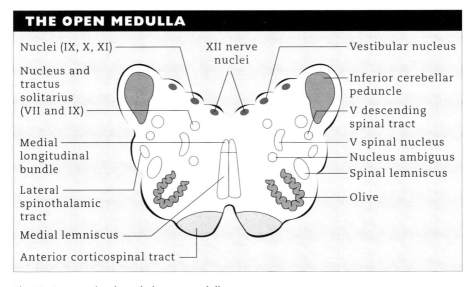

Nuclei (IX, X, XI)

Nucleus and tractus solitarius (VII and IX)

Medial longitudinal bundle

Lateral spinothalamic tract

Medial lemniscus

Anterior corticospinal tract

XII nerve nuclei

Vestibular nucleus

Inferior cerebellar peduncle

V descending spinal tract

V spinal nucleus

Nucleus ambiguus

Spinal lemniscus

Olive

Fig. 1.2 Cross-section through the open medulla.

- *Ptosis*
  (a) third nerve lesion (complete or partial ptosis);
  (b) sympathetic lesion (partial ptosis) as part of Horner syndrome; and
  (c) muscle weakness of myasthenia gravis (and, rarely, dystrophia myotonica, facio-scapulohumeral dystrophy, congenital and in taboparesis).
NB Ptosis is not caused by a 7th-nerve lesion.
- *Pupillary responses* (p. 8).

- *Visual fields* to confrontation (2nd nerve, p. 6).
- *External ocular movements* (3rd, 4th and 6th nerve, p. 7) and *nystagmus* (p. 10).
- The *fundi* (2nd nerve, p. 25).

Face (7th nerve)
- '*Screw up your eyes very tightly.*' Compare how deeply the eyelashes are buried on the two sides. Unilateral weakness is invariably caused by an LMN lesion.
- '*Grin.*' Compare the nasolabial grooves.

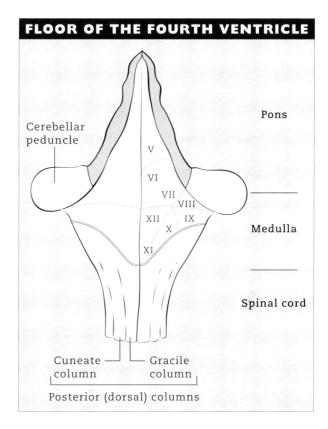

FLOOR OF THE FOURTH VENTRICLE

Cerebellar
peduncle

Pons

V

VI

VII

VIII

XII   IX

X

XI

Medulla

Spinal cord

Cuneate
column

Gracile
column

Posterior (dorsal) columns

Fig. 1.3 Floor of the fourth
ventricle showing cranial
nerve nuclei.

Mouth

• *'Clench your teeth'* (5th nerve, motor). Feel the masseters and test the jaw jerk if indicated. The jaw jerk is obtained from placing one finger horizontally across the front of the jaw and tapping the finger with a tendon hammer with the jaw relaxed and the mouth just open. An increased jaw jerk occurs in UMN lesions of the 5th cranial nerves (pseudobulbar palsy, p. 12).

• *'Open your mouth and keep it open'* (5th nerve, motor: pterygoids). You should not be able to force it closed—but do not push too hard. With a unilateral lesion, the jaw deviates towards the weaker side (the weak muscle cannot keep it open).

• *'Say aaah'* (9th and 10th nerves: both mixed, but the 9th is mainly sensory for the pharynx and palate, and the 10th motor). Normally the uvula and soft palate move upwards and remain central and the posterior pharyngeal wall moves little. With a unilateral lesion the soft palate is pulled away from the weaker side (there may also be 'curtain movement' of the posterior pharyngeal wall away from the weaker side).

• *'Put your tongue out'* (12th nerve). Look for wasting, fasciculation and whether it protrudes to one side (towards the weaker side because the weaker muscle cannot push it out).

Neck (11th nerve)

• *'Lift your head off the pillows'* or *'Put your chin on your right (or left) shoulder'* while you resist the movement. Look at and palpate the sternomastoids.

• *'Shrug your shoulders'* while you push them down. Look at and palpate the bulk of trapezius.

Ears (8th nerve)

Test hearing by whispering in each ear and perform Weber and Rinne tests (p. 9). You

VISUAL FIELD DEFECTS

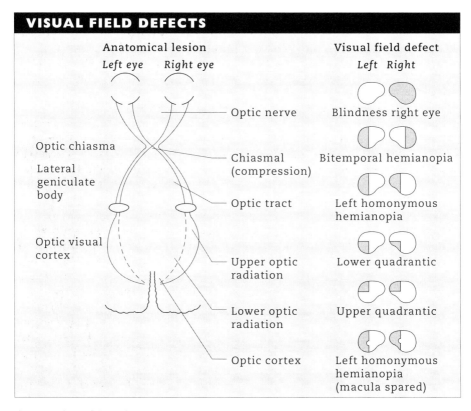

Fig. 1.4 Lesions of the optic nerve and tract and effects on visual fields. 'Macular sparing': the macula has extensive cortical representation and may be spared by lesions of the visual cortex.

should ask for an auriscope if indicated. The most common cause of conductive (air conduction) deafness is wax.

Facial sensation (5th nerve)

Test the three divisions on both sides with cotton wool. Check the corneal reflexes (often the first clinical deficit in 5th nerve lesions). Ask the patient if the sensation is equally unpleasant on the two sides.
NB It is frequently helpful to be able to draw cross-sections of the spinal cord and brainstem when considering lesions in those areas (see Figs 1.1–1.3).

Field defects

In principle you are comparing the patient's visual fields with your own. When testing the right eye, the patient should be level with you and look straight into your left eye with the patient's head held at arm's length. 'Keep looking at my eye and tell me when you first see my finger out of the corner of your eye.' Then bring your finger towards the centre of the field of vision from the four main directions (right, left, up, down). It is preferable to use a white-headed hatpin if you have one.

The nasal and superior fields are limited by the nose and eyebrow, respectively, but this is not often of clinical importance. Field defects (Fig. 1.4) are described by the side of the visual field which is lost, i.e. temporal field loss indicates loss of the temporal field of vision and denotes damage to the nasal retina or its connections back to the visual cortex. Perimetry will accurately define defects.

• *Temporal hemianopia* in one eye alone or in both eyes (bitemporal hemianopia) suggests a chiasmal compression, usually from a pituitary tumour.

• *Homonymous hemianopia* (loss of nasal field in one eye and temporal field in the other, i.e. to the same side of the body). This may occur with any postchiasmal lesion, most commonly following a vascular lesion affecting the occipital cortex (usually with macular sparing, because of the dual blood supply to the occipital cortex from the posterior and middle cerebral arteries). The side of the field loss is opposite to the side of the damaged cortex (i.e. a right-sided cerebral lesion produces a left homonymous hemianopia).
• *Upper quadrantic field loss* suggests a temporal lesion of the opposite cortex or optic radiation, and a lower quadrantic field loss suggests a parietal one. They are homonymous.
• *Central scotoma.* Loss of vision in the centre of the visual field is detected by passing a small-diameter white- or red-tipped pin across the front of the eyes, which are held looking forward. This occurs in acute retrobulbar neuritis most commonly caused by multiple sclerosis.
• Test for visual inattention—extinction and hemi-neglect—(p. 104) by presenting the stimulus simultaneously to both eyes. These suggest a right posterior parietal lesion.

Blindness

A history of transient blindness, total or partial (with specific field defects usually in one eye) is not uncommon in migraine. Carotid transient ischaemic attacks (TIAs) cause transient unilateral blindness (p. 90).

Sudden blindness also occurs with:
• retinal detachment;
• acute glaucoma;
• stroke involving the visual cortex;
• vitreous haemorrhage in diabetes;
• retinal artery or vein obstruction in temporal arteritis;
• fractures of the skull; and
• raised intracranial pressure.
NB The light reflex is absent except in cortical blindness.

Senile changes and *glaucoma* account for about two-thirds of blindness in the UK. Diabetes is the major non-ocular (systemic) cause (7–10%) chiefly as a result of vitreous haemorrhage, advanced retinopathy and cataract.

Trachoma is a common cause on a worldwide basis. *Hysterical blindness* is uncommon and should never be confidently assumed.

The blindness of *temporal arteritis* is preventable if steroid therapy is started in time.

Eye movements

These are controlled by the 3rd, 4th and 6th nerves. Conjugate movement is integrated by the medial longitudinal bundle, which connects the above nuclei together and to the cerebellum and the vestibular nuclei.

Squint (strabismus)

Congenital concomitant squints are present from childhood and are caused by a defect of one eye. The angle between the longitudinal axes of the eyes remains constant on testing extraocular movements, and there is no diplopia.

Paralytic squint is acquired and results from paralysis of one or more of the muscles that move the eye, or paralysis from proptosis. On testing external ocular movements, the angle between the eye axes varies and there is diplopia. The following rules should be borne in mind.
1 Diplopia is maximal when looking in the direction of action of the paralysed muscle.
2 The image further from the midline arises from the paralysed eye. This may be determined by covering up each eye in turn and asking which image has disappeared.
NB It is sometimes easier to test movements in each eye separately.

'*Do you see double?*' If so, ask in which direction it is worst. Move your forefinger in that direction and then ask if the two fingers that the patient sees are parallel to each other (lateral rectus palsy: 6th nerve) or at an angle (superior oblique palsy: 4th nerve). If the patient has not noticed diplopia, test the movements formally, right and left, up and down, and note if there is any nystagmus.

Apart from local lesions, such as pressure from tumour or aneurysm, isolated external ocular palsies may result from diabetes mellitus (ischaemia), multiple sclerosis, migraine, raised intracranial pressure, mononeuritis multiplex (e.g. polyarteritis) and, rarely, from sarcoidosis, syphilis (ischaemia) and meningitis (usually tuberculosis or pneumococcal).

Lateral rectus palsy (6th nerve)

This produces failure of lateral movement with convergent strabismus. It is the most common external ocular palsy. The diplopia is maximal on looking to the affected side. The images are parallel and separated horizontally. The outer-most image comes from the affected eye and disappears when that eye is covered. The palsy is produced as a false localizing sign in raised intracranial pressure or by direct involvement with tumour, aneurysm or, rarely, with acoustic neuroma (p. 104).

Superior oblique palsy (4th nerve)

This type is rare. Palsy produces diplopia that is maximal on downward gaze. The two images are then at an angle to each other when the palsied eye is abducted and one above the other when the eye is adducted. The diplopia is therefore noticed most on reading or descending stairs.

Third nerve palsy

It may not present with diplopia because there may be complete ptosis. When the lid is lifted the eye is seen to be 'down and out' (divergent strabismus) and there is severe (angulated) diplopia. The pupil may be dilated. It occurs with space-occupying lesions, brainstem vascular lesions (Weber syndrome) after surgery (e.g. for pituitary lesions) and aneurysm of the posterior communicating artery (painful).

The muscles themselves are involved in myasthenia gravis (p. 116) and in the ophthalmoplegia of thyrotoxicosis (p. 141), particularly looking up and out.

Pupillary reflexes

Pupil size is controlled by the balance between parasympathetic (constrictor) and sympathetic (dilator) tone.

Constriction of the pupil in response to light. This is relayed via the optic nerve, optic tract, lateral geniculate nuclei, the Edinger–Westphal nucleus

of the 3rd nerve and the ciliary ganglion. The cortex is not involved.

Constriction of the pupil with accommodation. Convergence originates within the cortex and is relayed to the pupil via the 3rd nerve nuclei. The optic nerve and tract and the lateral geniculate nucleus are not involved.

Therefore:
• if the direct light reflex is absent and the convergence reflex is present, a local lesion in the brainstem or ciliary ganglion is implied, possibly as a result of degeneration in the ciliary ganglia, e.g. the Argyll Robertson pupil of syphilis;
• if the convergence reflex is absent and the light reflex is present, a lesion of the cerebral cortex is implied, e.g. cortical blindness.

Examination of the pupillary reflexes should be performed in subdued light. The pupil should be positively inspected for irregularity. A torch is flashed twice at each eye (once for direct and once for consensual responses), preferably from the side so that the patient does not focus on it (and hence have an accommodation–convergence reflex).

If the pupil is constricted consider: Horner's syndrome (below), morphine, pilocarpine, pontine haemorrhage and Argyll Robertson pupil (must be irregular and have no light reflex). It also occurs in normal old age.

If the pupil is dilated consider: mydriatics (e.g. homatropine, tropicamide or cyclopentolate), a 3rd-nerve lesion, the Holmes–Adie syndrome (pupils constrict sluggishly to light, e.g. in half an hour in a bright room, and absent tendon reflexes) and congenital (ask the patient). In the unconscious patient a fixed dilated pupil (3rd-nerve lesion) may indicate temporal lobe herniation (from raised intracranial pressure) on the same side, intracranial bleeding, tumour or abscess.

Horner's syndrome

This is rare in practice but common in examinations. The syndrome comprises unilateral:
• ptosis (partial, i.e. sympathetic);
• miosis (constricted pupil) with normal reactions;

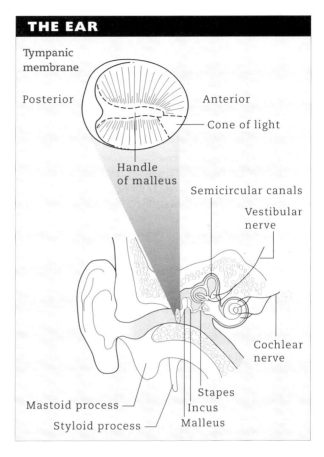

Fig. 1.5 The anatomy of the ear.

• anhidrosis (decreased sweating over face); and
• enophthalmos (indrawing of orbital contents), i.e. everything gets smaller or contracts.

The syndrome results from lesions of the sympathetic nerves to the eye, anywhere from the hypothalamus downwards through the sympathetic nucleus of the brainstem and during their passage through the cervical and upper thoracic cord, the anterior spinal first thoracic root, the sympathetic chain, stellate ganglion and carotid sympathetic plexus. It is essential to look for evidence of a T1 lesion and to palpate the neck and supraclavicular fossae for malignant glands.

Aetiology
• Carcinoma of the bronchus (T1, Pancoast tumour, p. 244).

• Cervical node secondary deposits.
• Cervical sympathectomy (look for the scar).
• Brainstem vascular disease (lateral medullary syndrome, p. 87) and demyelinating disease.
• Local neoplasms and trauma in the neck.
• Rarely, carotid or aortic aneurysms.
• Very rarely, syringomyelia and intrinsic cervical cord disease (vascular and neoplastic).

Hearing
The anatomy of the ear is shown in Fig. 1.5. Roughly assess auditory acuity in each ear in succession by blocking the sound in the other ear with a fingertip and then whispering at arm's length. Compare the two sides.

Weber test
A vibrating tuning fork is held in the middle of the forehead. In the absence of nerve deafness,

the sound is louder in the ear where air conduction is impaired, e.g. wax or otitis media. This sign can easily be checked by placing a vibrating tuning fork on one's own forehead and putting a finger in one ear.

Rinne test

Air conduction is normally better than bone conduction. The vibrating tuning fork is first placed behind the ear on the mastoid process and then rapidly held with its prongs in line with the external meatus. The patient is asked: 'Is it louder behind (with the tuning fork on the mastoid) or in front (with the tuning fork in line with the external meatus)?' Normally it is louder in front—this is termed Rinne-positive. Negative is abnormal and implies conductive (air) deafness in that ear—usually wax.

Dizziness and giddiness

Dizziness and giddiness are very common neurological presenting features.

The important clinical observation is to determine whether there is true vertigo or not (see below). If this is present, it strongly suggests a disorder of the brainstem (vascular or demyelinating) or its vestibular connections, e.g. labyrinthitis, Ménière disease (see below). Dizziness or unsteadiness without vertigo, particularly if intermittent, may suggest postural hypotension, which is relatively common in the elderly, in those on overenthusiastic hypotensive regimens and in those who stand stationary too long, particularly in warm weather. It may also suggest a cardiovascular disorder such as a transient cardiac arrhythmia including heart block or, less commonly, aortic stenosis or emboli, e.g. from carotid artery atheroma. Transient dizzy sensations may very rarely be a feature of temporal lobe epilepsy (p. 94). Usually no organic cause is found and the complaint may be a marker of emotional distress. NB 'Something wrong with the brain, think of the heart.'

Vertigo

Vertigo refers to unsteadiness with a subjective sensation of rotation of the patient or of the environment around. Vertigo results from disease of the inner ear, 8th cranial nerve or its connections in the brainstem.

Labyrinthine. Ménière disease, acute labyrinthitis.

Eighth nerve. Acoustic neuroma and other posterior fossa tumours, aminoglycosides (streptomycin and gentamicin).

Brainstem. Neoplasm, vascular disease (vertebrobasilar ischaemia, lateral medullary syndrome), demyelination (multiple sclerosis), migraine, aneurysms, degeneration (syringobulbia).

Ménière disease

The onset is usually in people over 40 years old with progressive deafness and tinnitus, usually only in one ear. There are attacks of vertigo, nausea and vomiting. Attacks cease when deafness is complete. Progression can be so slow that this may never occur. Examination shows a defect of 8th nerve conduction and abnormal results to caloric tests of vestibular function. Nystagmus is present during attacks of vertigo.

Treatment

Phenothiazines (e.g. prochlorperazine) and some antihistamines (e.g. promethazine) act as sedatives and against nausea during acute episodes. They may reduce the incidence and severity of attacks. Betahistine, a histamine analogue, may specifically help in this condition by reducing endolymph pressure. If very severe, ultrasonic destruction of the labyrinth should be considered, although it results in total deafness on that side.

Nystagmus

Nystagmus may result from any disturbance of either the 8th nerve and its connections in the brainstem or the cerebellum, and in phenytoin intoxication. Its direction is named after the quick phase (of 'saw-tooth' nystagmus). Nystagmus is usually more pronounced when the patient looks in the direction of the quick phase. Nystagmoid jerks may be produced in normal eyes by errors of examination technique—either holding the object too close to the patient or too far to one side.

Horizontal nystagmus

Vestibular nystagmus occurs following damage to the inner ear, 8th nerve or to its brainstem connections and is present only in the first few weeks after the damage because central compensation occurs. It is greater on looking *away* from the side of a destructive lesion. It may be caused by acute viral labyrinthitis, acute alcoholism, Ménière disease, middle-ear disease and surgery. It is usually associated with vertigo and often with vomiting, deafness and tinnitus. Multiple sclerosis, basilar artery ischaemia and syringobulbia cause less constitutional upset.

Cerebellar nystagmus occurs usually with lateral lobe lesions; even central (vermis) lesions causing severe truncal ataxia may cause no nystagmus. As cerebellar disease is frequently bilateral, nystagmus may occur to both sides. If it is unilateral it is greater *towards* the side of the *destructive* lesion.

Cerebellar lesions occur in multiple sclerosis, hereditary ataxias and vascular disease.

Nystagmus is often seen in patients who have taken high doses (although sometimes within the therapeutic range) of sedative drugs, especially phenytoin and barbiturates.

Ataxic nystagmus. The degree of nystagmus in the abducting eye is greater than in the adducting eye, which may fail to adduct completely. This is virtually pathognomonic of multiple sclerosis and is caused by damage to the medial longitudinal bundle.

Vertical nystagmus

The direction of jerks is vertical. Vertical gaze usually makes it more pronounced. It may be produced by sedative drugs (especially phenytoin) but otherwise localizes disease to the brainstem (although brainstem disorders more commonly produce horizontal nystagmus).

Pendular and rotary nystagmus

Unlike all the above, the phases of the nystagmus are equal in duration. It is secondary to an inability to fix objects and focus with one or both eyes because of partial blindness, e.g. albinism.

Facial palsy

In unilateral UMN lesions (e.g. stroke) movements of the upper face are retained because it is represented on both sides of the cerebral cortex. A flattened forehead and sagging lower eyelid are seen in complete LMN lesions (e.g. Bell's palsy and middle-ear surgery). Taste sensation from the tongue in the chorda tympani leaves the facial nerve in the middle ear, and therefore loss of taste over the anterior two-thirds of the tongue means that a facial nerve paresis must be caused by a lesion above this level, e.g. herpes zoster of the geniculate ganglion—the Ramsay Hunt syndrome. Lesions caused by tumours of the parotid gland do not give these signs. Facial palsy is a very late sign of acoustic neuroma. It may occur in an unusually extensive lateral medullary syndrome (p. 87).

Aetiology of cranial nerve palsies

The causes of single-nerve palsies include cerebral aneurysm, diabetes mellitus, trauma, surgery, cerebral tumour and multiple sclerosis. The various eponymous vascular lesions of the brainstem need not be separately remembered, but you should be able to discuss the localization of such lesions with the help of diagrams; they are relatively common causes of cranial nerve palsy. Polyarteritis nodosa, sarcoidosis, meningitis and Wernicke's encephalopathy are less common causes.

Speech disorders

'*Would you like to ask this patient some questions?*' It is likely that the patient has a speech disorder, but there may be some degree of dementia (p. 118).

• Ask name, age, occupation and address.

• Test orientation in time (date, season) and place, for dementia.

• If indicated, test memory and intellectual capacity.

• Test ability to name familiar objects (pen, coins, watch)—nominal dysphasia.

• Test articulation, e.g. 'baby hippopotamus', 'West Register Street'.

• If dysarthria is present, look in the mouth for local lesions and test the lower cranial nerves.

BULBAR AND PSEUDOBULBAR PALSIES

	Pseudobulbar (UMN lesion)	Bulbar (LMN lesion)
Emotions	Labile	Normal
Dysarthria	Donald Duck speech	Nasal
Tongue	Spastic, small for mouth	Flaccid, fasciculating
Jaw jerk	Increased	Normal or absent
Associated findings	Bilateral UMN lesions of limbs	Sometimes other evidence of MND, e.g. fasciculation in limbs

LMN, Lower motor neuron; MND, motor neuron disease; UMN, upper motor neuron.

Table 1.1 Clinical signs of bulbar and pseudobulbar palsies.

Dysphasia (or aphasia)

This is a disorder of the symbolic aspects of language, both written and spoken. In right-handed people and 50% of left-handed people, the left hemisphere is dominant in this respect. It usually follows cerebrovascular accidents and hence is common. Before assessing dysphasia it is important to exclude a dysarthria caused by a neuromuscular lesion affecting the muscles of speech. Depression and parkinsonism may cause slow responses but not a dysphasia.

Pure expressive (motor) dysphasia tends to result from lesions in the postero-inferior part of the frontal lobe (Broca's area, see Fig. 8.3, p. 82). Word finding is difficult, sometimes with no speech at all. Understanding can be preserved. A form of expressive dysphasia where patients cannot name objects while knowing what they are is called 'nominal dysphasia' (e.g. Ask when holding up a pen, 'What is this?' Pause. 'Is it a watch?' 'No.' 'Is it a key?' 'No.' 'Is it a pen?' 'Yes'). It is associated with spatial problems such as dressing and constructional apraxias.

Receptive (sensory) dysphasia results from lesions of the dominant temporo-parietal lobes (Wernicke's area, see Fig. 8.3, p. 82). There is a specific failure to understand the meaning of words which can produce 'fluent dysphasia' when the patient happily produces meaningless jargon.

Dysarthria

Inability to articulate properly because of local lesions in the mouth or disorders of the mus-cles of speech or their connections. There is no disorder of the content of speech.

- Paralysis of cranial nerves, e.g. Bell's palsy (7th), 9th, 10th or 12th nerves.
- Cerebellar disease—'scanning' speech or staccato, seen in multiple sclerosis.
- Parkinson disease: speech is slow, quiet, slurred and monotonous.
- Pseudobulbar palsy (spastic dysarthria): mono-tonous, high-pitched 'hot potato' speech (rare).
- Progressive bulbar palsy (rare).
- Stutter (usually physiological).

Bulbar and pseudobulbar palsies (Table 1.1)

Both forms are rare. The symptoms of dysarthria, dysphagia and nasal regurgitation result from paralysis of the 9th, 10th and 12th cranial nerves.

Pseudobulbar (UMN) palsy is more common than bulbar palsy and is caused by bilateral lesions of the internal capsule, most often the result of cerebrovascular accidents affecting both sides, usually sequentially. It can also occur in multiple sclerosis (p. 97). Bulbar (LMN) palsy is rare because motor neuron disease (MND), and the infective causes (poliomyelitis, Guillain–Barré), are rare.

Tests of higher cerebral functions

'*Would you like to have a few words with this patient?*' or '*Assess the higher cerebral functions*'

or 'Assess this patient's personality/mental state/ intellectual function'
This usually implies dysphasia, dysarthria or dementia (p. 118). You should have some all-purpose questions to ask such as 'What is your name?' 'Where do you live?' or 'What is your job?' The answers to these questions may give you some indication of the best lines for further questioning.

Orientation. Orientation in time and space is assessed by asking the patient his or her name, the date, and the place of the interview.

Motivation. Non-dominant lesions may cause loss of motivation.

Personality and mood. Subtle personality changes are best obtained from the relatives' history. Recent personality changes are common in depression, with feelings of exhaustion, guilt and self-deprecation and a tendency to cry when asked 'Are you depressed?'
  In dementia, the common personality changes are lack of social awareness, e.g. a previously religious person blaspheming in front of the vicar, lack of love for close and previously loved relatives and lack of interest in dress and appearance. In disseminated sclerosis, patients frequently appear happy despite serious disability. (This is also seen in other lesions of the frontal lobes.) Labile emotional expression with alternate laughing and crying for no obvious cause, and often without appropriate mood, is a feature of pseudobulbar palsy (see above).

Intellectual function. Intellectual function tests must be related to the patient's previous abilities.
  Loss of memory for recent events more than for distant events is a feature of organic cerebral disease and an early feature of dementia. Commonly used tests of intellectual function are as follow.
1 Naming the monarch, prime minister, members of favourite sports teams, famous places and capitals.
2 Serial 7s: the patient is asked to subtract successive 7s from 100.

3 Ability to remember numbers forward and backward. Most people can remember five or more forward and four or more backward.
4 Repetition of complex sentences, e.g. the Babcock sentence: 'The one thing a nation requires to be rich and famous is a large secure supply of wood.'
5 Interpretation of proverbs, e.g. 'People who live in glass houses should not throw stones.'

Dyslexia (difficulty in reading), dysgraphia (difficulty in writing) and dyscalculia (difficulty in calculating) are features of lesions in the posterior parietal lobe.

Agnosia is inability to understand or recognize objects and forms in the presence of normal peripheral sensation. Tactile agnosia is most common and tested by asking the patient to recognize and distinguish objects placed in the hand (astereognosis) or figures drawn on the palm with the eyes closed (dysgraphaesthesia).
  Agnosia denotes damage to the contralateral sensory cortex. Inability to recognize objects when viewed (visual agnosia) denotes a lesion of the occipital cortex.

Apraxia is the inability to perform complex and sequential actions to command in the presence of normal coordination, sensation and motor power. It occurs with lesions of the parietal cortices connected by the corpus callosum, e.g. inability to light a match (given the closed box); difficulty dressing (dressing dyspraxia) and inability to copy designs (constructional dyspraxia—most often seen in patients with hepatocellular failure).

Arms

Note: Figs 1.6 and 1.7 give an overview of the motor and sensory systems.

'*Examine this patient's arms (neurologically)*' You may be asked to look at a patient whose neurological syndrome involving the arm is part of a more central lesion such as a stroke or cerebral tumour (perhaps producing cortical sensory or motor loss), a cerebellar lesion,

MOTOR SYSTEM

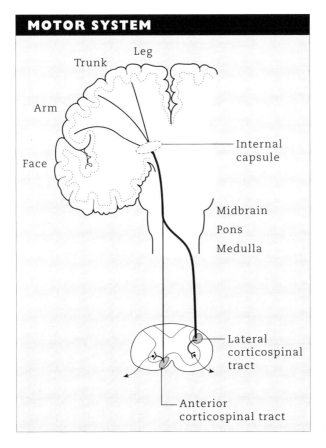

Fig. 1.6 Motor pathways.

brainstem involvement or cervical cord disease (e.g. vascular disease, tumour, syringomyelia). Isolated peripheral nerve lesions are common; peripheral neuropathies affecting the hands alone are not.

Amongst the most common neurological lesions of the arms are:
• *carpal tunnel syndrome* (median nerve palsy);
• *ulnar nerve palsy* (usually involved in the ulnar groove at the elbow—by osteoarthritis or trauma); and
• *cervical spondylosis* (usually affecting roots C5 and C6 but occasionally lower).
All three syndromes may present with motor and/or sensory signs and symptoms.

A mononeuropathy is usually a result of a mechanical cause or old injury and is only rarely caused by polyarteritis, diabetes mellitus, sarcoidosis or underlying carcinoma. Leprosy is very rare in the UK.

An examiner may indicate that neurological examination is required. If not, it is important to ensure that there are no obvious bone, soft-tissue or joint abnormalities. Quickly look at the face for parkinsonism or signs of a stroke. (Ask 'Are the arms or joints painful?') Then try to identify the problem more precisely by asking the patient 'Have you any loss of strength in your arms or hands?' and 'Have you had any numbness or tingling in your hands?' If you suspect a specific lesion, demonstrate the complete syndrome. If not, perform a methodical examination. The following scheme is recommended.

Motor system

'Examine the motor system'

Look for obvious muscle wasting and test the strength of the appropriate muscle if it is

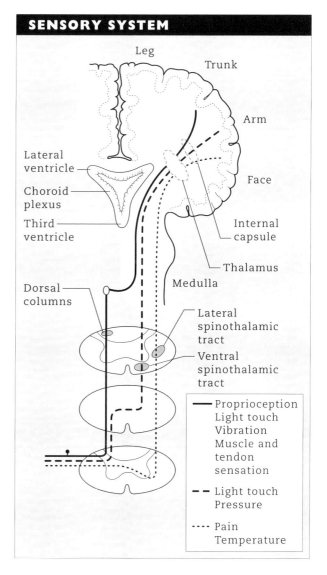

SENSORY SYSTEM

Leg

Trunk

Arm

Lateral
ventricle

Face

Choroid
plexus

Third
ventricle

Internal
capsule

Thalamus

Dorsal
columns

Medulla

Lateral
spinothalamic
tract

Ventral
spinothalamic
tract

——— Proprioception
Light touch
Vibration
Muscle and
tendon
sensation

- - Light touch
Pressure

···· Pain
Temperature

Fig. 1.7 Sensory pathways.

present. If there is wasting of the small hand muscles, note whether it is generalized (ulnar) or thenar (median). Note any fasciculation or tremor.

Test muscle tone—easiest at the elbow, although cogwheel rigidity may be more obvious at the wrist.

Test muscle power in groups (Table 1.2). 'I am going to test the strength of some of your muscles.'

• *Shoulder: C5.* 'Hold both arms out in front of you and close your eyes.' Look for drifting of one arm. This test checks not only weakness of the muscles at the shoulder but also for loss of position sense (when there is no evidence of weakness) and for lesions of the cerebral cortex (when the patient will not be aware of the drift, sometimes even with open eyes). You should also notice any winging of the scapula (nerve to serratus anterior, C5, 6, 7).

• *Elbow flexion: C5, 6, 7:* biceps. 'Bend your elbow up; don't let me straighten it.'

MOTOR ROOT VALUES

Joint	Movement	Roots	Muscles	Reflex
Shoulder	Abduction	C4, 5, 6	Supraspinatus, deltoid	
	External rotation	C4, 5, 6	Infraspinatus	
	Adduction	C6, 7, 8	Pectorals	+
Elbow	Flexion	C5, 6	Biceps	+
	Extension	C7, 8	Triceps	+
	Pronation	C6, 7		
	Supination	C5, 6	Biceps	+
Wrist	Flexion (palmar): radial	C6, 7		
	ulnar	C8		
	Extension (dorsiflexion)	C6, 7		
Fingers (long)	Flexion	C8		+
and thumb	Extension	C7		
Fingers (short)	Flexion	T1		
Hips	Flexion	L1, 2, 3	Iliopsoas	
	Extension	L5	Glutei	
		S1, 2		
	Adduction	L2, 3, 4	Adductors	+
	Abduction	L1, 4, 5	Glutei and tensor	
		S1	fascia lata	
Knee	Flexion	L5	Hamstrings	
		S1, 2		
	Extension	L3, 4	Quadriceps	+
Ankle	Dorsiflexion	L4, 5	Anterior tibial	
	Plantar flexion	S1, 2	Calf	+
	Eversion	L5	Peronei	
		S1		
	Inversion	L4	Anterior and	
			posterior tibial	
Toes	Flexion	S1, 2		
	Extension	L5		
		S1		
Anus		S2, 3, 4, 5		+
Cremaster		L1, 2		+

Notes

1 A simple *aide-mémoire* for reflexes and controlling muscle groups is: 12345678.

Ankle jerk	S1, 2
Knee jerk	L3, 4
Biceps jerk	C5, 6
Triceps jerk	C7, 8

2 All muscles on the back of the upper limb (triceps, wrist extensors and finger extensors) are innervated by C7.

3 T1 innervates the small muscles of the hand.

Table 1.2 Motor root values (including reflexes).

• *Elbow extension: C7: triceps.* 'Now straighten your elbows and push me away.'
• *Wrist and finger extension: C7.* 'Keep your wrist and fingers straight; don't let me bend them.'
• *Hand grip: C8, T1.* 'Squeeze my fingers hard and stop me pulling them out.'
Only allow the patient two of your fingers or they may be crushed.

Ulnar nerve tests (fingers)
Abduction of fingers ('Spread your fingers apart'). Try to squash them together and note how much effort this requires. Note also the bulk of the first dorsal interosseous muscle.

Adduction of fingers. Hold a piece of paper between straight fingers ('Don't let me pull it out').

Median nerve tests (thumb)
Abduction of thumb. The patient places the hand down flat with the palm upward and the thumb overlying the forefinger. Ask the patient to lift the thumb vertically against resistance.

Opposition of thumb. 'Put your thumb and little finger together and stop me pulling them apart with your forefinger'.
NB Thenar adduction is ulnar.

Reflexes
Details of the principal tendon reflexes are shown in Table 1.2. It is essential that the muscle involved is completely relaxed. If it is difficult to elicit, a tendon reflex may be 'reinforced' by asking the patient to concentrate on contracting muscles at a distant site (e.g. 'Grip your hands together').

Sensory system
Screening
For light touch (cotton wool) and pain (disposable pin). As a minimum, you should test once each on the front and back of the upper and lower arms and on each digit. Check vibration and position senses on a finger.

Coordination
Refer to the section on incoordination (p. 18).

Legs

'*Examine this patient's legs (neurologically)*' The most common neurological lesions affecting chiefly the legs are the following.
• *Peripheral neuropathy* (particularly diabetes mellitus).
• *Lumbar root lesions* (prolapsed intervertebral disc).
• *Lateral popliteal (common peroneal) nerve palsy.* Local pressure at the head of the fibula causes paralysis of the peroneal muscles and foot-drop. There may be sensory loss.
• *Spastic paraparesis.*
Try to identify the problem more precisely by asking the patient about any motor or sensory deficit. If no obvious lesion or syndrome is noted, perform systematic examination. The following scheme is recommended.

Motor system
Examination
Look for obvious muscle wasting and test the strength of the appropriate muscles if it is present. Note any fasciculation or tremor.

Test muscle tone. Lift the knee off the bed briskly while the patient is relaxed and see if the heel is lifted. Let it drop; observe how stiffly it falls. Then roll the leg to and fro, and see if the foot is rigid at the ankle or normally loose. Alternatively, bend the knee to and fro with an irregular rhythm (so that the patient cannot consistently resist the movement) or briskly abduct one leg to observe whether bilateral adductor spasm makes the other leg follow.

Test muscle power in groups. 'I am going to test the strength of some of your muscles.'
• *Hip flexion: L1, 2: iliopsoas.* 'Lift your leg up straight.' Push down on the patient's knee.
• *Hip extension: L5, S1: glutei.* 'Lift your leg up straight: push my hand down to the bed.' Push up to resist this.
• *Knee flexion: L5, S1, 2: hamstrings.* 'Bend your knee: don't let me straighten it.' Keep one hand above the patient's patella and pull up on the ankle.

• *Knee extension: L3, 4: quadriceps* (femoral nerve). 'Keep your knee straight: don't let me bend it.' Put your forearm behind the patient's knee and push down on the ankle.
• *Ankle plantar flexion: S1.* 'Push your foot down: don't let me push it up.'
• *Ankle dorsiflexion: L4, 5* (common peroneal nerve). 'Pull your foot up towards you and don't let me pull it down.'

Knee and ankle reflexes (p. 16)
Also examine ankle and patella clonus if these are brisk. Practise the technique. Clonus is a sustained rhythmical contraction of a spastic muscle, which undergoes sudden sustained stretching.

Plantar response
Gently but firmly draw a key or orange stick up the outer border of the sole and across the heads of the metatarsals.

Sensory system (Fig. 1.7, p. 15)
Light touch and pinprick
• once each on the medial and lateral sides of thigh and calf; and
• on the dorsum of the foot, tip of the big toe and lateral border of the foot.

Vibration sense at the medial malleolus and, if it is absent there, progress to the knee and hip.

Position sense. Test position sense at the big toes. If absent, check it at progressively more proximal joints.

Reduction or absence of vibration and position senses suggests not only dorsal column loss (usually caused by vitamin B_{12} deficiency) but also may be part of a peripheral neuropathy (usually diabetic). However, in peripheral neuropathy you expect the other modalities to be reduced (pin and touch). In a peripheral sensory neuropathy, a 'glove and stocking' distribution of loss is characteristic.

Coordination
Heel–shin test. 'Put your heel (touching the patient's heel) on your knee (touching the patient's knee) and slide it down your leg (slid-

ing your finger down the patient's shin).' This is primarily a test for intention tremor. If present, you should look for other signs of cerebellar disorders (arms, eyes, speech). Then ask the patient to stand and stand nearby yourself (to assist if the patient stumbles). Look for the following.
• *Rombergism* (more unsteady with the eyes closed than with them open), which indicates loss of position sense (posterior column lesion).
• *Truncal ataxia* while standing with feet together (cerebellar lesion).
• *Ataxic gait* on walking heel to toe—note direction of fall (ipsilateral cerebellar lesion).
• *Abnormalities of gait* on normal walking (including turning).

Abnormality of gait
(excluding orthopaedic disorders)

'Watch this patient walk'

Hemiplegia
The leg is rigid and describes a semicircle with the toe scraping the floor (circumduction). *Aetiology*: almost invariably a stroke.

Paraplegia
'Scissors' or 'wading through mud' gait. *Aetiology*: multiple sclerosis, cord compression; rarely, congenital spastic diplegia.

Festinant gait of parkinsonism
The patient is rigid, stooped and the gait shuffling. The arms tend to be held flexed and characteristically do not swing. The patient appears to be continually about to fall forwards and may show propulsion or retropulsion. Turning is poor. There may be 'freezing' in doorways.

Cerebellar gait
The patient walks on a wide base with the arms held wide with ataxia and veering and staggering towards the side of the disease. *Aetiology*: usually multiple sclerosis. Cerebellar tumour (primary or secondary), the cerebellar syndrome of carcinoma (non-metastatic) and familial degenerations should be remembered.

Sensory (dorsal column) ataxia

A stepping and stamping gait. The patient walks on a wide base and looks at the ground. The patient tends to fall if he or she closes the eyes (rombergism).

Aetiology: diabetic pseudotabes, subacute combined degeneration of the cord, Friedreich's ataxia, tabes dorsalis. Ataxia in multiple sclerosis may very rarely be of this kind (it is usually cerebellar).

Steppage (drop-foot) gait

There is no dorsiflexion of the foot as it leaves the ground and the affected legs (or leg) are lifted high to avoid scraping the toe.

Aetiology: usually lateral popliteal nerve palsy (trauma or diabetic). Less commonly, poliomyelitis or peroneal muscular atrophy. Very rarely, heavy metal (lead, arsenic) poisoning.

Waddling gait

The pelvis drops on each side as the leg leaves the ground.

Aetiology: wasting disorders of the muscles of the pelvic girdle and proximal lower limb muscles and osteomalacia.

Notes

Sensory testing (vibration and position, touch, pain, temperature)

It is important that the patient understands what sensations you are testing and what is an appropriate response. No person is entirely consistent in sensory testing and a few discrepant responses are to be expected and ignored. Increasingly inconsistent responses are often caused by wandering attention. Two of the stimuli conventionally used (vibration and position senses) are strange ones and the patient quickly needs to be taught about them. If you already have a good and professional system the following suggested scheme will be unnecessary.

Vibration sense

Ensure that the patient can recognize vibration by placing the vibrating tuning fork on the patient's sternum. Then stop the vibration to allow the patient to recognize the difference. 'Now with your eyes closed tell me if you can feel the vibration.' Start at the big toes and work proximally to the medial malleoli, patellae and anterior superior iliac spines, comparing right with left (and with yourself if necessary).

Position sense

With the patient looking, hold a big toe or a finger by its sides (holding the top and bottom introduces touch and pressure sensations). Move the toe away from the patient—'this is down'—and then towards the patient—'this is up'. 'Now with your eyes closed tell me whether I move the toe (finger) up or down.'

Light touch (cotton wool) and pinprick

These stimuli should be familiar to the patient. Appropriate instructions might be: 'With your eyes closed, say *now* every time I touch you', and/or 'Say *pin* when you feel a pinprick'. Areas of anaesthesia are easily produced by suggestion. If the patient finds it difficult, try the 'finger plus pin' technique. A pin is held against the examiner's forefinger and, while testing, slid down at irregular times to touch the patient so that the patient will sometimes feel just a finger and at other times a finger plus the pin: 'Tell me when you feel the sharpness'. This keeps the patient's attention, if not yours. The pin should be safely discarded after use on one patient because of the risks of transmission of blood-borne viruses, especially human immunodeficiency virus (HIV) and hepatitis B.

Ask the patient to outline for you the extent of any numbness or tingling; you may then confirm and define the extent of sensory loss with the cotton wool or a pin.

You must have an approximate idea of the dermatomes (Fig. 1.8). The following points may be found useful:

- C4 and T2 are the neighbouring dermatomes over the front of the chest at the level of the first and second ribs;
- C5, 6, 7, 8 and T1 supply the upper limb;
- C7 supplies the middle finger front and back;
- T7 supplies the lower ribs;

SENSORY DERMATOMES

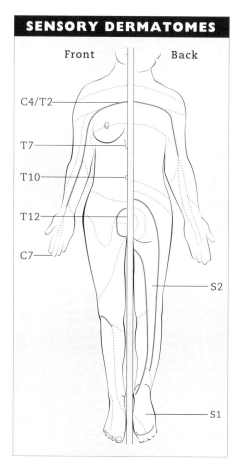

Fig. 1.8 Sensory dermatomes.

- T10 supplies the umbilical region;
- T12 is the lowest nerve of the anterior abdominal wall;
- L1 supplies the inguinal region;
- L2 and 3 supply the anterior thigh (lateral and medial);
- L4 and 5 supply the anterior shin (medial and lateral); and
- S1 supplies the lateral border of the foot and sole, and the back of the calf up to the knee.

Temperature

Coldness and warmth are familiar to the patient. Appropriate instructions might be: 'With your eyes closed tell me whether this is cold or warm'. A quick check can be performed using the side of a forefinger and the prongs of the tuning fork as comparatively 'warm' and 'cold'.

Patterns of sensory loss in limbs

Peripheral sensory neuropathy (p. 105)

All modalities tend to be lost symmetrically starting distally (at the periphery). The loss is more marked in the lower limbs. This pattern is seen in diabetes mellitus, carcinomatous neuropathy, vitamin B_{12} deficiency, and with some drugs or chemicals.

Spinal cord lesions

See Fig. 1.1 (p. 4) for a cross-section of the spinal cord. Dissociated sensory loss is a feature of spinal cord lesions. Classically, vibration and position sense are carried in the dorsal columns, which decussate in the medulla.

All other sensations are carried in the lateral spinothalamic tracts, which decussate at the level of the origin in the cord or just above it. NB Do not confuse them with the lateral columns, which are the pyramidal tracts.

Dorsal column loss without spinothalamic loss occurs in both legs in vitamin B_{12} deficiency. (It also occurs in the ipsilateral leg in hemisection of the cord—Brown-Séquard syndrome.)

Spinothalamic loss without dorsal column loss (dissociated anaesthesia) occurs in syringomyelia, usually in the arms. (It also occurs in the contralateral leg in hemisection of the cord.)

Cerebral cortical lesions

Astereognosis and dysgraphaesthesia occur with parietal sensory loss. They are tested by asking the patient to recognize, with the eyes closed, respectively objects placed in the hands, or numbers drawn on the palm. Two-point discrimination is also a sensitive test of parietal cortical function.

Motor testing (involuntary movement, tone, power, wasting, coordination)

First look for *involuntary movements* at rest—fasciculation, tremor (p. 23) or choreoathetosis.

Then test *muscle tone* (before testing for power, because this may leave the patient tense). Engage the patient in conversation so that he or she is relaxed. Tone is most easily assessed at the elbow (although cogwheel rigidity may be more obvious at the wrist) and at the knee. Move the joint to and fro with an irregular rhythm and to a variable extent so that the patient cannot consistently resist the movement.

Ask the patient which movements were weak and then try to confirm these observations and look for related deficiencies.

Test *muscle power* in groups. Make your instructions slow and precise. Look at and feel the bulk of the muscles as you test their strength. You must have an approximate idea of the root values of at least certain movements so that you can perform a rapid 'motor root' screen (upper and lower limb, Table 1.2, p. 16).

You must know the root values of the common reflexes (see Table 1.2, p. 16).

Patterns of motor loss in limbs
Lower motor neuron lesion
There is reduced or absent power with marked muscle wasting in the established lesion. The muscles are flaccid and the reflexes absent. In the foot there is no plantar response. The lesion affects the motor distribution of the spinal root or peripheral nerve.

Upper motor neuron lesion
There is reduced or absent power with relatively little wasting. The muscle tone and reflexes are increased and clonus is often present. In the foot the plantar response is upgoing.

There tends to be a characteristic distribution of weakness:
• in the arms, weakness is more marked in elbow extension than flexion and wrist dorsiflexion than palmar flexion;
• in the legs, weakness is more marked in hip flexion, knee flexion and ankle dorsiflexion than in their antagonist movements.

These are most easily remembered by recalling the posture of the limbs in the hemiplegic patient when walking.

Proximal myopathy
Proximal muscle wasting and weakness also occur in polymyositis, carcinomatous neuromyopathy, hereditary muscular dystrophies, Cushing syndrome usually from steroid therapy, thyrotoxicosis, osteomalacia and diabetes

(amyotrophy, p. 157). The statin drugs and *Trichinella spiralis* infection of muscles may produce acute myositis.

Isolated peripheral nerve lesions
Median nerve lesion (e.g. carpal tunnel syndrome)
Patients with carpal tunnel syndrome may complain of tingling and numbness of the fingers and/or weakness of the thumb, which are at their worst on waking. It is often unilateral at the time of presentation and remains so if idiopathic. Pain at the flexor aspect of the wrist may occasionally radiate up to the elbow and, exceptionally, as far as the shoulder.

You should examine for:
• *motor loss*: thenar wasting and weakness of thumb abduction and opposition;
• *sensory loss*: palmar surface only, on the thumb and two and a half fingers (i.e. to the middle of the ring finger);
• *Tinel's sign*: percuss over the flexor retinaculum to elicit tingling in the same sensory area; and
• *evidence of pregnancy myxoedema, rheumatoid arthritis* and *acromegaly.*
It is most common in overweight middle-aged women with none of these.
NB Bilateral carpal tunnel syndrome is commonly caused by rheumatoid arthritis and also occurs in long term dialysis patients (amyloid deposits of β_2-microglobulin). In the examination also consider cervical spondylosis (T1 lesion), MND and syringomyelia if you are in doubt about the diagnosis.

Ulnar nerve lesion
The ulnar nerve supplies all the small muscles of the hand except three of the four muscles of the thenar eminence (i.e. it supplies adductor pollicis). It may be compressed in the ulnar tunnel at the wrist or in the ulnar groove at the elbow (e.g. if the arm has been incorrectly positioned in general anaesthesia). These patients may complain of tingling or deadness and/or weakness of the ring and little fingers.

You should examine for the following.
• Motor loss with flattening of the contours of the hand caused by muscle wasting. The ring and little fingers are held slightly flexed, and

there is loss of power in abduction and adduction of the fingers (claw hand).

• Sensory loss, back and front, over the one and a half ulnar fingers (i.e. little finger and half the ring finger).

• 'Filling in' of the ulnar groove at the elbow and limitation of movement at the elbow. X-rays of the elbow may show osteoarthritis or local fracture.

NB In 2–3% of people, the ulnar nerve supplies *all* the hand muscles. If you are in doubt about the diagnosis consider a lesion in the neck and look for restricted movements of the cervical spine (T1 lesion).

Radial nerve lesion

This is rare and usually results from prolonged local pressure to the nerve (e.g. an arm over the back of a chair—'Saturday night palsy'). It causes wrist-drop. Sensory loss may be very limited because the median and ulnar nerve territories overlap the radial territory.

Lateral cutaneous nerve of the thigh

Compression causes meralgia paraesthetica, a syndrome characterized by hyperalgesia, burning pain and numbness in the lateral aspect of the thigh and is associated with tight jeans or obesity.

Lateral popliteal palsy

The lateral popliteal (common peroneal) nerve supplies the peroneal muscles which dorsiflex and evert the foot. The nerve may be damaged as it passes over the head of the fibula, resulting in foot-drop. There may be sensory loss over the outer aspect of the leg and foot.

Wasting of the small hand muscles

These are innervated by the T1 root. Wasting of the muscles in both hands occurs with:

• old age and cachexia;
• rheumatoid arthritis;
• bilateral cervical ribs;
• MND;
• syringomyelia; and
• bilateral median and ulnar nerve lesions.

If present in one hand only, the following should also be considered:

• cervical cord lesions, including tumours;
• brachial plexus trauma; and
• a Pancoast tumour (p. 244).

Proximal myopathy

This characteristically produces difficulty in standing from the sitting position and difficulty in raising the arms above the head. It occurs (often slight) in thyrotoxicosis, diabetes mellitus, polymyositis, carcinomatous neuromyopathy, osteomalacia, Cushing syndrome (usually iatrogenic) and in the hereditary muscular dystrophies.

Mixed motor and sensory neuropathy

See peripheral neuropathy and mononeuritis multiplex (p. 105).

Incoordination

There are two chief patterns of incoordination: one dominated by a failure in controlling accurate limb movements (cerebellar) and the other dominated by an ignorance of limb position when visual and cutaneous clues are excluded (proprioceptive).

Cerebellar incoordination

'*Demonstrate some cerebellar signs.*' The signs are ipsilateral to a destructive lesion.

Finger–nose test. The patient is asked to point alternately to his or her own nose and to your finger held in front of him or her. The intention tremor is more marked when the patient has to stretch to reach your finger. If you keep your finger still and then ask the patient to repeat the test with the eyes closed, you may bring out past-pointing—deviation of the patient's finger consistently to one side of your own (the same side as the cerebellar lesion). The tremor is not altered by closing the eyes. The heel–shin test has similar significance. Remember that muscular weakness alone may make the patient unsteady in these tests, and that this may resemble an intention tremor.

Dysdiadochokinesia. ('Tap rapidly on the back of your hand like this . . . and now the other side.') The test is more sensitive if the patient taps alternately with the front and backs of his fingers, i.e. pronates and supinates. Rapid repetitive alternating movements of the wrists are irregular in both force and rate in cerebellar disease. There also tends to be abnormal movement at elbow and shoulder. Supination/pronation tests are more sensitive than flexion/extension ones.

Nystagmus, typically horizontal, is more marked on looking towards the side of the lesion. Do not get the patient to focus on an object too far laterally or too near the eyes.

Dysarthria is slurred and explosive, sometimes as if drunk.

Truncal ataxia. The gait is reeling and staggering as if drunk with a tendency to fall to the side of the lesion. Heel–toe walking may accentuate the sign. It may be the sole cerebellar sign in midline (vermis) cerebellar lesions.

Causes of cerebellar signs
• Multiple sclerosis.
• Brainstem vascular disease.
• Anticonvulsant therapy may produce gross nystagmus.
• Rarely, brainstem tumours, posterior fossa tumours (especially acoustic neuroma), degenerative disorders (e.g. alcoholism and hereditary ataxias), the cerebellar syndrome of bronchial carcinoma and (very rarely) hypothyroidism.

Proprioceptive incoordination

(dorsal column loss)
The signs are ipsilateral to the lesion. When there is loss of proprioception, the patient can still place the limbs accurately by looking at them. Incoordination is therefore only obviously present when the eyes are closed. Tests are performed with the eyes open and the eyes closed. When the patient's coordination is worse with the eyes closed than with them open, he or she is said to have loss of position sense (dorsal column loss or proprioceptive loss). If there is dorsal column loss (vibration and position senses) but no spinothalamic loss

(pain and temperature senses), there is said to be a dissociated sensory loss. (This term also describes the rarer reverse situation of spinothalamic loss without dorsal column loss.) Dissociated sensory loss is evidence of spinal cord disease.

Finger–nose and heel–shin tests are normal when the patient can see but incoordinate when he or she cannot. Rombergism is present when the patient, standing with the feet together, is unsteadier with the eyes closed than when they are open. The gait is ataxic and the patient walks on a wide base with high steps. Muscle tone and the tendon reflexes may be diminished (or increased in vitamin B_{12}-deficiency myelopathy).

Causes of dorsal (posterior) column loss
Subacute combined degeneration of the cord (p. 114). This may progress sufficiently to give dorsal column loss—peripheral neuropathy is the earliest manifestation. It is very rare in the clinic but patients treated with vitamin B_{12} may be seen in examinations (when the peripheral neuropathy may be considerably recovered, although the spinal cord lesions are not).

Tabes dorsalis. This is now exceedingly rare.

Hemisection of the cord (see Fig. 1.1 (p. 4), Fig. 1.6 (p. 14), Fig. 1.7 (p. 15) and p. 20).

Tremor

'*Look at this patient's tremor*' There are four common tremors.
1 The resting tremor of parkinsonism, maximal at rest and with emotion and inhibited by movement. It is best demonstrated by passive, slow flexion–extension movements at the wrist. It is mainly distal and asymmetrical.
2 Essential tremor. This is an accentuation of physiological tremor present at rest and brought out by placing a sheet of paper on the outstretched fingers. It increases with age and, unlike parkinsonism, does not involve the legs or gait. It is faster when associated with β_2-adrenergic stimulation (bronchodilators), caffeine, anxiety, after exercise and hypoglycaemia. In thyrotoxicosis it is associated with

warm moist palms, tachycardia and eye signs of Graves disease. There is a family history in 50%. It may improve with β-blockade and ethanol. In alcoholics, the tremor is exacerbated by withdrawal of alcohol.

3 The intention tremor of cerebellar disease. It is reduced or absent at rest and associated with past-pointing, nystagmus, dysarthria and ataxia, including truncal ataxia. It is rare except in multiple sclerosis.

4 Flapping tremor occurs in hepatic precoma and in the carbon dioxide retention of respiratory failure.

Athetosis refers to slow sinuous, writhing movements of the face and limbs, especially the distal parts. In torsion spasm (dystonia) the movements are similar but slower and affect the proximal parts of the limbs. The movements are purposeless. Both occur in lesions of the extrapyramidal system. They are rare.

Choreiform movements are non-repetitive, involuntary, abrupt, jerky movements of face, tongue and limbs. They may be localized or generalized (both are rare). They occur in lesions of the extrapyramidal system and with phenothiazine toxicity and occasionally in pregnancy or those taking an oral contraceptive. Rheumatic chorea (Sydenham chorea, p. 103) is now very rare. Huntington chorea is an inherited triplet repeat disease (p. 103).

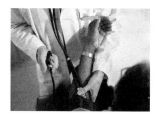

Eyes

'*Look at these eyes*' 'Unless specifically instructed (e.g. '*Look at the pupils*' or '*Look at the fundi*'), a complete examination is required. There may be obvious exophthalmos (p. 142) or squint (p. 7): otherwise follow the scheme in Table 2.1.

Optic fundus

First check that the ophthalmoscope is adjusted to suit your own eyes (usually no lens) and that the light beam is circular and bright by shining it on your other hand. It is useful to start by observing the patient's eye through the ophthalmoscope from about 1 m to see if there is any loss of the red light reflex (indicating opacities is the translucent media which may cause difficulty when trying to inspect the retina). You should interpret the fundal findings in the light of the patient's refractive errors (you may discover this from a quick look at the patient's glasses) and you should use a similar lens in the ophthalmoscope. Short-sighted (myopic) patients have a negative (concave) lens in their glasses (objects look smaller through them) and tend to have a deep optic cup and some temporal pallor of the disc. Long-sighted patients (hypermetropic) have a positive lens in their glasses (convex, magnifying) and their optic disc tends to look small and have ill-defined margins. You should be able to recognize and comment on the following.

Myelinated nerve fibres
A normal variant in which there are bright white streaky irregular patches, usually adjacent to the disc margin and radiating from it.

Diabetic fundus
This is characterized by:
• Background retinopathy (capillary leak of proteins, lipids, red cells); microaneurysms (dots), most frequent temporal to the macula; retinal haemorrhages (blots); hard exudates. Retinal vein dilatation.
• Maculopathy: oedema and/or background changes at the macula, associated with reduced visual acuity, exacerbated when looking through a pinhole.
• Preproliferative (secondary to retinal ischaemia): cotton-wool spots (soft exudates) of retinal oedema; venous beading and reduplication.
• Proliferative (response to severe retinal ischaemia): new vessel formation; pre-retinal haemorrhage; vitreous haemorrhage, which obscures the retina.
• Advanced (secondary to fibrosis): fibrous proliferation; traction retinal detachment.
• Results of treatment (photocoagulation): spots of retinal burns.
NB Glaucoma and cataract are more common in diabetes than in the general population.

Hypertensive fundus
There are usually the changes of arteriosclerosis (grades 1 and 2, including tortuosity, arterial nipping, silver wiring, varying vessel calibre). Hypertension produces haemorrhages and exudates (grade 3) and more severe disease in addition produces papilloedema (grade 4, malignant hypertension). Note that the subhyaloid haemorrhage sometimes seen in subarachnoid haemorrhage may indicate underlying hypertension.

EYE EXAMINATION

Observe	For	Clinical association
Eyes and eyelids (from in front)	Squint (congenital or acquired) Xanthelasma	Diabetes, atheroma, myxoedema, primary biliary cirrhosis (p. 211)
	Ptosis (partial, i.e. 3rd nerve or sympathetic, or complete, i.e. 3rd nerve)	If bilateral: myasthenia dystrophia myotonica
Cornea	Corneal arcus Calcification Kayser–Fleischer rings	Age and hyperlipidaemias Hypercalcaemia (rare) Wilson disease (very rare)
Visual acuity (Snellen chart)		May pick up early change in diabetes
Visual fields to confrontation (p. 6)		
Eye movements (p. 7)	Failure of lateral movements Failure of down and in movement Failure of other movements (with ptosis and fixed dilatation of pupil) Failure of all movements Nystagmus (p. 10)	6th-nerve palsy 4th-nerve palsy 3rd-nerve palsy Usually myasthenia, glass eye Cerebellar, vestibular or brainstem lesion
Pupils	Dilatation	Homatropine or part of 3rd-nerve lesion, Holmes–Adie syndrome
	Constriction	Horner syndrome, Argyll Robertson pupil, morphine, pilocarpine
NB *Check light and accommodation reflexes* (p. 8) (*Glass eyes have neither*).		
Iris (with ophthalmoscope)	Iritis (p. 28)	
Lens	Lens opacities or cataract (shine light obliquely across lens); this is often missed and may make examination of the fundus difficult or impossible	Senility, diabetes, trauma Rare causes include congenital rubella syndrome, parathyroidism, dystrophia myotonica and drugs (chloroquine, amiodarone and steroids)
Fundus (p. 25)		

Table 2.1 Examination of the eyes.

Papilloedema

The earliest findings are redness of the disc and blurring of the nasal margin. Small vessels may appear to dip over the swollen edge, and the optic cup disappears. Later, small haemorrhages appear. The blind spot may enlarge. The main causes are:

• raised intracranial pressure (tumour, abscess, meningitis, and the rare benign intracranial hypertension found chiefly in young overweight women);

• malignant hypertension; and

• rarely, optic retrobulbar neuritis, venous obstruction and the hypercapnia of respiratory failure.

NB Papillitis should be distinguished from

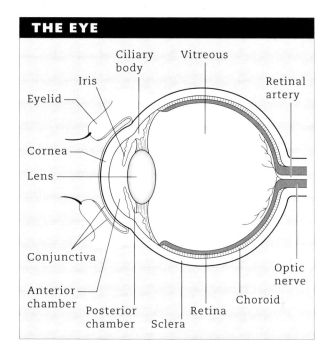

THE EYE

Fig. 2.1 Anatomy of the eye, showing the uveal tract.

papilloedema. It is usually caused by multiple sclerosis. There may be impaired colour vision and acuity, a central scotoma and pain. The disc is red and swollen with a blurred margin, exudates and haemorrhages.

Optic atrophy
• Glaucoma.
• Secondary to papilloedema (disc edge blurred)—rare.

• Primary (disc margin sharp with cup and cribriform plate well-defined) occurs after papillitis (almost invariably multiple sclerosis), from optic nerve pressure and in retinal artery thrombosis. Rarely, methanol abuse, vitamin B_{12} deficiency and the hereditary ataxias.

Exudates and haemorrhages
Chiefly in hypertension and diabetes mellitus but also in uraemia, acute leukaemia, raised

CAUSES OF IRITIS AND CHOROIDITIS

Iritis	Choroiditis
Diabetes	Idiopathic (i.e. unexplained), the most frequent in the UK
Sarcoid	
Ankylosing spondylitis	Toxoplasmosis (invariably acquired)
Reiter syndrome	
Ulcerative colitis and Crohn disease	Diabetes
Still disease	Sarcoid
(Rare causes include gonorrhoea, *Toxoplasma*, *Brucella*, tuberculosis, syphilis)	(Rare causes include *Toxocara*, tuberculosis, syphilis)

Table 2.2 Causes of iritis and choroiditis.

intracranial pressure, severe anaemia and carbon dioxide retention.

Uveitis, iritis and choroiditis

The uveal tract comprises the choroid (posterior uvea), the ciliary body and the iris (anterior uvea) (Fig. 2.1). Uveitis occurs alone or as part of other generalized diseases, some of which tend to involve either the iris (iritis, or anterior uveitis) or the choroid (choroiditis or posterior uveitis), although virtually all may involve both. Iritis is recognized by ocular pain and blurring of vision with vascularization around the corneal limbus and a 'muddy' iris. It is usually unilateral. The causes are listed in Table 2.2.

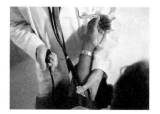

Limbs (joints and peripheral vascular disease)

Legs

In the legs the usual abnormalities are neurological, vascular or rashes (cellulitis, psoriasis, erythema nodosum). Diabetes mellitus is very common and may cause both, and you may be presented with a 'diabetic foot' (ischaemia, peripheral sensory neuropathy with ulceration and deformity; see Charcot joints, p. 157). Many neurological diseases such as multiple sclerosis and strokes are chronic and appear in examinations. Paget disease (rare) causes an enlarged, bowed tibia, but also check the face and skull for bony enlargment. Erythema nodosum occasionally appears in examinations because, although it is short-lived, it is fairly common. Pretibial myxoedema (very rare) is occasionally shown. Relatively rare cases include the results of spinal injury or prolapsed intervertebral discs (cervical or lumbar), peripheral nerve damage and subacute combined degeneration of the spinal cord. Patients with motor neuron disease or a carcinomatous neuropathy may be well enough to be included. Syringomyelia and the myopathies are rare but these patients have a better prognosis and are often available for examinations.

'Examine the legs' Unless attention is directed towards a particular part of the legs, such as the feet or knees, the following scheme is recommended.
1 Look for obvious *joint deformity*. Also note *bone deformity*, leg shortening and external rotation of fractured neck of femur, Paget disease, previous rickets (rare except in the elderly), the results of previous poliomyelitis, Charcot joints of diabetes and, very rarely, syphilis. Note if *oedema* is present.

2 Look at the *skin* (purpura, rash, ulcer) and note cyanosed or necrotic toes.
3 Examine *abnormal joints*.
4 *Peripheral vasculature*. Compare and assess the temperature of the dorsa of both feet, noting asymmetry and any interdigital infection and loss of hair. If the feet are cold, feel the dorsalis pedis and posterior tibial pulses and, if these are absent, proceed to feel for the popliteal and femoral pulses, and listen for arterial bruits over both. Ask the patient about a history of intermittent claudication. If there are ulcers, ask the patient if they are painful; if not, there is a neuropathy, most frequently diabetic.
5 Then examine the legs neurologically (p. 17).

Arms

In the arms the usual abnormalities seen are of the joints or the nervous system. The most common neurological conditions in the upper limbs are the results of multiple sclerosis, stroke or peripheral nerve compression. Less common conditions, which may be seen in examinations, are the results of pressure on the cord or brachial plexus (remember cervical spondylosis and cervical rib), motor neuron disease, syringomyelia and dystrophia myotonica.

'Examine the arms' (upper limb, hands) This may mean primarily the hand, which should always be inspected first, or the joints (including elbow or wrist). Usually it means a neurological examination (wasting, nerve palsies, root lesions) but:
• observe any tremor at rest (parkinsonism, familial, alcohol withdrawal);

• observe the skin for purpura (p. 309) and signs of liver disease (liver palms, spider naevi) and Dupuytren's contracture;
• look at the fingers and nails for clubbing (p. 49), cyanosis, nicotine staining, anaemia and the splinter haemorrhages and Osler nodes of subacute bacterial endocarditis (splinter haemorrhages are often occupational and not diagnostic, and Osler nodes are very rare);
• glance at the patient's face as this may provide a further clue, e.g. pallor, exophthalmos, parkinsonian facies, acromegaly, spider naevi, and tophi on the ears in gout;
• note any joint swelling (ask if the joints are painful before touching them) and any associated muscle wasting (often marked in rheumatoid arthritis) and examine abnormal joints; and
• then examine the arms neurologically (p. 13).

Notes

If there is evidence of joint disease, look for the conditions listed below.

Rheumatoid arthritis (p. 130)

This is usually symmetrical, with ulnar deviation at the metacarpophalangeal joints, spindling of the fingers, nail fold infarcts, muscle wasting and swelling of the joints, except the terminal interphalangeal joints. Look for the changes of psoriatic arthritis, including pitting of the nails and onycholysis with involvement of the terminal interphalangeal joints, psoriasis at the elbows and for the skin changes of steroid therapy. Rheumatoid arthritis may produce gross deformity. Nodules (20%) may be present at the elbow and down the radial border of the forearm. Note characteristic proximal interphalangeal deformities: boutonnière (flexion) and swan-neck (hyperextension).

Osteoarthritis (osteoarthrosis, p. 138)

This is asymmetrical and most frequently seen in the elderly as Heberden nodes—osteophytes around the terminal interphalangeal joints. Any joint of the hand may be involved, but it involves especially the terminal interphalangeal and first carpometacarpal joints.

Gout (p. 182)

Gout may attack any joint of the body. It may be monoarticular or polyarticular. Usually, the metatarsophalangeal joint of the big toe is involved first. It becomes red, hot, shiny and tender. There is often marked soft-tissue swelling and there may be superficial tophi over joints and in the cartilage of the ear. Ask about thiazide diuretics and note any polycythaemia.

NB Osteo-, rheumatoid and gouty arthritis may mimic each other but rheumatoid is usually symmetrical.

Acute arthritis may well be septic: joint aspiration and blood culture are essential.

Head and Neck

Head

'Look at this patient's face' This somewhat unsatisfactory request usually implies either that the patient has an abnormal facies (or neck), or that he or she has abnormal facial movements, or poverty of movement (parkinsonism and myxoedema). If the abnormality is not immediately obvious, the following checklist of the systems which may be involved might be found useful.

Endocrine and metabolic
- Cushing, usually iatrogenic otherwise rare.
- Myxoedema; thyrotoxicosis.
- Acromegaly.
- Pagetic skull.

Neurological
- Facial palsy from stroke or Bell's palsy.
- Ptosis and ocular palsies (3rd nerve, sympathetic in Horner syndrome and myasthenia gravis).
- Parkinsonism.
- Myopathy (including dystrophia myotonica with cataract and frontal baldness).
- Ophthalmic herpes (zoster), including the conjunctiva.

Figure 4.1 shows the sensory dermatomes in the head and neck.

Cardiorespiratory
- Cyanosis of lips (look at the tongue) of chronic obstructive airway (note pursing lips on expiration, and poor expansion), or cardiac failure.
- Elevated jugular venous pressure of heart failure (or fluid overload). Kussmaul's sign may be present with cardiac tamponade. There will be no pulse wave in the extremely elevated pressure because of mediastinal obstruction. Obstructive airways disease gives elevation of the jugular venous pressure during expiration (in proportion to the obstruction).

Gastrointestinal
- Jaundice and spider naevi.
- Peutz–Jeghers syndrome (p. 25).
- Hereditary haemorrhagic telangiectasia.
- Anaemia (white hair, and glossitis of pernicious anaemia).
- Angular cheilitis is usually caused by over-closure from aged dentures and mandibular resorption rather than anaemia.

Auto-immune disease
- Systemic lupus erythematosus (butterfly rash).
- Scleroderma (tight mouth and shiny tight skin of fingers).
- Dermatomyositis (periorbital rash).

Skin diseases
- Acne vulgaris.
- Rosacea.
- Psoriasis.
- Port wine stain (of Sturge–Weber syndrome).

Neck

'Examine the neck' This usually means that there is enlargement of the lymph glands, or that a goitre is present, or that the jugular venous pressure is raised (see Table 7.2, p. 59).

Cervical lymphadenopathy
This is often easier to feel from behind.

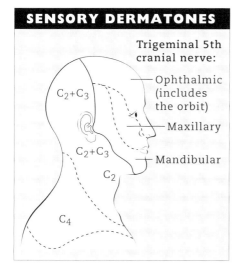

SENSORY DERMATONES

Trigeminal 5th
cranial nerve:

C_2+C_3

Ophthalmic
(includes
the orbit)

Maxillary

C_2+C_3

Mandibular

C_2

C_4

Fig. 4.1 Sensory dermatomes of the head
and neck.

Cervical lymphadenopathy may be the presenting symptom of a generalized lymphadenopathy, so further examination should include all lymph gland groups and palpation for enlargement of the liver and spleen. Generalized lymphadenopathy usually results from:
• infectious mononucleosis and rubella;
• reticuloendothelial disorders;
• chronic lymphatic leukaemia;
• other less common causes include granulomatous disorders including toxoplasmosis, tuberculosis, sarcoidosis and brucellosis.

When examining the neck glands, do not forget the occipital group. If lymphadenopathy is present, check for local infection or neoplasm over the whole head and neck. Remember to look into the mouth and pharynx, and check the thyroid. Check the nose for blood, discharge and patency. Tuberculosis must be considered in all cervical lymphadenopathy. This is also a common site for stage I Hodgkin disease, and also for neoplastic secondary deposits from the lung, testis, breast and nasopharyngeal carcinomas.

Glands in the root of the neck may be symptomatic of pulmonary, abdominal (including the testes) or breast malignancy.

Localized lymphadenopathy usually results from:
• local infection (any age);
• carcinoma (usually over 45 years old);
• Hodgkin disease (usually patients under 35 years, p. 311); and
• non-Hodgkin lymphoma.

Enlarged thyroid (p. 140)

'Look at this patient's thyroid gland' This means the patient has a goitre. It is unlikely that the patient is hyperthyroid but this must first be excluded by looking for the evidence, such as fine finger tremor, hyperkinesia, eye signs of Graves disease (lid lag, lid retraction, exophthalmos), tachycardia or fast atrial fibrillation and hot sweaty hands. Similarly, check for the characteristic facies, slow movements, dry thick skin, hair changes and croaking voice of hypothyroidism and proceed to test the ankle jerks if indicated.

Look at the patient's neck and ask him or her to swallow. Palpate the gland first from behind and then from the front. The patient's chin should be flexed to relax the tissues (untrained patients invariably extend the neck). If the patient has to swallow more than two or three times, give a glass of water. Pay special attention to the following.
• *Character.* Diffuse or multinodular. The gland is diffusely enlarged in Graves disease, Hashimoto thyroiditis, iodine deficiency and dyshormonogenesis. Patients with multinodular goitres are usually non-toxic (euthyroid). The usual clinical problem is their bulk, which may produce compression (of trachea, oesophagus or laryngeal nerve) and cause distress from their appearance. Single nodules should be regarded as malignant (although most are not), and removed or biopsied.
• *Tenderness.* This is unusual except in viral thyroiditis (rare) and occasionally in autoimmune thyroiditis and carcinoma.
• *Mobility.* Attachment to surrounding tissues suggests carcinoma.
• *Retrosternal extension.* Feel in the suprasternal notch and percuss the upper sternum for dullness.
• *Lymph glands.* An enlarged chain of lymph glands suggests papillary thyroid carcinoma.

- *Trachea* central or displaced.
- *Thyroidectomy scar*. If present, you should suspect hypothyroidism or hypoparathyroidism. Elicit Chvostek sign (may be present in normal people) and perform Trousseau test (p. 182).
- Auscultate over the gland for a systolic bruit. Look for vitiligo, acropachy and pretibial myxoedema if autoimmune thyroid disease is suspected.

You should ask about pressure symptoms of dyspnoea, any drugs (especially medicines containing iodine) and take a family history for inborn enzyme deficiency (dyshormonogenesis). If you are asked to suggest investigations you should consider the following.

- Thyroid function tests. These should include as appropriate (and available) serum free thyroxine, free triiodothyronine and thyroid-stimulating (thyrotrophic) hormone.
- Tests for thyroid microsomal autoantibodies.
- X-rays for tracheal deviation or compression.
- Laryngoscopy to observe vocal cords if the voice has changed.
- Radioiodine scan (for cold nodules) and ultrasound (to distinguish solid from cystic masses) are not sufficiently reliable so perform needle biopsy of isolated nodules for cytology, or total removal.

NB The observed incidence of simple goitre, autoimmune thyroiditis and carcinoma in one series was 89, 10 and 1%, respectively. Carcinoma is suggested by a hard fixed gland, lymph gland enlargement, pressure symptoms, vocal cord paralysis, rapid increase in size and evidence of metastasis to bone (p. 144).

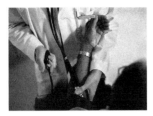

Abdomen

Examination

'Examine this patient's abdomen' (Fig. 5.1) The most usual abnormality seen in examinations is a palpable mass or the presence of free fluid, or both. These are relatively rare in the clinic, where the clinician more commonly elicits only areas of maximum tenderness. The most common conditions suitable for examination purposes are diseases that are chronic and that produce enlargement of the spleen or liver, such as the chronic leukaemias, myelofibrosis or chronic liver disorders. Other palpable masses include renal swellings, especially polycystic kidneys. Neoplastic or inflammatory swellings may be present and it is usually not possible to distinguish between these on physical examination alone. Patients with acute abdominal disease virtually never appear in clinical examinations. Remember always to look before palpation, to have warm hands and to palpate gently so as to gain the patient's confidence and to avoid hurting him or her. You should ask the patient to let you know if you are hurting them. Check this by looking at the patient's face periodically during palpation, especially if you elicit guarding or rebound tenderness.

A complete examination of the alimentary system involves inspection of the tongue, mouth, teeth and throat but this is rarely required in examinations. Loss of weight, clubbing, jaundice, anaemia and spider naevi should always be looked for.

• Look at the hands especially for clubbing, leukonychia, tobacco staining, liver palms, spider naevi and Dupuytren's contracture.
• Palpate the neck, supraclavicular fossae, axillae and groins for lymph nodes (the testes drain to the para-aortic and cervical glands).
• Inspect the eyes and conjunctivae for anaemia and jaundice.
• Lie the patient flat (one pillow) with arms by the sides.
• Observe the abdomen for:
  (a) general swelling with eversion of the umbilicus in ascites and visible enlargement of internal organs (liver, spleen, kidneys, gall bladder, stomach (in pyloric stenosis), urinary bladder and pelvic organs);
  (b) abnormal veins or abnormally distended veins usually in cirrhosis with the direction of flow away from the umbilicus (portal hypertension). The flow is upwards from the groin in inferior vena cava obstruction (Fig. 5.2);
  (c) scars of previous operations, striae, skin rashes and purpura;
  (d) pigmentation localized or generalized; and
  (e) visible peristalsis suggests obstruction except in very thin patients.
• Palpate for internal organs and masses. It is often of value to percuss the liver and spleen areas initially to avoid missing the lower border of a very large liver or spleen. It is essential to start palpation in the right iliac fossa and work upwards towards the hepatic and splenic areas, first superficially and then deeper. Ascites may obscure a liver edge, but firm 'dipping' on to an enlarged liver should always be attempted unless it causes pain.

The 'scratch test' can often help *roughly* to define the extent of hepatomegaly. Place the stethoscope firmly just below the xiphisternal cartilage; the liver lies beneath this in normal people. Sound is conducted through solid

THE ABDOMEN

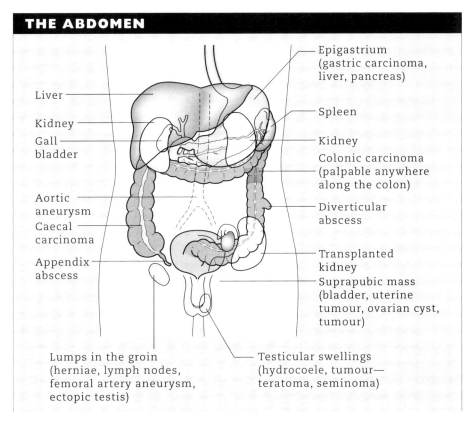

Liver

Kidney

Gall
bladder

Aortic
aneurysm

Caecal
carcinoma

Appendix
abscess

Epigastrium
(gastric carcinoma,
liver, pancreas)

Spleen

Kidney

Colonic carcinoma
(palpable anywhere
along the colon)

Diverticular
abscess

Transplanted
kidney

Suprapubic mass
(bladder, uterine
tumour, ovarian cyst,
tumour)

Lumps in the groin
(herniae, lymph nodes,
femoral artery aneurysm,
ectopic testis)

Testicular swellings
(hydrocoele, tumour—
teratoma, seminoma)

Fig. 5.1 Examination of the abdomen: (i) gently palpate all quadrants for tenderness and masses; (ii) feel for enlarged liver, spleen or kidneys, and for masses arising from the bowel (in the left and right iliac fossae), the epigastrium (stomach and pancreas), the aorta (aneurysm), or the pelvis (uterus, bladder and ovaries); (iii) percuss and auscultate over enlarged organs or masses; (iv) examine hernial orifices and external genitalia in men; and (v) perform a rectal examination.

objects, so firm stroking of the skin progressing from the right costal margin downwards will be audible until the liver edge is reached.

Liver

The upper border is in the fourth to fifth space on percussion. It moves down on inspiration. If enlarged, the edge may be tender, regular or irregular, hard, firm or soft. Note if it is pulsatile (tricuspid incompetence). The liver may be of normal size but low because of hyper-inflated lungs in chronic obstructive airway disease.

Spleen

Smooth rounded swelling in left subcostal region, usually with a distinct lower edge (as compared with the kidney). It enlarges diagonally downward and across the abdomen in line with the ninth rib. The examining hand cannot get above the swelling. Percussion over it is dull. There is a notch on the swelling. It may occasionally be more easily palpated with the patient lying on the right side.

Kidneys

They are palpated in the loin bimanually, i.e. most easily felt by pushing the kidney forwards from behind on to the anterior palpating hand. They move slightly downwards on inspiration. Percussion is resonant over the kidney. The examining hand can easily get between the

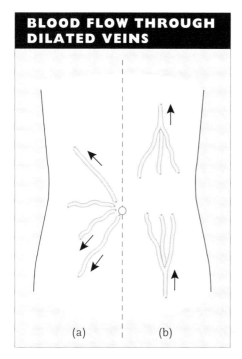

BLOOD FLOW THROUGH DILATED VEINS

(a)   (b)

Fig. 5.2 Blood flow through dilated anterior abdominal wall veins. Portal vein and inferior vena caval occlusion can be distinguished by the different directions of flow below the umbilicus. (a) Direction of flow in portal vein occlusion. (b) Direction of flow in inferior vena caval occlusion.

swelling and the costal margin. The lower pole of the right kidney can often be felt in thin normal persons.

Abnormal masses

Palpate for abnormal masses particularly in the epigastrium (gastric carcinoma) and suprapubic region (an overfilled bladder and ovarian and uterine masses are often missed) and note colonic swellings. The descending colon is commonly palpable in the left iliac fossa (faeces may be indented). The abdominal aorta, which is pulsatile and bifurcates at the level of the umbilicus (L4), is easily palpable in thin and lordotic patients. This is very seldom the only evidence of aortic aneurysm.

If general swelling is present, suspect ascites and examine for shifting dullness and ballottement of the liver (dipping). A fluid thrill may be demonstrable in large, tense effusions.

Complete the examination by feeling for inguinal and, if relevant, cervical glands (the drainage from the testes is to the para-aortic and cervical glands), the femoral pulses, checking for leg oedema, and listening for renal bruits and bowel sounds. Do not forget the hernial orifices—inguinal and femoral—and check for a cough impulse.

External genitalia

It is essential to examine them in practice but rarely required in examinations. Seminoma is a treatable and curable disease of the relatively young and, very rarely, left-sided varicocoele may suggest a left renal carcinoma.

Rectal examination

Essential in practice as rectal carcinoma is common but should not be performed in examinations unless suggested by the examiner. Some examiners will expect the candidate to comment on its desirability, particularly in the presence of gastrointestinal disease.

Notes

Splenomegaly

There are two common causes of a very large spleen:
• chronic myeloid leukaemia; and
• myelofibrosis.

NB Other causes, rare in the UK but very common on a worldwide basis, are malaria and kala-azar (visceral Leishmaniasis).

There are two additional causes of a moderately enlarged spleen (4–8 cm):
• lymphoproliferative disorder, e.g. Hodgkin's disease and chronic lymphatic leukaemia; and
• cirrhosis with portal hypertension.

However, there are many causes of a slightly enlarged spleen:
• any of the above;
• glandular fever, *Brucella* and infectious hepatitis (unlikely in the examination); and
• many subacute and chronic infections, including subacute bacterial endocarditis and in many infections.

Other rare causes include amyloid (rheumatoid arthritis is the most common cause; chronic sepsis is less common), Felty syndrome (p. 135), multiple myeloma, sarcoid, collagen disease and storage diseases. Other blood disorders which can give splenic enlargement are idiopathic thrombocytopenia, pernicious anaemia, congenital spherocytosis and polycythaemia rubra vera.

Hepatomegaly

There are three common causes:
• congestive cardiac failure;
• secondary carcinomatous deposits; and
• cirrhosis (usually alcoholic).
  Other causes include:
• infections—glandular fever, infectious hepatitis;
• leukaemia and reticuloendothelial disorders;
• tumours (primary hepatoma, amoebic and hydatid cysts);
• amyloid, sarcoid and storage diseases;
• primary biliary cirrhosis (large regular liver in women with jaundice and xanthelasmas); and
• haemochromatosis (look for pigmentation).

Hepatosplenomegaly

The list is much the same as for splenomegaly alone because the most common causes are chronic leukaemia, cirrhosis with portal hypertension, lymphoproliferative disorder and myelofibrosis, but each of these is usually associated with other clinical signs.

Palpable kidneys

The left kidney is nearly always impalpable but the lower pole of a normal right kidney may be felt in thin people. *Unilateral enlargement* may result from a local lesion, e.g. carcinoma, hydronephrosis, cysts or from hypertrophy of a single functioning kidney. *Bilateral enlargement*, occurs in polycystic disease (the liver may also be enlarged) and very rarely in bilateral hydronephrosis and amyloidosis. Following *renal transplantation* a kidney may be palpable in the iliac fossa, and the patient may be cushingoid in appearance as a result of steroid therapy. Look for scars of previous surgery and arteriovenous shunts.

Mass in right subcostal region

It may be difficult to decide the nature of a mass in this region which may be derived from the liver (including Riedel's lobe), colon, kidney or, occasionally, gall bladder. If you are uncertain, say so, giving the most likely possibilities and the reasons for your conclusions. This will determine the approach to further investigation, which should start with simple studies:
• urine for haematuria and proteinuria;
• stool for occult bleeding; and
• ultrasound for solid or cystic masses.
  Then proceed as indicated by clinical suspicion and the results of studies of one or more of the following.
• *Liver*—liver function tests, ultrasound scan and biopsy.
• *Kidney*—ultrasound, computed tomography (CT) scan or intravenous urogram.
• *Colon*—sigmoidoscopy, barium enema and colonoscopy.
• *Gall bladder*—ultrasound.
• CT scan may be helpful for masses which remain obscure and which arise from the pelvis.

Ascites

The clinical features are abdominal distension, dullness to percussion in the flanks, shifting dullness and a fluid thrill.
  The common causes are:
• intra-abdominal neoplasms (remember gynaecological lesions);
• hepatic cirrhosis with portal hypertension (relatively late in the disease, p. 213);
• congestive cardiac failure and, rarely, constrictive pericarditis;
• nephrotic syndrome (and other low albumin states); and
• tuberculous peritonitis (rare in this country, but should be suspected in Asian and Irish patients).
  Paracentesis of a few millilitres of fluid for diagnosis is simple. The specimen should be examined for:
• protein content (> 30 g/l suggests an exudate; less, a transudate);
• microscopy and bacterial culture (including tuberculosis); and
• cytology for malignant cells.

Paracentesis may occasionally be required for the relief of severe symptoms but not otherwise because the fluid tends to reaccumulate, and repeated paracentesis leads to excessive protein loss.

The suprapubic region is often neglected by physicians examining the abdomen. The more common causes of a suprapubic mass are the distended bladder (retention from prostatic hypertrophy, tricyclic antidepressants), pregnancy, uterine and ovarian tumours (ovarian fibroids, ovarian cysts, carcinoma).

NB See p. 214 for management of ascites.

Jaundice

Yellow coloration of the skin and sclerae is usually only apparent when the serum bilirubin is over 35 µmol/l. The sclerae are not coloured in those with yellow skin caused by hyper-carotinaemia. Keep in mind the three basic causes of jaundice (haemolytic, hepatocellular and obstructive) but remember that most cases are caused by:
• acute viral hepatitis (p. 207)—most of these patients are not admitted to hospital unless they are very ill, recovery is unduly prolonged, or intrahepatic cholestasis persists;
• bile duct obstruction from gallstones or carcinoma of the head of the pancreas;
• drugs (p. 216);
• multiple secondary deposits of carcinoma in the liver (clinical jaundice is not common when the patient presents but the bilirubin is frequently slightly raised);
• intrahepatic cholestasis (drugs, viral hepatitis, ascending cholangitis and primary biliary cirrhosis);
• infectious mononucleosis;
• Gilbert syndrome (p. 42) is intermittent and harmless; and
• less common causes include: haemolytic anaemia, congenital hyperbilirubinaemia, stricture or carcinoma of the major bile ducts or ampulla.

'Would you like to ask this (jaundiced) patient some questions?'

Ask about
• *Age*. As a cause of jaundice, carcinoma becomes more common and hepatitis less common the older the patient.
• *Injections or transfusions* in the last 6 months (virus hepatitis), including drug addicts. Look for evidence of injections.
• *Contacts* with jaundice and residence abroad.
• *Occupation*. Farm and sewage workers are at risk from leptospirosis.
• *Presence of dark urine and pale stools* of biliary obstruction.
• *Recent drug therapy*, especially phenothiazines and the contraceptive pill.
• *Period of onset* from first symptoms to jaundice. In general, hepatitis A is short (1–3 weeks), carcinoma is medium (1–2 months) and cirrhosis is long. Hepatitis B is from 6 weeks to 6 months.
• *Alcohol consumption*.
• *Recent abdominal pain*, or a history of chronic dyspepsia may suggest cholecystitis, cholangitis, gallstones or pancreatic carcinoma.
• *Recent surgery*, anaesthesia (halothane).
• *Family history* if Gilbert syndrome is suspected.

'Would you like to examine this (jaundiced) patient?'

Examine
Skin of the face and abdomen and assess the degree of jaundice—deep green suggests long-standing obstruction and pale lemon suggests haemolysis. The sclerae often show minor degrees of jaundice not evident elsewhere.

Face, upper chest and hands for spider naevi and the hands for Dupuytren's contracture, liver palms and clubbing. Note that xanthelasmas with deep jaundice in a middle-aged woman probably indicate primary biliary cirrhosis.

Neck for lymph node enlargement as a result of secondary spread of abdominal carcinoma.

Abdomen for the following.
• Recent operation scars which suggest cholecystectomy or surgery for intra-abdominal carcinoma.
• Hepatomegaly. Irregular when infiltrated with

carcinoma, tender in infectious and acute alcoholic hepatitis (and when enlarged in congestive
heart failure) and sometimes with carcinoma.
• Splenomegaly in portal hypertension (and
spherocytosis and infectious mononucleosis).
• Palpable enlarged gall bladder suggesting bile
duct obstruction caused by carcinoma of the
pancreas (rather than gallstones).
• Ascites, which is probably more often caused
by gynaecological malignancy than to the portal
hypertension of cirrhosis, where it occurs late.

'What investigations would you perform?' The
aims of investigation are:
• to discover the site of any obstruction to
the outflow of bile and to determine whether
operative interference is necessary;
• to determine the degree of impairment of
liver cell function and its cause, and to observe
its course; and
• to eliminate rare causes such as haemolysis.

Haematology
Including a reticulocyte count and Coombs'
test, which may give evidence of haemolytic
anaemia. A normal reticulocyte count virtually
excludes haemolytic jaundice. Leukocytosis
may indicate infection (cholangitis) or carcinoma. Abnormal mononuclear cells suggest
infectious mononucleosis (Paul–Bunnell) or,
possibly, viral hepatitis.

Urine analysis
In obstructive jaundice the difficulty is usually
to distinguish between benign causes (gallstone
obstruction) and malignant causes (carcinoma
of the head of the pancreas). Remember that
hepatitis A and B, which usually occur in younger
patients, and drug jaundice, often present with
the typical clinical picture of obstructive jaundice from intrahepatic cholestasis and that this
may occasionally be persistent.
  Drug jaundice should always be reconsidered.

Conjugated bilirubin renders the urine yellow.

Urobilinogen is colourless but on standing the
urine turns brown as urobilinogen is converted
to urobilin by oxidation.

Haemolytic jaundice is acholuric (no bilirubin in
the urine) but the urine contains excess urobilinogen because excess bilirubin reaches the
intestine and is re-excreted as urobilinogen.

Obstructive jaundice gives urine coloured dark
brown with excess bilirubin but a reduction
of urinary urobilinogen, because little or no
bilirubin reaches the gut because of the
obstruction and therefore cannot be reabsorbed and re-excreted. In the early stages of
hepatocelluar jaundice in acute viral hepatitis,
excess urobilinogen may sometimes be present before clinical jaundice becomes apparent.
This is a result of failure of the liver to take up
the excess urobilinogen absorbed from the gut.
With increasing severity, biliary obstruction
develops and, as bilirubin (conjugated) appears
in the urine, it disappears from the gut and therefore urobilinogen disappears from the urine. The
reciprocal effect also occurs during recovery.

Liver function tests
Liver function tests either measure the ability of
the liver to perform normal functions (e.g. serum
albumin is a measure of protein synthesis; prothrombin time is a measure of the ability to synthesize clotting factors; bilirubin is a measure of
bile salt conjugation and excretion), or measure
liver enzymes (alkaline phosphatase, transaminases), which are indicators of liver cell damage.

Serum bilirubin
Bilirubin from red cell breakdown is transported to the liver where it is conjugated
to glucuronic acid. Conjugated bilirubin is
secreted in the bile and degraded in the gut by
bacteria to urobilinogen. Urobilinogen is either
excreted in the stool or reabsorbed from the
gut and excreted by the kidneys. Jaundice
becomes clinically detectable if bilirubin is
> 35 μmol/l. Serum bilirubin is predominantly
unconjugated in haemolytic jaundice and the
other liver function tests are usually normal.
It is mainly conjugated in obstructive jaundice.

Causes of increased bilirubin
• Hepatocellular failure.
• Biliary obstruction.

• Haemolysis—chiefly unconjugated and hence acholuric (no bile in the urine).
• Gilbert disease (autosomal dominant)— impaired conjugation of bilirubin. Bilirubin increases on fasting. Other liver function tests are normal.

Alkaline phosphatase

Alkaline phosphatase is found in high levels in biliary canaliculi, osteoblasts, intestinal mucosa and placenta. Serum alkaline phosphatase is characteristically greatly elevated in obstructive jaundice and less so in hepatocellular jaundice. A raised level in the absence of other signs of liver disease or abnormal liver function tests suggests the presence of malignant secondary deposits in the liver (or bone) or Paget's disease. It is very seldom raised in myeloma (see below). The normal range is higher in growing adolescents and in pregnancy.

Causes of increased alkaline phosphatase
• Liver cholestasis
• Obstructive jaundice (e.g. stone, carcinoma).
• Intrahepatic cholestasis (e.g. drugs such as chlorpromazine, cholangitis, primary biliary cirrhosis).
• Obstructive phase of hepatitis.
• Bone (osteoblastic activity):
   (a) Paget's disease;
   (b) bone metastases (markedly raised if prostatic in origin);
   (c) vitamin D deficiency;
   (d) hyperparathyroidism;
   (e) growth in children (particularly puberty); and
   (f) bone fractures.

Normal alkaline phosphatase
Alkaline phosphatase is usually normal in:
• alcohol consumption, unless very excessive;
• Gilbert syndrome; and
• myeloma (lesions are destructive without osteoblastic activity).

Hepatocellular damage

Shown by raised serum level of liver enzymes (transaminases). Very high values suggest viral hepatitis or toxic damage. Slight elevation is consistent with obstructive jaundice. γ-glutamyl transferase, an inducible microsomal enzyme, is probably the most sensitive index of alcohol ingestion, but it is raised in most forms of liver disease including acute and chronic hepatitis and cirrhosis (or large bile ducts in obstruction) and drugs which induce microsomal enzymes, e.g. phenytoin.

Serum gamma-glutamyl transferase
Causes of increase
It is increased in liver disease but not bone disease (it very seldom arises from an extra-hepatic source). It is therefore used to check the origin of raised alkaline phosphatase. It is:
• induced by drugs, particularly alcohol (even with moderate intake) and phenytoin; and
• increased in liver cholestasis.

Serum aspartate aminotransferase
Increased aspartate aminotransferase occurs in the following.
• Active liver cell damage, including hepatitis (viral, drug-induced), metastatic infiltration.
• Acute myocardial infarction (peaks at 24–48 h, may fall to normal by 72 h). The degree of elevation reflects the amount of muscle damage.
• Acute pancreatitis.
• Haemolysis.

Serum alanine aminotransferase
This usually parallels the aspartate aminotransferase.

Serology
Always check viral hepatitis antibody serology, particularly in patients with jaundice of unknown cause. Antimitochondrial antibodies are detected in 90% of cases of primary biliary cirrhosis. Antinuclear factor and smooth-muscle antibodies are detected in over 50% of cases of chronic active hepatitis.

Radiology of abdomen
X-ray and ultrasound may show gallstones and will put on record the size of the liver and spleen. *Isotopic liver scans* may demonstrate 'holes' caused by carcinomatous secondaries (or large bile ducts in obstruction). *Ultrasound and CT scans* (Fig. 5.3) may show primary

CT OF UPPER ABDOMEN

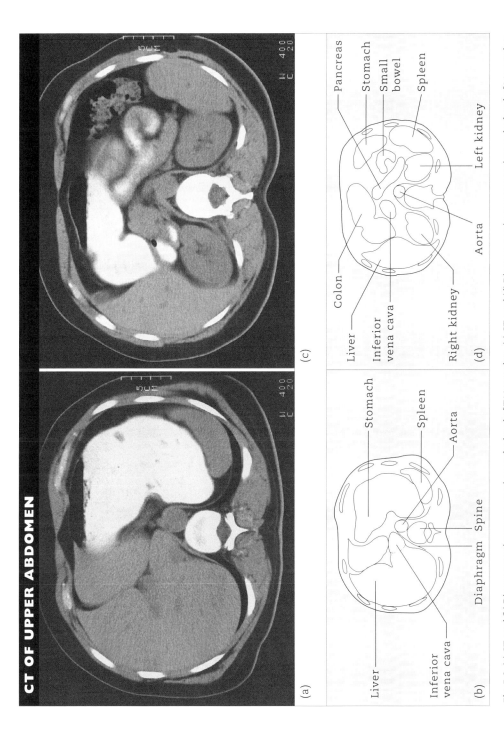

(a)

(b)

Liver

Inferior
vena cava

Diaphragm   Spine

Stomach

Spleen

Aorta

(c)

(d)

Pancreas

Stomach

Small
bowel

Spleen

Left kidney

Aorta

Right kidney

Inferior
vena cava

Liver

Colon

Fig. 5.3 (a) CT, and (b) Diagrammatic representation at the level of T11 vertebra. (c) CT, and (d) Diagrammatic representation at the level of L1 vertebra.

or secondary tumour, pancreatic carcinoma, stones in the gall bladder and dilatated ducts in obstruction (not always shown when the obstruction is caused by stones).

Needle liver biopsy

Biliary obstruction is a relative contraindication because of the potential danger of causing biliary peritonitis. Ultrasound and CT-guided biopsy may provide the histological diagnosis in focal lesions. In experienced hands it is a safe procedure provided the prothrombin concentration and platelet counts are normal. Fresh frozen plasma will quickly reverse the prothrombin time for the duration of the procedure.

Other investigation procedures which may be helpful.
• For hepatoma: α-fetoprotein and selenomethionine scan.
• For obstructive jaundice: endoscopic retrograde cholangiopancreatography (ERCP) is valuable to define obstruction of the pancreaticoduodenal tree for sphincterotomy, to release stones and to relieve obstruction by insertion of a stent.
NB In obstructive jaundice if the cause is not clinically obvious:
• retake the drug history;
• perform blood and urine tests as above;
• perform ultrasound, or abdominal CT scan for large ducts, pancreatic carcinoma, stones, secondary carcinoma; and
• liver biopsy if the ducts are not enlarged on ultrasound or CT.

Congenital non-haemolytic hyperbilirubinaemias

These may explain persistent jaundice in the young after viral hepatitis or slight jaundice in the healthy.

Gilbert syndrome (autosomal dominant)
• This is the only common congenital hyperbilirubinaemia (1–2% of the population). There is impaired glucuronidation of bilirubin (reduced uridine diphosphate glucuronyl trans-

ferase (UDPGT)) resulting in a raised unconjugated plasma bilirubin and acholuria. About 40% have a reduced red cell survival with a consequent increase in bilirubin production.
• The plasma bilirubin is usually < 35 μmol/l.
• Diagnosis is by exclusion: there is no haemolysis and the other liver function tests are normal. Fasting and intravenous nicotinic acid produce a rise in plasma bilirubin.
• Liver biopsy is very rarely indicated (unless the diagnosis is uncertain) and the liver is histologically normal.
• The prognosis is excellent and treatment unnecessary. It is important because it should not be confused with serious liver disease.

Dubin–Johnson syndrome
(autosomal recessive)
A rare benign disorder, usually in adolescents, of failure to excrete conjugated bilirubin. The plasma bilirubin is conjugated. The liver is stained black by centrilobular melanin and there is a late rise in the bromsulphalein (BSP) test elimination curve at 90 min.

Uraemia

'This patient is uraemic. Would you ask him some questions and examine him?'

Ask about
• Symptoms of renal failure—thirst, polyuria and nocturia, anorexia, nausea and vomiting, fatigue and itching.
• Symptoms of urinary tract infection (dysuria), prostatism (poor stream), renal stone, glomerulonephritis (haematuria) and nephrotic syndrome (ankle oedema).
• Drug therapy, analgesics.
• Past history: nephritis, diabetes, hypertension and, in women, pelvic surgery (ureteric obstruction) and pre-eclampsia.
• Family history: hypertension, polycystic kidneys, familial nephritis and gout.

Examine for
• Brownish pallor of uraemia.
• Bruising.

- Hypertension and its consequences, especially cardiac enlargement or failure.
- Hypotension (especially postural) and reduced tissue turgor from dehydration.
- Hyperventilation from acidosis (Kussmaul's respiration).
- Palpable bladder in outflow obstruction.
- Palpable kidneys (polycystic disease and hydronephrosis).
- Ankle (or sacral) oedema of nephrotic syndrome or fluid overload.
- Signs of dialysis (arteriovenous fistula, continuous ambulatory peritoneal dialysis (CAPD) catheter).
- Peripheral neuropathy.
- Pericarditis is a late event in uraemia.
- Muscular twitching, hiccup, fall in blood pressure and uraemic frost are rare terminal manifestations.
- Rectal examination for prostatic hypertrophy or carcinoma must be performed in practice.

Investigate initially
- Urine for microscopy, protein and glucose.
- Blood for urea, creatinine, potassium and bicarbonate.
- Ultrasound for pelvic dilatation of outflow obstruction and for renal size.

Urea and creatinine (p. 196)
Production rate of urea varies, making it a less useful measure of renal function than creatinine, which is produced at a roughly constant rate proportional to skeletal muscle mass.

Serum urea increased
- *Decreased excretion*: renal failure (prerenal, renal or postrenal, p. 193).
- *Increased protein catabolism*: steroids, surgery, cytotoxic therapy, trauma, infection.
- *Increased protein intake*: dietary, gastrointestinal haemorrhage.

Serum urea decreased
- *Decreased synthesis*: extensive liver disease, low protein intake (malnutrition or malabsorption).
- *Increased excretion*: pregnancy (glomerular filtration rate (GFR) increases).

- *Dilution*: inappropriate anti-diuretic hormone (ADH) secretion, overenthusiastic intravenous fluids.

Serum creatinine increased
Impaired kidney function: 50% loss of renal function is needed before the serum creatinine rises above the normal range; it is therefore not a sensitive indicator of mild to moderate renal injury.

Creatinine clearance provides a more accurate assessment (if performed correctly). The patient performs a 24-h collection of urine (the first urine passed on waking is discarded, and all urine passed, up until and including emptying the bladder the following morning, is collected). A single measurement of plasma creatinine is made during this time. Creatinine clearance is measured as:

(urine creatinine concentration ÷ plasma creatinine) × urine volume per minute.

In addition to being filtered by the glomerulus, small quantities of creatinine are excreted by the tubules. The creatinine clearance therefore slightly overestimates the GFR. Chromium-51 ethylenediamine tetra-acetic acid ($[^{51}Cr]$ EDTA) clearance more accurately reflects the GFR. It is calculated from the rate of disappearance of a bolus injection of $[^{51}Cr]$ EDTA from the blood.

Serum creatinine decreased
Loss of muscle mass, including muscular dystrophies.

Dysphagia

'This patient complains of dysphagia; please question and examine him' This term includes both difficulty with swallowing and pain on swallowing. The former symptom is more prominent in obstruction and the latter with inflammatory lesions.

The history should be taken of the more common causes, remembering that previous reflux oesophagitis suggests peptic stricture and that recurrent chest infections occur with achalasia, bronchial carcinoma or pharyngeal pouches.

Examine the mouth and pharynx (pallor, carcinoma, neurological abnormalities), neck (goitre, and glands from carcinoma) and abdomen (carcinoma) with an initial glance at the hands for koilonychia of iron deficiency (Plummer–Vinson syndrome, see below).

Most common causes

Carcinoma of the oesophagus and gastric fundus usually gives a history of increasing painless difficulty with swallowing foods for the previous 2–3 months. The patient is often reduced to taking only soups and drinks by the time of presentation.

Peptic oesophagitis (with pain) proceeds to stricture with difficulty in swallowing.

Rarer causes

• Achalasia of the cardia, mainly in the relatively young. Food 'sticks' and is regurgitated unchanged a short while later (without acid); 25% present with recurrent pulmonary infection.
• External pressure. Because the oesophagus is slippery, symptoms of pressure from outside masses (especially carcinoma of the bronchus) are very seldom presenting ones. A retrosternal goitre large enough to produce dysphagia is usually obvious.
• The elderly may develop a dysmotility syndrome which may resolve spontaneously.

Very rare causes

Neurological disease: myasthenia gravis (p. 116) and bulbar palsies (p. 12).

Plummer–Vinson syndrome (Paterson–Brown–Kelly) usually occurs in middle-aged women who have iron-deficiency anaemia, koilonychia and glossitis. It may be associated with a postcricoid oesophageal web, which is associated with a 10% incidence of local cancer.

Investigations

If you are asked to discuss investigations, suggest:
• haemoglobin, serum iron and ferritin;
• barium swallow (Fig. 5.4); and

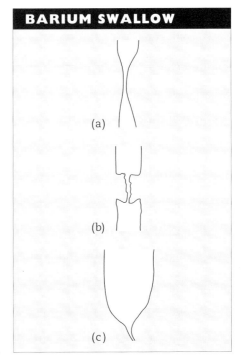

BARIUM SWALLOW

Fig. 5.4 Barium swallow X-ray. (a) Benign peptic stricture—smooth narrowing, usually at lower end of oesophagus in association with reflux or hiatus hernia. (b) Malignant stricture—irregular narrowing with shouldered edges. (c) Achalasia—smooth narrowing of the lower end of the oesophagus with dilatation above.

• endoscopy with biopsy to differentiate between benign peptic stricture and carcinoma.
NB The postcricoid web occurs in the anterior oesophageal wall and appears on barium swallow as an anterior indentation at the top of the oesophagus at the level of the cricoid cartilage.

Diarrhoea

Acute gastroenteritis with diarrhoea and vomiting is the second most common group of disorders affecting the community (second only to acute respiratory infections).

Aetiology

Infectious diarrhoea
This is usually *acute* and viral. None of the

common enteroviruses (Coxsackie, polio, echoviruses) can be confidently incriminated. Infant diarrhoea is usually caused by a rotavirus. Some outbreaks of diarrhoea are caused by specific serotypes of *Escherichia coli* to which the local population is not immune. The vast majority of patients are successfully treated symptomatically.

Food poisoning. *Salmonella typhimurium* is responsible for 75% of bacterial food poisoning. *S. enteritidis* infection from eggs and poultry is common. Staphylococcal food poisoning results from eating precooked meats and dairy foods, and is produced by the bacterial toxin.

Enteric fevers. Typhoid and paratyphoid must also be considered in patients returning from endemic areas.

Dysentery (p. 232). Results from ingestion of organisms of the genus *Shigella* (bacillary dysentery). Amoebic dysentry and giardiasis should also be considered in patients recently returned from the tropics.

Campylobacter infection is one of the most common causes of bacterial gastroenteritis in the UK. It is carried and communicated by cattle (milk), pets and is common in poultry. Incubation takes up to a week, followed by fever, myalgia and cramping diarrhoea, occasionally bloody.

Clostridium difficile infection (pseudomembranous colitis, p. 221) usually follows antibiotic therapy.

Cryptosporidium causes severe and sometimes intractable diarrhoea in acquired immunodeficiency syndrome (AIDS).

Non-infectious diarrhoea
The following conditions must be considered:
• drugs, including purgatives (common);
• diverticulitis (common);
• colonic carcinoma, sometimes with spurious diarrhoea secondary to partial obstruction (usually alternates with spells of constipation);

• irritable bowel syndrome (p. 229) (common);
• ulcerative colitis and Crohn disease;
• malabsorption syndromes; and
• diabetes, thyrotoxicosis (rare).

'This patient has developed diarrhoea. Would you question and examine him?' In hospital, the acute diarrhoeas are seen less frequently than in general practice. It is important to determine whether the recent attack is an isolated one or part of a chronic or recurrent history. If it is isolated and acute, ask about travel and residence abroad, contact history, previous antibiotic therapy and, if food poisoning is suspected, the time relationship to previous food and its effect on other eaters. If the diarrhoea is recurrent or chronic, ask about appetite, weight loss, abdominal pain, blood or mucus in the stools, drug ingestion including purgatives and operations.

Examination

In practice a complete medical examination is required. In examinations, note particularly weight loss, anaemia and clubbing (Crohn disease, p. 221). Look for abnormal abdominal masses (usually carcinoma, but Crohn disease should be suspected in young patients). Rectal examination and sigmoidoscopy should invariably be performed in chronic and recurrent diarrhoeas but these should not be attempted in examinations (although the examiner should be told of their necessity).

Investigation

'How would you investigate this patient?' If it is a single episode of acute diarrhoea and has not settled within 5−7 days or if the patient is ill, perform the following.
• Full blood count for anaemia and blood cultures for *Salmonella typhi*, *S. paratyphi* and *S. enteritidis*, particularly in travellers from abroad.
• Stool to laboratory for examination for cysts, ova and parasites (amoeba, *Giardia*) and for culture (typhoid and paratyphoid, *Campylobacter*, *Clostridium difficile*).
• Sigmoidoscopy, particularly in suspected ulcerative colitis or carcinoma (or amoebic colitis). Biopsy and histology may be diagnostic.

If acute diarrhoea remains undiagnosed or fails to respond to simple symptomatic remedies within 1–2 weeks or in chronic diarrhoea, it is usually necessary (if not previously indicated) to proceed to further investigation, including sigmoidoscopy with biopsy followed after a few days (to allow healing) by barium enema. If the history suggests malabsorption (p. 225), perform endoscopic duodenal biopsy and, if Crohn disease is suspected, obtain small-bowel barium studies.

Bloody diarrhoea suggests:

- colonic carcinoma;
- diverticular disease;
- ulcerative colitis;
- dysentery;
- ischaemic colitis; or
- *Campylobacter* enteritis, usually from uncooked chicken.

If the cause is not obvious, rectal bleeding needs full investigation with sigmoidoscopy and barium enema, proceeding to colonoscopy if necessary. However, the most common cause of rectal bleeding is haemorrhoids and fissures.

NB Dysentery (bacillary and amoebic), typhoid and paratyphoid, and cholera are notifiable to the public health authorities in the UK.

Respiratory System

The most usual types of clinical case seen in examinations are those secondary to carcinoma of the bronchus or caused by long-standing chronic disease. Asthma and chronic bronchitis are very common chronic disabilities. Bronchiectasis is still sufficiently common to appear in examinations. Pleural effusions are usually secondary to underlying carcinoma (primary or secondary) or to infection.

Examination

'*Examine the chest*' or '*Examine the lungs*' This means '*Examine the respiratory system*' unless otherwise specified.

If asked to question the patient, enquire about smoking, occupation, dyspnoea, chest pain, cough, sputum and haemoptysis, allergy, family history of allergy and an occupational history (e.g. asbestosis, mining). The diagnosis of chronic bronchitis is made on the history of 3 months' productive cough in 2 consecutive years.

Observation
• On approaching the patient note dyspnoea and cyanosis and any evidence of loss of weight.
• Examine the hands for clubbing, tobacco staining and feel for the bounding pulse of carbon dioxide retention if you suspect respiratory failure.
• Quickly check the height of the jugular venous pressure, and the tongue for cyanosis.
• Remove all patient's clothes above the waist and observe the shape of the chest and spine, any scars (NB Carcinoma of the breast) and the movements for symmetry and expansion (subtle differences are best seen from the end of the bed), and the use of accessory muscles

in the neck and shoulders. Enlarged lymph glands may be visible in the neck.
• Count the respiratory rate.

Palpation
The anterior surface markings of the lungs are shown in Fig. 6.1. Palpate for chest expansion. Always compare the movements of the two sides. *Diminished movement on one side means pathology on that side* (Table 6.1).

Palpate the trachea in the suprasternal notch (easier with the patient's head partially extended). Deviation denotes fibrosis or collapse of the upper lobe or whole lung in the direction of the deviation, or pneumothorax (or, very rarely, a large pleural effusion) on the other side. NB Local causes may produce deviation in the absence of lung disease, e.g. a goitre or spinal asymmetry. The position of the heart apex beat is of no help in assessing lung disease except if there is marked mediastinal shift.

Palpate for cervical lymphadenopathy.

Percussion
Percuss by moving down the chest comparing both sides. Stony dullness in the axilla usually indicates pleural effusion. Pleural thickening and collapse, consolidation or fibrosis of the lung also give dullness .
NB Upper-lobe fibrosis in an otherwise fit elderly patient is probably a result of old tuberculosis.

Diminished movement with resonance on one side usually means pneumothorax (or, occasionally, a large bulla).

Auscultation
Bronchial breathing occurs with consolidation, including that at the top of an effusion.

SURFACE MARKINGS OF THE LUNGS

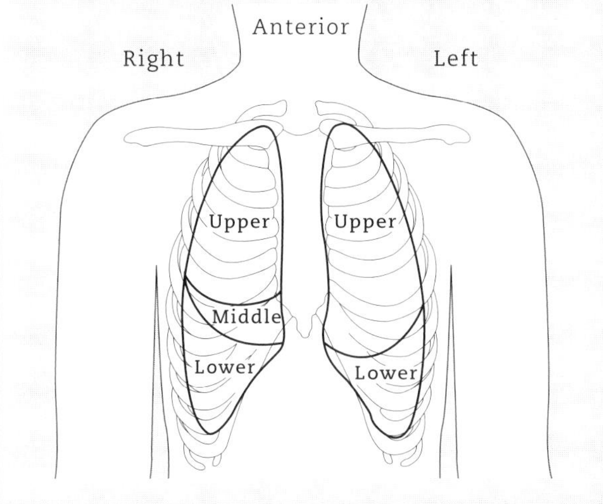

Anterior

Right

Left

Upper   Upper

Middle

Lower   Lower

Fig. 6.1 Oblique fissures run along the line of the fifth/sixth rib; a horizontal fissure runs from the fourth costal cartilage to the sixth rib in the mid-axillary line. Note: posteriorly you are listening mainly to lower lobes. Anteriorly you are listening mainly to upper lobes and on the right the middle lobe.

PHYSICAL SIGNS

	Movements on side of lesion	Trachea	Percussion	Breath sounds	Tactile fremitus and vocal resonance
Pleural effusion	Diminished	Usually central May be deviated away from lesion if very large	Dull (stony)	Diminished, often with bronchial breathing at top of effusion	Diminished
Pneumothorax	Diminished	Usually central May be deviated away if very large	Hyperresonant	Diminished	Diminished
Consolidation (pneumonia)	Diminished	Central or deviated towards side of lesion if associated with collapse	Dull	Bronchial (tubular) if airway open Absent if airway obstructed, e.g. carcinoma	Increased if airway open Diminished if airway obstructed
Fibrosis	Diminished	Deviated towards fibrosis if upper lobe affected	Dull	Bronchial	Increased
Chronic obstructive pulmonary disease		Central, possibly with tug	Normal or hyperresonant	Scattered added sounds	Normal

NB All the signs—bronchial breathing, increased vocal resonance, increased tactile fremitus, whispering pectoriloquy—occur in consolidation.

Table 6.1 Physical signs in lung disease.

Diminished breath sounds occur overlying an effusion, pleural thickening, pneumothorax and, in the obese, as a result of interposition of abnormal features between the lung surface and the stethoscope. Diminished breath sounds can also occur with obstructed airways (e.g. in severe asthma).

Added sounds are either wheezes (*rhonchi*) or crackles (*crepitations*—sounds like rubbing strands of hair between finger and thumb behind the ear). Wheezing is common in asthma and bronchitis but sometimes occurs in left ventricular failure ('cardiac asthma'). Crackles are 'fine' in pulmonary congestion and fibrosing alveolitis, and 'coarse' in the presence of excess bronchial secretions. Vocal resonance is increased over areas of consolidation. Friction rubs occur with pleurisy.

Whispering pectoriloquy occurs in association with consolidation. The patient is asked to whisper (not phonate) '1–2–3–4' and this is heard by the exploring stethoscope on the chest wall overlying the consolidation. (It can be imitated by whispering with both ears blocked with index fingers.)

Notes

Clubbing
Associated with diseases in the lungs, heart and abdomen:
• Carcinoma of bronchus (the only common cause).
• Pus in the pleura (empyema), lung (abscess) or bronchi (bronchiectasis, cystic fibrosis).
• Fibrosing alveolitis.
• Cyanotic congenital heart disease.
• Subacute bacterial endocarditis.
• Crohn disease (less commonly, ulcerative colitis or cirrhosis).

Haemoptysis
Aetiology
Common
• Bronchial carcinoma (or, rarely, other vascular tumours).
• Tuberculosis (active or healed).
• Pulmonary embolism with infarction.

• Infection (pneumococcal pneumonia, lung abscess and *Klebsiella pneumoniae*).
The presence of chronic bronchitis, a common cause of slight haemoptysis, does not exclude any of the above.

Uncommon
• Foreign body—history of general anaesthetic, visit to dentist or inhalation of food, especially peanuts.
• Coagulation disorders.
• Bronchiectatic cavities or chronic bronchitis.
• Mitral stenosis.
• Wegener's granulomatosis (a generalized vasculitis which may present with rhinitis and round lung shadows with or without ear, nose and throat masses and/or renal failure, p. 125).
• Goodpasture syndrome (glomerulonephritis with haemoptysis, p. 201).

Investigation
The usual clinical problem is to exclude carcinoma and tuberculosis. A full history and clinical examination will usually identify pulmonary infarction, foreign body, bronchiectasis, mitral stenosis and pulmonary oedema.
• *Sputum for culture*, including tuberculosis and cytology for malignant cells.
• *Chest X-ray*.
• *CT or MRI scan* may define the site and nature of the lesions seen on chest X-ray.
• *Bronchoscopy* with biopsy for cytology and culture. Visible lesions are biopsied—this is essential in all patients suspected of early bronchial carcinoma, which is amenable to surgery only if diagnosed early.
• *CT guided biopsy* of mass lesions.
• *Isotope (V/Q) lung scan* if pulmonary embolism is suspected.
NB About 40% of patients with haemoptysis have no demonstrable cause. Patients who have had a single small haemoptysis, no other symptoms and a normal chest X-ray (posteroanterior and lateral) probably do not require further investigation, but a follow-up appointment with a chest X-ray is advisable after 1–2 months. Patients who have more than one small haemoptysis should be regarded as having carcinoma or tuberculosis

until proved otherwise, and be referred for bronchoscopy.

Pleural effusion

Aetiology
• Carcinoma: primary bronchus (the effusion implies pleural involvement) or secondary (commonly breast).
• Cardiac failure.
• Pulmonary embolus and infarction.
• Tuberculosis.
• Other infections (pneumonia).
• Rarely, lymphomas, systemic lupus erythematosus, rheumatoid arthritis and transdiaphragmatic spread of ascites including peritoneal dialysis and Meigs syndrome (usually a right-sided transudate from benign ovarian fibroma).
NB Aspiration of the fluid is usually necessary both for treatment and to assist diagnosis. A pleural biopsy should be performed at the same time. Specimens are sent to the laboratory for:
• microscopy;
• bacterial culture, including tuberculosis;
• histology;
• cytology for malignant cells; and
• protein content: 30 g/l approximately divides exudates from transudates.

Cyanosis

'Cyanosis' is a clinical description and refers to the blue colour of a patient's lips, tongue (central) or fingers (peripheral). Central cyanosis is almost always caused by the presence of an excess of reduced haemoglobin in the capillaries. Over 3 g/dl is usually present before cyanosis is apparent. Thus, in anaemia, severe hypoxaemia may be present without cyanosis.

'*Look at this (cyanosed) patient*' It is often difficult to tell whether cyanosis is present or not. Comparison of the colour of the patient's tongue or nail beds with your own nail beds (presumed to be normal) may help if both hands are warm.

Look at the patient's tongue. If it is cyanosed, the cyanosis is central in origin and secondary to:
• chronic bronchitis and emphysema, often with cor pulmonale;

• congenital heart disease (cyanosis may be present only after exercise);
• polycythaemia; or
• massive pulmonary embolism.
In central cyanosis there is always cyanosis at the periphery.

If the tongue is not cyanosed but the fingers, toes or ear lobes are, the cyanosis is peripheral:
• physiological caused by cold; and
• pathological in peripheral vascular disease (the cyanosed parts feel cold).
NB Left ventricular failure may produce cyanosis that is partly central (pulmonary) and partly peripheral (poor peripheral circulation).

A rare cause of cyanosis, which is not caused by increased circulating reduced haemoglobin, is the presence of methaemoglobin (and/or sulphaemoglobin). The patient is relatively well and not necessarily dyspnoeic. *Methaemoglobinaemia* is usually the result of taking certain drugs, e.g. sulphonamides, primaquine (an 8-amino quinoline) or nitrites.

Cyanosis is an unreliable guide to the degree of hypoxaemia.

Chest radiology

Normal chest X-rays are shown in Fig. 6.2 (posteroanterior) and 6.3 (lateral). Fig. 6.4 is a radiological chest diagram of lobar collapse. CT chest scans are shown in Fig. 6.5. CT scanning is more sensitive and may be useful in detecting interstitial disease, cavitation or empyema. Chest X-ray findings in cardiovascular disease are described on p. 78.

Blood gases

'*Comment on these blood gases*' The normal arterial values are:

P_{O_2}	12–14 kPa
P_{CO_2}	4.7–6.0 kPa
pH	7.37–7.42
Standard HCO_3^-	23–27 mmol/l

Look at the pH to diagnose an acidosis or alkalosis.

LATERAL CHEST X-RAY

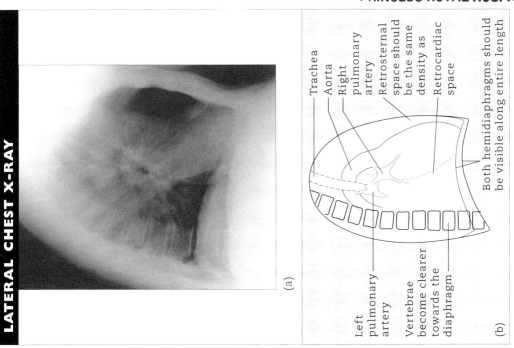

Fig. 6.3 (a) X-ray. (b) Diagrammatic representation.

NORMAL PA CHEST X-RAY

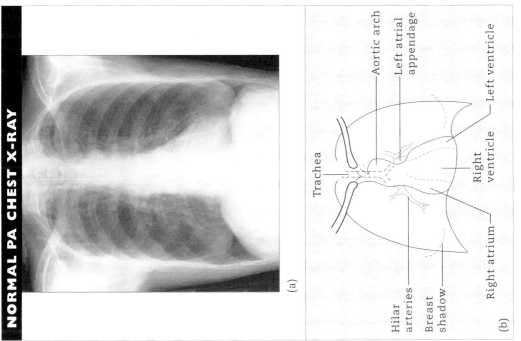

Fig. 6.2 (a) X-ray. (b) Diagrammatic representation.

LOBAR COLLAPSE

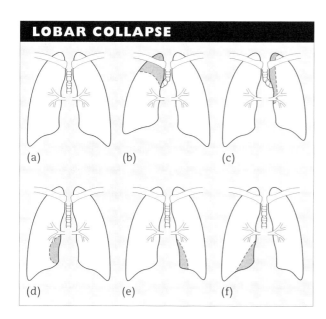

(a)   (b)   (c)

(d)   (e)   (f)

Fig. 6.4 Diagrammatic representation of radiological appearance of lobar collapse. (a) Normal. (b) Right upper lobe: trachea deviated to right, right diaphragm and hilium elevated. (c) Left upper lobe: trachea deviated to left, left hilium and diaphragm elevated. (d) Right middle lobe: right heart border lost. (e) Left lower lobe: trachea may deviate to left, shadow behind heart. (f) Right lower lobe: trachea may deviate to right, outline of right diaphragm lost.

Look at the P_{CO_2}. If it is raised this may account for an acidosis of respiratory origin (respiratory failure). If it is reduced this may account for an alkalosis as a result of hyperventilation (pain, stiff lungs, anxiety and hysterical hyperventilation or artificial ventilation).

Look at 'standard HCO_3^-' (measured at a normal P_{CO_2}, i.e. with simulated normal ventilation). If it is raised this accounts for a metabolic alkalosis. If it is reduced it accounts for a metabolic acidosis (usually renal or diabetic ketosis).

Look at the P_{O_2}. If it is high, the patient is on added oxygen. If low, the patient has either lung disease (the P_{CO_2} is usually high) or a right-to-left shunt.

Interpretation
• P_{CO_2} reflects alveolar ventilation.
• P_{O_2} reflects ventilation/perfusion imbalance, gas transfer or venous-to-arterial shunts.

Arterial gas patterns
High P_{CO_2}, *low* P_{O_2}. Respiratory failure resulting from chronic obstructive pulmonary disease, asthma or chest wall disease (e.g. ankylosing spondylitis or neuromuscular disorders).

Normal or low P_{CO_2}, *low* P_{O_2}. Hypoxia as a result of parenchymal lung disease with normal airways. These patients hyperventilate and hence lower the P_{CO_2} because of hypoxia (and 'stiff lungs'), e.g. pulmonary embolism, fibrosing alveolitis. Another cause is venous admixture from right-to-left shunts (e.g. tetralogy of Fallot, p. 283).

Low P_{CO_2}, *normal* P_{O_2}. A common pattern usually seen after painful arterial puncture (causing hyperventilation), and in hysterical hyperventilation.

Causes of hypoxaemia
• Hypoventilation because of sedative drugs, central nervous system disease, neuromuscular disease, crushed chest/or obstructive sleep apnoea. The arterial P_{CO_2} is characteristically high.
• Ventilation/perfusion imbalance. Hyperventilation of some alveoli cannot compensate for the hypoxaemia which results from the hypoventilation of other alveoli. This is the usual cause of a reduced transfer factor.
• Physiological shunt (venous admixture) when deoxygenated blood passes straight to the left heart without perfusing ventilated alveoli. This occurs in cyanotic congenital heart disease.

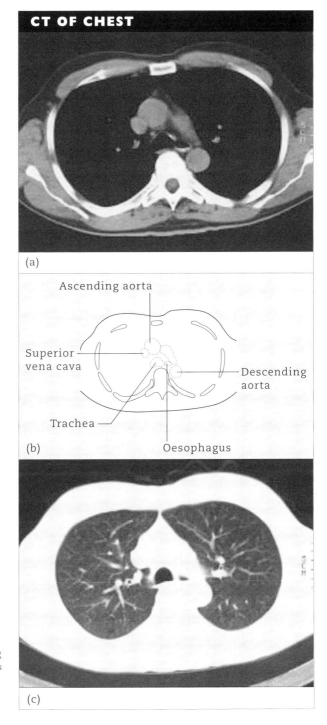

Fig. 6.5 (a) CT of chest at the level of T4 vertebra. (b) Diagrammatic representation. (c) The same CT in which a different window setting has been used to visualize the lung markings (the window settings determine the range of densities displayed by the computer).

The arterial Po_2 is not significantly improved by the administration of 2 l oxygen/min.

• Low inspired oxygen concentration because of altitude or faulty apparatus.

Type 1 respiratory failure ($Po_2 < 8$ kPa; CO_2 normal) refers to patients with a lung disease that produces hypoxaemia as well as hyperventilation (low CO_2), e.g. pulmonary oedema, pneumonia, asthma, pulmonary fibrosis and pulmonary thromboembolism.

Type 2 respiratory failure ($Po_2 < 8$ kPa; $CO_2 > 6.6$ kPa) with hypoxaemia and a high Pco_2 implies a defect in ventilation with obstructed airways, reduced chest wall compliance, or central nervous system disease because otherwise the excess carbon dioxide would be blown off.

Pulmonary function tests

The simplest tests of lung function are spirometric. If a patient exhales as fast and as long as possible from full inspiration into a spirometer, the volume expired in the first second is the forced expiratory volume in 1 s (FEV_1) and the total expired is the forced vital capacity (FVC). Relaxed (slow) vital capacity may provide a better measure of trapped gas volume in chronic airways obstruction and is as easy to

Fig. 6.6 Spirometric patterns. (a) Normal (elderly man) forced expiratory volume/ forced vital capacity (FEV/FVC) = 3.0/4.0 = 75%. (b) Restrictive, FEV/FVC = 1.8/2.0 = 90%. (c) Obstructive, FEV/FVC = 1.4/3.5 = 40%.

measure as these other values. Constriction of the major airways (e.g. asthma) reduces the FEV_1 more than the FVC. Restriction of the lungs (e.g. by fibrosis) reduces the FVC and, to a lesser degree, the FEV_1. The $FEV_1 : FVC$ ($FEV\%$) ratio thus tends to be low in obstructive airways disease (e.g. chronic bronchitis and asthma) and normal or high in fibrosing alveolitis (p. 253). It is best to see the shape of the actual curve as well as the figures derived from it (Fig. 6.6). Spirometry is often performed before and after bronchodilatation.

The peak expiratory flow rate (PEFR) measures the rate of flow of exhaled air at the start of a forced expiration. It gives similar information to the FEV_1.

Normal values for all these tests vary with age, sex, size and race, and suitable nomograms should be consulted unless the changes observed are gross.

Transfer factor

The patient must have a vital capacity of over 1 litre and be able to hold the breath for 15 s. This test measures the transfer of a small concentration of carbon monoxide in the inspired air on to haemoglobin. It is reduced in diseases that reduce ventilation or perfusion or alters the balance between them, and increased in pulmonary haemorrhage. Correction must be made for haemoglobin concentration, because the transfer factor varies directly with haemoglobin. Its chief value is for monitoring progression in interstitial disease, including fibrosing alveolitis and confirming a diagnosis of pulmonary haemorrhage.

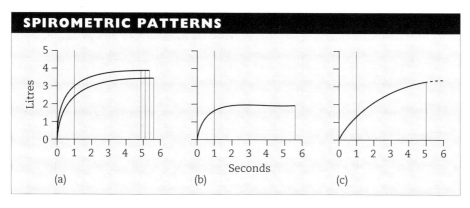

SPIROMETRIC PATTERNS

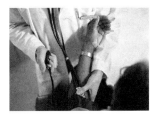

Cardiovascular System

There is no shortage of patients with cardio-vascular disease who are suitable for inclusion in examinations. Patients with ischaemic heart disease have few physical signs and the diagnosis of angina of effort will be made on symptoms alone. Valvular disease, whether acquired or congenital, and septal defects often give rise to murmurs which may be diagnostic. The penalties for failing to elicit and describe and interpret these correctly are often disproportionate to their real importance in diagnosis and treatment. A cardiologist rarely reaches a final decision on physical signs alone unsupported by an electrocardiogram, chest X-ray and echocardiogram. Patients with congestive heart failure and cases of myocardial infarction are very common in hospital and during the recovery phase may be sufficiently well to be included in an examination list.

Arterial pulse

'Examine the (arterial) pulse' If you are asked this, there is frequently an arrhythmia (often atrial fibrillation or multiple ectopic beats). Less commonly, you may feel the very slow regular pulse of complete heart block. There may be a tachycardia, such as that associated with thyrotoxicosis, anaemia or anxiety.

Do not attempt to estimate the blood pressure from the pulse.

Examine a carotid, brachial or radial pulse, whichever you are familiar with assessing. Describe as follows.

Approximate rate

Glance at the jugular venous pressure while counting, because this may give valuable addi-tional information about cardiac rhythm and failure (see below).

Rhythm

This is regular, basically regular with extra or dropped beats, or completely irregular. If it is clinically atrial fibrillation, remember that the pulse rate is different from the heart rate, so listen at the apex as well.

Volume and character (Table 7.1)

These abnormalities fall into three categories:

1 useful to confirm or assess other findings in the cardiovascular system (plateau, collapsing, small volume);

2 rare and/or difficult (alternans, bisferiens and paradoxus); and

3 examination 'catch' (absent radial).

NB The rate and rhythm are relatively easy to assess but the character of the pulse is extremely difficult to evaluate.

Neck veins

'Look at the veins of the neck' ('Examine the jugular venous pressure or pulse')

Raised jugular venous pressure and pulse (Table 7.2 and Fig. 7.1)

You should comment on the *vertical* height of the top of the column of blood above the sternal angle. The patient should be lying at 45° and the neck relaxed. Illumination, perhaps from your pocket torch (on which you can usefully place a centimetre scale), should be across the area. The sternal angle is about 5 cm above the left atrium when the patient is lying at 45°. The normal central venous pressure (CVP) is

SPECIAL PULSES

Type	Character	Seen in
Plateau	Low amplitude, slow rise, slow fall	Aortic valve stenosis
Collapsing (water hammer)	Large amplitude, rapid rise, rapid fall	Aortic regurgitation. Also severe anaemia, hyperthyroidism arteriovenous shunt, heart block, patent ductus arteriosus
Small volume	Thready	Low cardiac output because of obstruction: valve stenosis (tricuspid, pulmonary, mitral, aortic) or pulmonary hypertension
		Shock
Alternans	Alternate large- and small- amplitude beats rarely noted in pulse; usually on taking blood pressure (note doubling in rate as mercury falls)	Left ventricular failure
Bisferiens	Double-topped	Aortic stenosis with aortic regurgitation
Paradoxus	Pulse volume decreases excessively with inspiration (of little diagnostic value)	Cardiac tamponade, constrictive pericarditis, severe inspiratory airways obstruction (chronic bronchitis and asthma)
Absent radial		Congenital anomaly (check brachials and blood pressure)
		Tied off at surgery or catheterization
		Arterial embolism (usually atrial fibrillation)

Notes
1 The state of one vessel wall does not necessarily correlate with the state of the arteries elsewhere.
2 It takes little time to check if the other radial (or brachial) pulse is present.
3 If you think the patient may have hypertension, you should look for radial femoral delay (aortic coarctation).
4 If the character of the pulse is abnormal you should ask whether you may take the blood pressure, to estimate the pulse pressure (and to check alternans).

Table 7.1 Abnormalities of the arterial pulse.

< 7 cm and therefore the jugular vein is normally just visible.

In the neck, the venous pulse differs from the arterial pulse:
• its height varies with posture, it is impalpable and low pressure means that it is easily abolished by light finger pressure;
• the height varies with respiration (fall in inspiration and rise with expiration); and
• there are two peaks with each pulsation, 'a' and 'v'.

The deep venous pulse is seen welling up between the heads of sternomastoid in the front of the neck on expiration, and is a better guide to right atrial pressure than the superficial venous pulse which can be obstructed by the soft tissues of the neck. If you can find neither then proceed as follows.
• Look at the other side of the neck.
• Suspect a low level: unless the liver is tender, press on the abdomen gently but firmly. This 'hepatojugular reflux' (not 'reflex') has no

RAISED JUGULAR VENOUS PRESSURE

Character	Compression of neck and abdomen	Conclusion
Non-pulsatile	No change in jugular venous pressure	Superior mediastinal obstruction (usually carcinoma of bronchus), platysmal compression or large goitre
Pulsatile	Jugular vein fills and empties	Right heart failure Expiratory airways obstruction (asthma and bronchitis) Fluid overload Cardiac tamponade (very rare)

Note: There is no 'a' wave in atrial fibrillation.

Table 7.2   Raised jugular venous pressure (JVP).

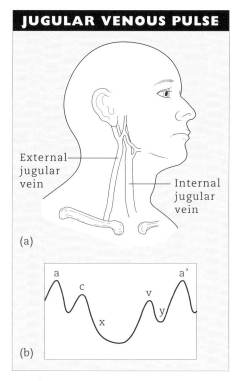

JUGULAR VENOUS PULSE

External jugular vein

Internal jugular vein

(a)

a

c

a'

v

x

y

(b)

Fig. 7.1 (a) Surface markings of the internal and external jugular veins. (b) Jugular venous pulse waveform.

pathophysiological significance and the sole purpose of this manoeuvre is to demonstrate the vein and to show that it can be filled (i.e. that the pressure is not high).

• Suspect a high level: the top of the column may be above the mastoid. Check if the ear lobes move with the cardiac cycle and sit the patient vertical to get a greater length of visible jugular vein above the right atrium. The venous pressure can sometimes be demonstrated in dilatated veins of an arm or handheld at a suitable height above the right atrium. The level at which pulsation occurs should be determined.

If the jugular venous pressure is raised (especially if > 10 cm).

• A large 'a' wave (corresponds with atrial systole) occurs in conditions where the right atrial pressure is raised, e.g. tricuspid stenosis, pulmonary hypertension, pulmonary stenosis and mitral stenosis. A cannon wave is a massive 'a' wave occurring in complete heart block when the right atrium contracts against a closed tricuspid valve. There is no 'a' wave in atrial fibrillation because there is no atrial systole.

• Look for a large 'v' wave (corresponds with ventricular systole) indicating tricuspid regurgitation (usually secondary to marked heart failure): a murmur may be audible on auscultation of the heart.

• Examine the abdomen for an enlarged, tender, pulsatile liver.

• Check the ankles for oedema and then sit the patient up and examine the back of the chest for crepitations and for pleural effusions (unilateral or bilateral) and for sacral oedema. These should be carried out even if the jugular

venous pressure is not raised because oedema of cardiac failure may persist after jugular venous pressure has been reduced by treatment.
• Examine for the underlying cause, e.g. heart valve lesion or fluid overload.

Heart

'*Examine the heart*' Most heart cases in an examination have a murmur. Such patients make it easy for an examiner to assess the candidate's ability to elicit and describe accurately the physical signs that are present. You may be watched throughout your examination and you must therefore have devised a system of examination that is second nature to you, even in this stressful situation.

A full examination of the heart is not advisable without examining the arterial and venous pulses and this is usually performed first. It is important to know not only the auscultatory features of the various heart abnormalities but also to know which of them are found in association with each other and to examine for these with particular care. Thus, a patient in whom you have diagnosed mitral stenosis should be examined with special attention to the aortic valve.

Chronic rheumatic heart disease is still the most common type of heart case in examinations, although most have had cardiac surgery. It is becoming progressively less common in clinical practice because rheumatic fever is now a rare disorder. You may see patients with ventricular septal defects; the smaller lesions may not require surgery and often produce loud murmurs. For similar reasons you may be shown a patient with an atrial septal defect (ASD)—often not diagnosed until middle age—but the auscultatory findings may be difficult to elicit. Beware of coarctation of the aorta where loud murmurs may originate in collateral vessels over the chest wall.

On approaching the patient note any cyanosis, dyspnoea or malar flush.
• Examine the arterial pulses and look for clubbing.
• Examine the jugular venous pulse.
• Examine the front of the chest. First look for the scars of previous surgery and then for the localized thrusting apex beat of left ventricular hypertrophy and the parasternal lift of right ventricular hypertrophy. Then palpate for these phenomena and for thrills (palpable murmurs). Note that a tapping apex is thought to be an accentuated mitral first sound and in subsequent examination you will be trying to substantiate a diagnosis of mitral stenosis. Finally, listen to the heart, starting at the apex (Fig. 7.2). It may be difficult to establish which are the first and second sounds, but an experienced clinician recognizes them by their quality. A thumb on the right carotid artery can help to time the first sound. A third heart sound heard just after the second is common in young people, but abnormal over the age of 40 when it implies ventricular disease. The fourth heart sound, heard just before the first side, occurs in hypertension, aortic stenosis and myocardial infarction.
• Examine each part of the cardiac cycle for murmurs. Listen actively and positively, aware of what might be there, e.g. a high-pitched blowing murmur just after the first sound at the base of the heart (aortic regurgitation), or a low-pitched murmur starting well after the second sound internal to the apex (mitral stenosis, MS). There is no alternative to experience for this; it is essential to know the character of the murmurs of the more common cardiac lesions. Their description is formalized and stereotyped so that if you say there is a rumbling diastolic murmur at the apex, you have diagnosed mitral stenosis. You should attempt to make whatever you hear fit one of the known patterns (Table 7.3). Remember to listen for a friction rub of pericarditis over the lower sternum, and for a triple rhythm of cardiac failure. These are easily missed.
• Listen to the lungs, especially at the bases posteriorly for fine crackles. Look for sacral and ankle oedema. Establish the blood pressure.

Continuous murmurs

These are murmurs maximal in systole and pass through the second sound into diastole. They are caused by:
• patent ductus arteriosus (best heard in second left intercostal space);

LISTENING TO HEART VALVES

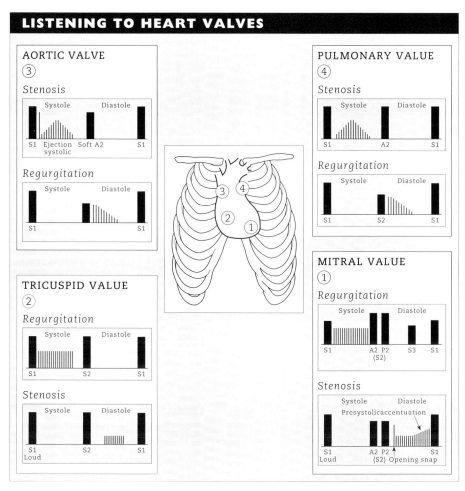

Fig. 7.2 Suggested stethoscopic route (1–4) for listening to heart valves. 1, apex; 2, lower right sternal edge; 3, right second intercostal space; 4, left second intercostal space. See Valvular heart disease, pp. 276–80.

• coarctation of the aorta (the murmur comes from flow in intercostal collateral arteries);
• arteriovenous malformation in the lung;
• coronary arteriovenous fistula; and
• ruptured sinus of Valsalva (the pockets behind each leaflet of the aortic valve)—a high-pitched murmur because of high pressure.
NB The unsatisfactory question, '*listen here or listen at this point*', usually the apex or aortic area is used to ensure that the candidate roll the patient on to the left side for mitral stenotic murmurs, or sits the patient forward and asks him or her to exhale fully for aortic regurgitation.

Heart failure (p. 265)

The signs of left ventricular failure are tachycardia, triple rhythm, fine basal crackles of pulmonary oedema and pleural effusion usually associated with signs of right ventricular failure, i.e. raised jugular venous pressure, hepatomegaly, ankle and sacral oedema.

If right ventricular failure is secondary to lung disease (cor pulmonale), there is usually clinical evidence to suggest chronic obstructive pulmonary disease (p. 233) or, less commonly, pulmonary embolism (p. 250). Other rare causes include bronchiectasis, fibrosing alveolitis, cystic fibrosis and primary pulmonary hypertension. Treatment is discussed on p. 267.

CHARACTERISTICS OF MURMURS

Lesion	Murmur and position	Radiation and notes
Aortic stenosis (often with aortic regurgitation)	Basal mid systolic, often loud and with a thrill. Possible ejection click	Maximal in second RICS and radiating into neck. Also at apex
Pulmonary stenosis (may be part of Fallot's tetralogy)	Basal mid systolic with click if stenosis is valvar	Maximal in second LICS. Increase on inspiration (with increased blood flow). Pulmonary component of second sound is quiet and delayed
Aortic regurgitation (often accompanying mitral stenosis in the UK because syphilis is now rare)	Early immediate blowing diastolic murmur	Usually maximal in third LICS or, less often, in second RICS. Radiation between right carotid and cardiac apex. Look for Argyll Robertson pupils, etc.
Pulmonary regurgitation very rare	Early immediate blowing diastolic murmur	Maximal in second and third LICS
Mitral stenosis	Mid or late rumbling diastolic murmur at apex	Loud mitral first sound. Opening snap. Turn patient on left side (and exercise) to accentuate murmur. Presystolic accentuation if in sinus rhythm
Mitral regurgitation mitral stenosis is present as well)	Pansystolic at apex	Radiation to axilla (but often heard parasternally)
Tricuspid regurgitation	Pansystolic and lower sternum	'v' wave in neck and pulsatile liver
Ventricular septal defect (small ones are common, severe are rare)	Rough, loud and pansystolic. Maximal at third to fourth LICS parasternally	
Atrial septal defect	Pulmonary systolic murmur with fixed split second sound (no murmur from blood flow through the defect)	Possible diastolic murmur from tricuspid valve if atrial septal defect flow is large
Patent ductus arteriosus	Machinery murmur, maximal in late systole and extending into diastole. Maximal in second to third LICS in mid-clavicular line	Also audible posteriorly
Coarctation	Loud rough murmur in systole, maximum over apex of left lung both posteriorly and anteriorly	Murmurs of scapular and internal mammary shunt collaterals. Radial femoral delay. Hypertension in arms
Friction rub	Scratchy noise, usually systole and diastole	Varies with posture and breathing

Notes
1 'Base' denotes the first and second intercostal spaces.
2 RICS and LICS refer to right and left intercostal spaces, respectively.

Table 7.3 Characteristics of murmurs.

Hypertension (p. 269)

'This person has hypertension—please examine him or her to demonstrate the key signs' If you are allowed to question the patient, ask about anginal chest pain, intermittent claudication, headaches, visual changes, family history, salt intake, breathlessness and drugs taken (especially the contraceptive pill, cold cures containing sympathomimetic drugs and monoamine oxidase inhibitors). A patient on ACE inhibitors may have a dry cough.

Slight or moderate hypertension usually gives no abnormalities detectable on physical examination. In long-standing or severe hypertension there will usually be left ventricular hypertrophy and a loud aortic second sound. The other consequences of sustained hypertension should be looked for—hypertensive retinopathy, heart failure, renal failure, cerebrovascular disease. It is essential to think of the less common causes of hypertension and therefore to consider the following.
• Observe the face for evidence of Cushing syndrome—usually resulting from steroids.
• Feel both radial arteries and take the blood pressure in both arms for coarctation.
• Examine for aortic coarctation (radial–femoral arterial pulse delay, weak femoral pulses and the bruits of the coarctation and of the scapular anastomoses and visible pulsation of the anastomoses).
• The kidneys are palpable in polycystic disease.
• A renal artery bruit may be present in the epigastrium in renal artery stenosis.
• Think also of chronic renal diseases (test the urine), of phaeochromocytoma (rare) and of primary hyperaldosteronism (very rare).

Myocardial infarction (p. 255)

'This patient has had a myocardial infarction: would you ask him some questions?' The patient will be in the recovery stage. The history is more important than the physical signs. Symptoms (pain or fatigue) are often present in the preceding weeks.

Ask about
• *Pain.* Onset (rest or exercise), quality (compressing), distribution (including radiation), duration (usually over half an hour). Tearing interscapular pain suggests dissecting aneurysm. NB Intensity is no guide to the extent of the infarct, especially in the elderly where pain may be absent.
• *Breathlessness.* About one-quarter of all cases describe an acute attack of dyspnoea as a feature of the attack and in the elderly it may be the only feature.
• *Cold sweat.* Also common, and often associated with nausea and vomiting.
• *Pallor.* Normally reported by witnesses.
• *Previous attacks of angina.* If they have had a previous infarct or angina their new pain will usually resemble that which they have had previously.
• *Past history* of hypertension, strokes, symptoms of peripheral vascular disease and, in young women, whether they have diabetes mellitus or are on the contraceptive pill.
• *Family history* of heart attacks, especially if young; diabetes; hypertension; raised cholesterol; gout.
• *Other risk factors*, e.g. smoking, occupation.

Examination
'Would you like to examine him?'
• Evidence of a low cardiac output (hypotension and small-volume rapid pulse).
• Signs of cardiac failure, including crackles at the lung bases.
• Arrhythmias, tachycardia, bradycardia.
• Pericardial friction (immediate and postinfarction Dressler syndrome).
• Evidence of mitral regurgitation (papillary muscle dysfunction).
• Evidence of a cardiac aneurysm (double impulse)—rare.
• Evidence of septal perforation (acquired ventricular septal defect, VSD)—rare and acute.
• Deep venous thrombosis—a complication of immobilization.
• Evidence of hyperlipidaemia, especially xanthelasmas and tendon xanthomas.
• Evidence of associated diseases: hypothyroidism, diabetes mellitus, gout, cigarette smoking (smell and finger-staining).

• Evidence of the relevant alternatives in the differential diagnosis, especially pulmonary embolism, pericarditis, dissecting aneurysm, pleurisy, cholecystitis, reflux oesophagitis, radicular pain.

Investigations

'*What investigations would you perform?*' Ask for an electrocardiogram (ECG) series and a cardiac enzyme series, e.g. troponin or creatine kinase (CK) isoenzyme (p. 259). You may note rises in the white cell count, erythrocyte sedimentation rate and temperature. A chest X-ray is necessary in all cardiac investigations.

Management

'*Discuss the management*' The following aspects should be considered:
• aspirin;
• thrombolytic therapy (p. 260);
• bed rest;
• analgesia and sedation;
• oxygen therapy;
• anticoagulants;
• β blockade;
• complications (cardiac failure and shock, arrhythmias, rupture of septum, papillary muscle dysfunction and cardiac aneurysm);
• smoking;
• obesity;
• statins for hyperlipidaemia (p. 168); and
• advice on discharge from hospital, i.e. work, driving, sexual activities (p. 264).

Arrhythmias (Table 7.4)

Supraventricular tachycardias

Supraventricular tachycardias arise from the atria or atrioventricular junction. QRS complex is normal unless there is also bundle branch block.

Sinus tachycardia

Sinus rhythm, rate > 100 beats/min. An underlying cause (anxiety, exercise, fever, anaemia, heart failure, thyrotoxicosis) can usually be identified.

Atrial fibrillation

Atrial fibrillation (AF) is predominantly a disease of the elderly, occurring in 0.2% of men aged 47–56 and 3% of those aged 77–86 (Framingham study, 1949).

Rheumatic AF occurs in association with rheumatic valve disease, whereas in nonrheumatic AF there is an underlying metabolic disorder or other form of cardiac disease.

Lone AF occurs in the absence of valvular, myocardial or other identifiable disease.

The common causes are:
• ischaemic heart disease;
• thyrotoxicosis;
• mitral valve disease; and
• cardiomyopathy.

Management

Check serum potassium, echocardiogram and thyroid function. The aims are to restore sinus rhythm or control the ventricular rate and minimize the risk of embolization.

Direct current (DC) cardioversion establishes sinus rhythm in 90% of patients, but relapse is common. Long-term amiodarone reduces the frequency of relapse, although side-effects can limit its use.
NB Side-effects of amiodarone are reversible corneal microdeposits, photosensitivity, skin discoloration, hypothyroidism, hyperthyroidism, diffuse pulmonary alveolitis and fibrosis, peripheral neuropathy and myopathy.

Medical therapy
Quinine, flecainide and amiodarone have all been used to restore and maintain sinus rhythm.

Digoxin does not restore sinus rhythm, but is effective in controlling the ventricular rate, either alone or in combination with β-blockers.

The incidence of ischaemic stroke (embolic or thrombotic) is increased in patients with AF. Five prospective trials have shown that using warfarin is effective in reducing the risk of stroke (see Trial Box 7.1). When warfarin is contraindicated, aspirin 75–150 mg/day is effective, although less so.

Atrial flutter

The atria discharge at around 300/min, giving the characteristic 'saw-tooth' baseline on ECG (see Fig. 7.15, p. 74). There is usually atrioventricular block, leading to a ventricular rate of

CARDIAC ARRHYTHMIAS

Rhythm	Rate Atrial	Ventricular	Diagnosis	Underlying diseases	Therapy (pp. 62–65)
Regular	90+	90+	Sinus tachycardia	Anxiety, cardiac failure, thyrotoxicosis, fever, anaemia	Treat underlying disease
	120–200	120–200	Supraventricular tachycardia	None (60%), thyrotoxicosis, digitalis, tobacco, caffeine, Wolff–Parkinson–White syndrome	Vagal stimulation (pressure on the carotid sinus), β-blocker or verapamil or digoxin
	200–400	100–200	Atrial flutter with block	Ischaemic heart disease, thyrotoxicosis (digitalis)	Digoxin, DC cardioversion, verapamil
	80+	30–45	Complete heart block with cannon 'a' waves in jugular vein pulse, variable intensity first sound, wide pulse pressure	Postinfarction, idiopathic, digitalis, cardiomyopathy	Nil if asymptomatic Atropine or cardiac pacemaker
	40–50	40–50	Sinus bradycardia	Athletes, myocardial infarction, myxoedema, hypothermia, sinoatrial disease	As heart block if following infarction
Irregular			Multiple ectopics (including coupled beats) ECG basically regular	Ischaemia, digitalis, thyrotoxicosis, cardiomyopathy	Stop digitalis and give potassium if necessary. β-blocker if resulting from digitalis
	60–100 treated 100+ untreated		Atrial flutter with varying block Atrial fibrillation (apex rate is only guide to true heart rate. ECG essential)	Ischaemia, rheumatic heart disease (MS), thyrotoxicosis. Rarely, pulmonary embolism, constructive pericarditis, cardiomyopathy or bronchial carcinoma	Digoxin, or DC cardioversion following myocardial infarction and following treated mitral stenosis and thyrotoxicosis
Cardiac arrest	120–200		Ventricular tachycardia	Myocardial infarction and ischaemia (p. 255)	
		No peripheral pulse	Ventricular fibrillation and sometimes ventricular tachycardia Ventricular asystole		

DC, Direct current; ECG, electrocardiogram; MS, mitral stenosis.

Table 7.4 Cardiac arrhythmias.

150/min (2 : 1) or 100/min (3 : 1). The rate is basically regular, although affected by 2 : 1, 3 : 1 and variable block.

The causes are similar to AF, although atrial flutter is less common.

Management

Drugs such as sotalol, amiodarone, propafenone and flecainide can be effective in restoring sinus rhythm. DC cardioversion can also be used to terminate atrial flutter.

TRIALS BOX 7.1

Atrial Fibrillation Aspirin Anticoagulation (**AFASAK**) studied 1007 patients with chronic non-rheumatic atrial fibrillation (AF). A total of 335 patients received warfarin openly (international normalized ratio (INR) 2.8–4.2), and in a double-blind study 336 received aspirin 75 mg/day or placebo. The incidence of thromboembolic complications and vascular mortality was significantly lower in the warfarin group than in the aspirin or placebo groups, which did not differ significantly. *Lancet* 1989; **i**: 175–179.

Boston Area Anticoagulation Trial for Atrial Fibrillation (**BAATAF**) compared warfarin (INR 1.5–2.7) with placebo in 420 patients. Warfarin reduced the risk of stroke by 14%. *N Engl J Med* 1990; **323**: 1505–1511.

Stroke Prevention in Atrial Fibrillation (**SPAF**) studied 1330 patients with constant or intermittent AF. Systemic embolization was reduced by 42% in patients receiving aspirin, and 67% in a subgroup of patients eligible to receive warfarin (INR 1.3–1.8). *Circulation* 1991; **84**: 527–539.

The **Stroke Prevention in Atrial Fibrillation (SPAF) III study** compared low-dose warfarin (initial INR 1.2–1.5) plus aspirin with adjusted-dose warfarin (INR 2.0–3.0) in 1044 patients with AF and other risk factors for thromboembolism (left ventricular dysfunction, hypertension, previous thromboembolism). Dose-adjusted warfarin was significantly better at preventing stroke. *Lancet* 1996; **348**: 633–638.

Canadian Atrial Fibrillation Anticoagulation (**CAFA**) compared warfarin (INR 2–3) and placebo in 378 patients. Warfarin reduced the risk of stroke by 79%. *J Am Coll Cardiol* 1991; **18**: 349–355.

Veterans Affairs Stroke Prevention (**VASP**) in non-rheumatic AF compared warfarin (INR 1.2–1.5) and placebo in 571 men with chronic AF. Warfarin reduced the risk of stroke by 79%. *N Engl J Med* 1992; **327**: 1406–1412.

European Atrial Fibrillation Trial (**EAFT**) compared warfarin and placebo in patients with non-rheumatic AF and a history of minor ischaemic stroke or transient ischaemic attack within the previous 3 months. Warfarin reduced the risk of subsequent stroke by 67%. *N Engl J Med* 1995; **333**: 5–10.

Atrial tachycardia

The atrial rate is slower than in atrial flutter, being between 120 and 200/min. The ECG shows abnormally shaped P waves (see Fig. 7.14, p. 74). There is often a degree of atrioventricular (AV) block.

Management

Atrial tachycardia is commonly caused by digoxin toxicity, which should be stopped. If not, digoxin, verapamil or β-blockers may be used to control the ventricular rate. Sinus rhythm may be restored by DC cardioversion.

Pre-excitation syndromes

In addition to the AV node, an additional connection (accessory pathway) between the atria and ventricles allows atrial impulse to be transmitted more quickly to the ventricles—hence the term pre-excitation syndrome. The main types are Wolff–Parkinson–White and Lown–Ganong–Levine syndromes.

Wolff–Parkinson–White syndrome is caused by an accessory pathway (bundle of Kent) that bypasses the AV junction. It is characterized by a short PR interval and a widened QRS complex because of the presence of a δ wave (see Fig. 7.7, p. 71). In type A, the ventricular complex is positive in lead V1; in type B, it is negative.

Two main arrhythmias occur.
• In *re-entrant tachycardia* the normal (AV node) conduction pathway and the accessory pathway form a circuit through which impulses repeatedly circulate. The δ wave is lost. Drugs that block the AV node (e.g. adenosine, verapamil) usually restore sinus rhythm.
• In *atrial fibrillation* most ventricular complexes are broad because of the presence of large δ waves. AV nodal blocking drugs may increase the ventricular rate and should be avoided. DC cardioversion usually terminates AF. Amiodarone may be used to slow conduction in the accessory pathway.

Lown–Ganong–Levine is also characterized

by a short PR interval but has a normal QRS, i.e. without a δ wave. It is also complicated by paroxysmal tachycardia.

Ventricular tachycardia

The ventricular rate is usually 120–200/min. It usually reflects serious underlying myocardial disease. It is often self-limiting, but if sustained may cause hypotension and shock. The ECG shows a broad-complex tachycardia, and P waves dissociated from the ventricular activity may be seen (see Fig. 7.17, p. 75). The axis is often bizarre.

Management

Lidocaine (lignocaine) may terminate ventricular tachycardia (p. 263). Amiodarone can be used if lidocaine fails, but DC cardioversion should be performed if there is shock.

In *torsade de pointes* the QRS axis progressively changes so that the complexes appear to twist continuously. There is QT prolongation in sinus rhythm. Underlying causes should be identified and treated (antiarrhythmic drugs, hypokalaemia, hypomagnesaemia, tricyclic antidepressants). Antiarrhythmic agents may aggravate the condition. DC cardioversion or pacing is often effective in terminating attacks.

Ventricular fibrillation

See cardiac arrest.

Heart block (see Fig. 7.6, p. 71)

In *first-degree block* the PR interval is prolonged.

In *second-degree block* the normal 1 : 1 ratio of P : QRS complexes is lost but a relationship between P waves and QRS complexes still exists. The relationship may be either progressive lengthening of the PR interval until one QRS complex is dropped (Mobitz type I or Wenckebach) or dropped QRS complexes without a change in the PR interval.

If there is complete dissociation between P waves and QRS complexes *third-degree heart block* exists. The QRS complex rate (and hence ventricular rate) is usually slow (15–50/min) and regular. Cardiac pacing is often required.

Cardiorespiratory arrest
Clinical features
- Sudden loss of consciousness.

- Absent carotid and femoral pulses.
- Respiratory arrest follows shortly after.

Aetiology
- Almost invariably cardiac arrhythmia (ventricular fibrillation (VF), ventricular tachycardia (VT) or asystole)
- Rarely, the primary event is respiratory arrest (e.g. severe asthmatic attack).

Management
- Watch patient for 1–2 s to ensure correct diagnosis (observe for fluttering and opening of eyelids or return of consciousness).
- Recheck carotid pulse.
- If absent, call cardiac arrest team and strike sternum hard.
- Carry out external cardiac massage and ventilation through Brooke's airway.
- Establish intravenous line.
- Defibrillate as soon as machine arrives with 200 J (ensure everyone is away from the bed or trolley).
- Continue until the cardiac arrest team arrives, then:
  (a) intubate and ventilate;
  (b) check rhythm on ECG monitor; and
  (c) treat according to Fig. 7.3, p. 66.

Electrocardiograms
Hints and facts (Fig. 7.4, p. 68)
- 1 little square is 0.04 s; 1 big square is 0.2 s.
- 1 little square vertically is 1 mV.
- Normal PR interval is 0.12–0.2 s (three small squares to one big square).
- Normal QRS duration is up to 0.12 s (three small squares).

The QT interval varies with rate. Upper limits of normal are approximately:
- rate 60/min QT 0.43 s
- rate 75/min QT 0.39 s
- rate 100/min QT 0.34 s.

When presented with an ECG, check that it is labelled correctly (patient's name, date, leads for each group of complexes) and then assess the rate and rhythm.

Rate
Assess the rate by counting the large squares between two QRS complexes and dividing into

CARDIOPULMONARY RESUSCITATION (CPR)

Unresponsive

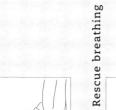

"Are you alright?"

Airway

Open airway

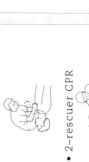

No breathing

Breathing

Rescue breathing

No pulse

Circulation

CPR

2:15

Call for help

Including:
- defibrillator
- airway adjuncts
- oxygen
- emergency kit

Consider:
- precordial thump *in witnessed or monitored arrest*

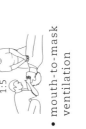

- 2-rescuer CPR

1:5

- mouth-to-mask ventilation

(a)

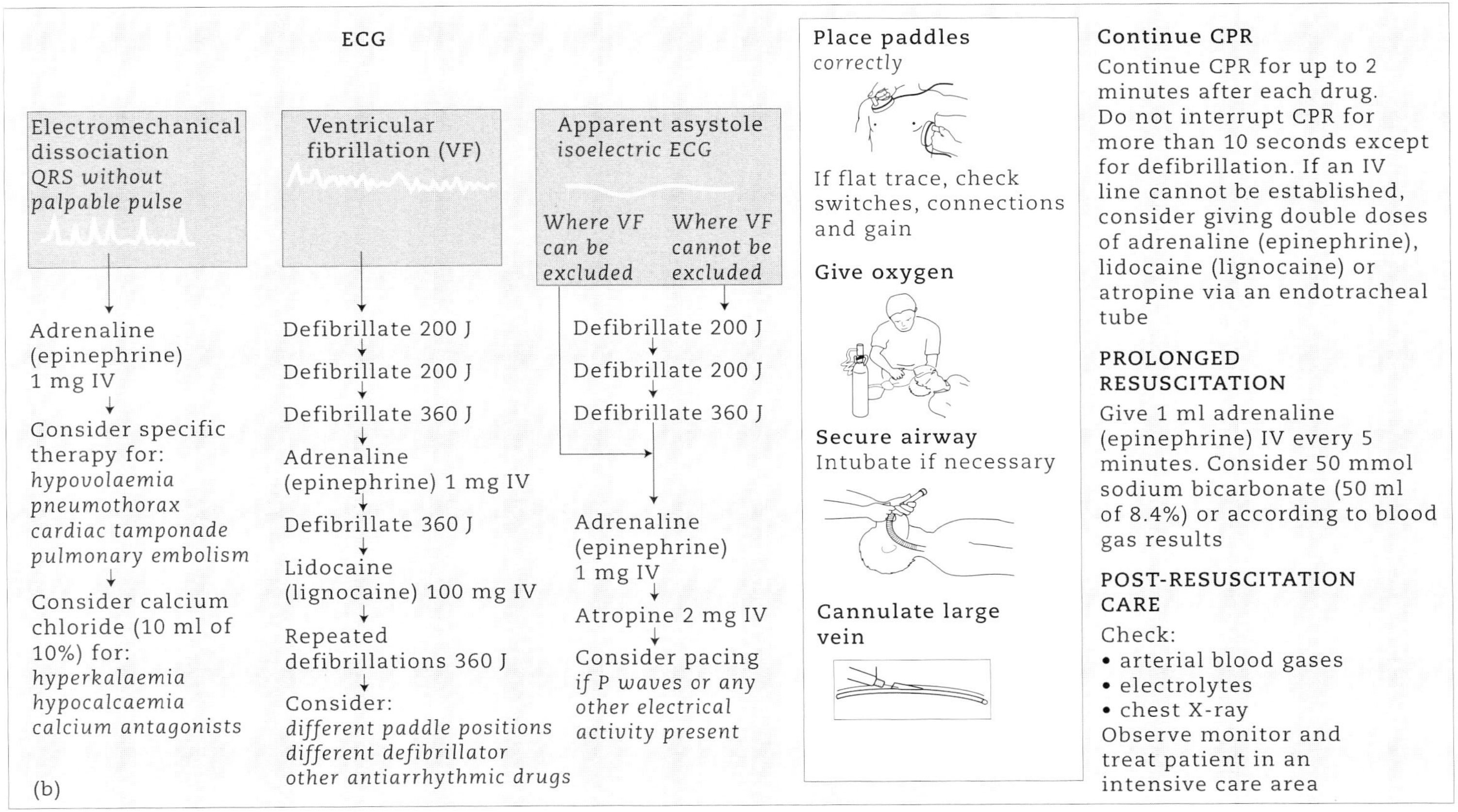

ECG

Electromechanical dissociation QRS without palpable pulse	Ventricular fibrillation (VF)	Apparent asystole isoelectric ECG			Place paddles correctly	Continue CPR

ECG

Electromechanical dissociation QRS without palpable pulse

→ Adrenaline (epinephrine) 1 mg IV

→ Consider specific therapy for:
hypovolaemia
pneumothorax
cardiac tamponade
pulmonary embolism

→ Consider calcium chloride (10 ml of 10%) for:
hyperkalaemia
hypocalcaemia
calcium antagonists

Ventricular fibrillation (VF)

→ Defibrillate 200 J
→ Defibrillate 200 J
→ Defibrillate 360 J
→ Adrenaline (epinephrine) 1 mg IV
→ Defibrillate 360 J
→ Lidocaine (lignocaine) 100 mg IV
→ Repeated defibrillations 360 J
→ Consider:
different paddle positions
different defibrillator
other antiarrhythmic drugs

Apparent asystole isoelectric ECG

Where VF can be excluded / *Where VF cannot be excluded*

→ Defibrillate 200 J
→ Defibrillate 200 J
→ Defibrillate 360 J

Adrenaline (epinephrine) 1 mg IV
→ Atropine 2 mg IV
→ Consider pacing if P waves or any other electrical activity present

Place paddles correctly

If flat trace, check switches, connections and gain

Give oxygen

Secure airway
Intubate if necessary

Cannulate large vein

Continue CPR

Continue CPR for up to 2 minutes after each drug. Do not interrupt CPR for more than 10 seconds except for defibrillation. If an IV line cannot be established, consider giving double doses of adrenaline (epinephrine), lidocaine (lignocaine) or atropine via an endotracheal tube

PROLONGED RESUSCITATION

Give 1 ml adrenaline (epinephrine) IV every 5 minutes. Consider 50 mmol sodium bicarbonate (50 ml of 8.4%) or according to blood gas results

POST-RESUSCITATION CARE

Check:
• arterial blood gases
• electrolytes
• chest X-ray
Observe monitor and treat patient in an intensive care area

(b)

Fig. 7.3 Cardiopulmonary resuscitation (CPR).

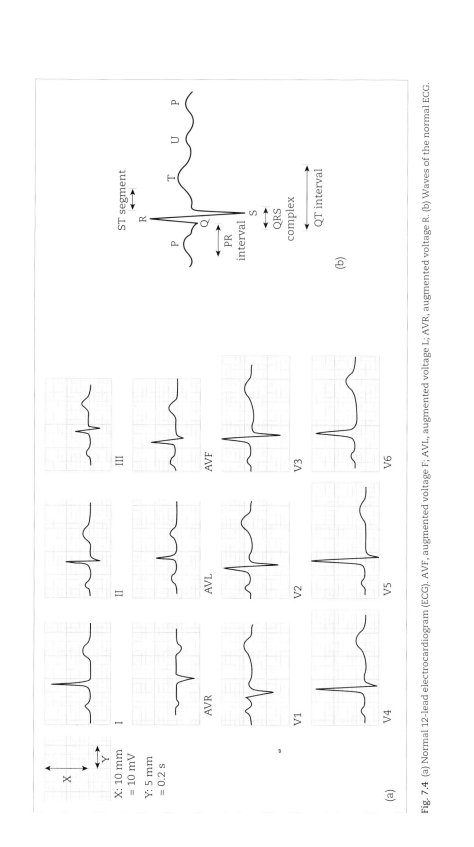

Fig. 7.4 (a) Normal 12-lead electrocardiogram (ECG). AVF, augmented voltage F; AVL, augmented voltage L; AVR, augmented voltage R. (b) Waves of the normal ECG.

300 (i.e. if two squares, the rate is 150/min; three squares, 100/min; four squares, 75/min; five squares, 60/min). If the rate is less than 60/min the patient has a bradycardia; if greater than 100/min, a tachycardia.

Regularity

Use the edge of a piece of paper to mark off a series of R waves, and then shift the paper along one or more complexes. The marks on the paper will still correspond with the R waves if the rhythm is regular. Total irregularity is almost always caused by AF. Proceed as always, quickly and methodically to the following.

Check the mean frontal QRS axis (Fig. 7.5)
Use the limb leads, and remember the angles at which these leads 'see' the heart (lead $I = 0°$). To gain a rough idea of the axis, find the lead with the maximum net positive deflection (sum of the positive R wave and negative Q and S waves)—the axis lies close to this. Then calculate the total deflection (R wave minus Q and S waves) in leads I and AVF which are perpendicular to each other (at 0 and 90° respectively). Add these together as vectors (use the squares on the ECG paper)—the net vector is the axis (see Fig. 7.5).

The normal range is 0–90°.

Causes of axis deviation
Left—left ventricular strain or hypertrophy (e.g. hypertension, aortic stenosis), ostium primum atrial septal defect.
Right—right ventricular strain or hypertrophy (e.g. pulmonary embolus, chronic lung disease, pulmonary valve stenosis), ostium secundum, ASD.

Check individual waves
Do this in order (i.e. P wave, PR interval, QRS complex, ST segment, QT interval, T wave) for their presence, shape and duration. This always needs to be performed for each lead in turn, although you will come to recognize certain patterns (e.g. bundle branch block, myocardial infarction). It is usually safe to ignore augmented voltage R (AVR).

P wave (atrial depolarization)
Most easily seen in VI and V2. It is peaked in right atrial hypertrophy, and bifid in left atrial hypertrophy (left atrial depolarization occurs slightly later than right, giving a second peak). It may be 'lost' (in the QRS complex) in nodal rhythm (originates from the AV node).

PR interval
If the PR interval is longer than 0.2 s (one large square), first-degree heart block is present (Fig. 7.6a).

If the normal 1 : 1 ratio of P : QRS complexes is lost but a relationship between P waves and QRS complexes still exists, second-degree heart block is present (Fig. 7.6b). The relationship may be either progressive lengthening of the PR interval until one QRS complex is dropped (Mobitz type 1 or Wenckebach) or dropped QRS complexes without a change in the PR interval.

If there is complete dissociation between P waves and QRS complexes, third-degree heart block exists (Fig. 7.6c). The QRS complex rate (and hence ventricular rate) is usually slow (15–50/min) and regular. Cardiac pacing is often required.

A short PR interval occurs in the Wolff–Parkinson–White syndrome in which an abnormal AV conduction pathway (bundle of Kent) predisposes to arrhythmias. The PR interval is short and the QRS complex slurred by a δ wave at the beginning (Fig. 7.7, p. 71).

QRS complex
If the QRS complex is longer than 0.12 s (three small squares), bundle branch block exists. In left bundle branch block (LBBB) the complex is negative (V- or W-shaped) in VI (Fig. 7.8). In right bundle branch block (RBBB) the complex is positive (M-shaped) in VI (Fig. 7.9).

Pathological (broad, deep) Q waves are greater than 0.04 s (1 small square) wide and greater than 0.2 mV (two small squares deep). They may be normal in AVR or VI. In the absence of bundle branch block, ventricular rhythms and the Wolff–Parkinson–White syndrome they indicate myocardial infarction. The site of such pathological Q waves indicates the site of the myocardial infarction—inferior if in AVF, III (the inferior leads) (Fig. 7.10), anterior if in the chest leads (Fig. 7.11, p. 72).

POSITION OF THE LIMB LEADS

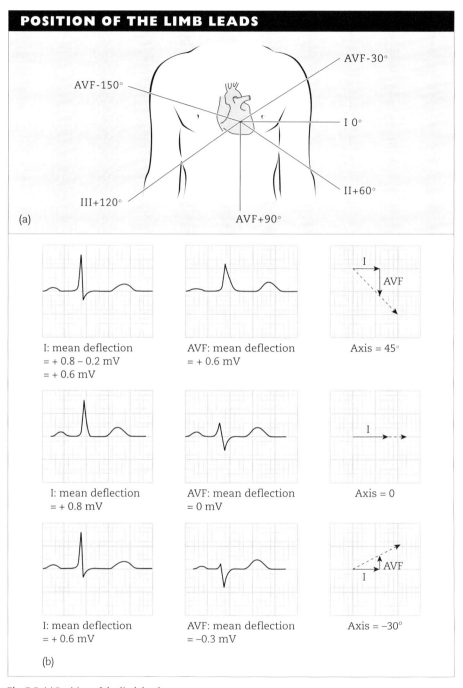

Fig. 7.5 (a) Position of the limb leads.
(b) Calculation of the cardiac axis.

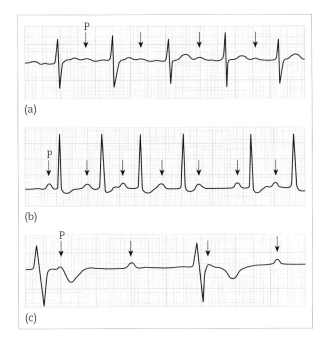

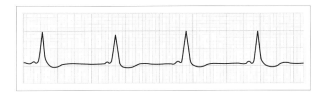

Fig. 7.6 (a) First-degree heart block. PR interval 0.30 s. (b) Second-degree heart block (Wenckebach or Mobitz type I). (c) Third-degree heart block (complete). Atrioventricular dissociation.

Fig. 7.7 Wolff–Parkinson–White (WPW) syndrome. Short PR interval and δ waves. Lown–Ganong–Levine (LGL) has no δ wave but is otherwise identical.

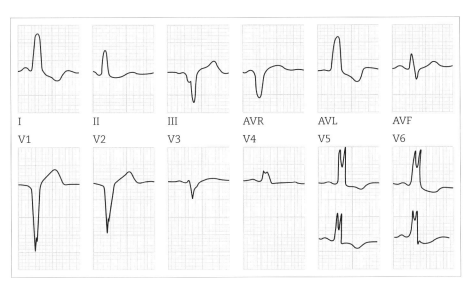

Fig. 7.8 Left bundle branch block. RSR (M-shaped QRS complex) is visible in some of the left ventricular leads, I, AVL and V4–6, and notched QS complexes in the right ventricular lead, V1–2.

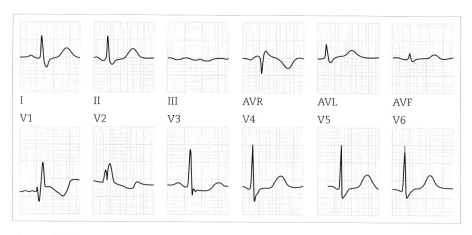

Fig. 7.9 Right bundle branch block. RSR in the
right ventricular leads V1–2 and slurred S waves
in the left ventricular leads I, AVL and V4–6.

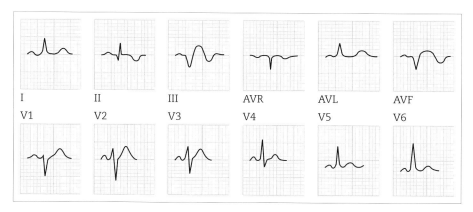

Fig. 7.10 Inferior myocardial infarction.

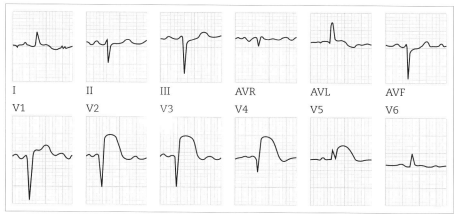

Fig. 7.11 Anterior myocardial infarction.

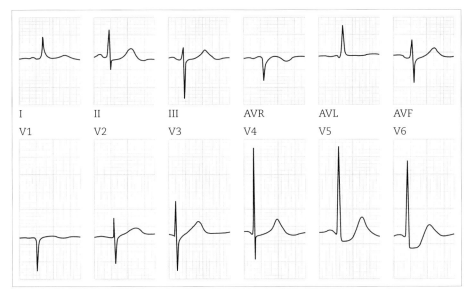

Fig. 7.12 Myocardial ischaemia (clinical history essential). The main characteristic is a depressed ST segment in leads standard II, V5 and V6. Also note inverted U waves in II, III, AVF and V4–6.

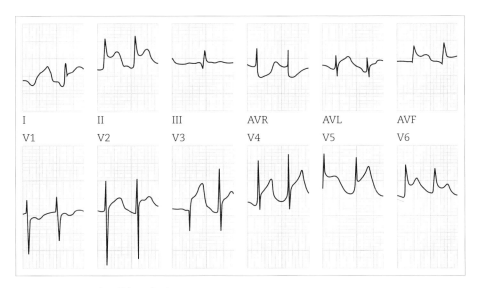

Fig. 7.13 Acute pericarditis. Raised concave-upwards ST segments in most leads, maximal in leads II and V5–6.

ST segment

The ST segment is depressed in myocardial ischaemia (Fig. 7.12), digoxin therapy and left ventricular hypertrophy.

It is raised in myocardial infarction (convex or domed—see Figs 7.10 and 7.11) and pericarditis (concave, Fig. 7.13).

T wave

The T wave is peaked in hyperkalaemia (see

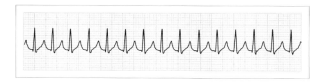

Fig. 7.14 Supraventricular tachycardia.

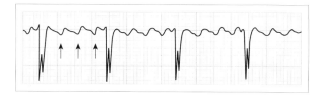

Fig. 7.15 Atrial flutter with 'saw-tooth' atrial waves and 4:1 block.

below) and sometimes acutely in myocardial infarction.

It is inverted in ventricular strain or hypertrophy, myocardial ischaemia and infarction (as with myocardial infarction, the leads indicate the site), bundle branch block, digoxin therapy and cardiomyopathies (abnormalities of cardiac muscle which may be ischaemic, drug or alcohol, familial or idiopathic in origin).

U wave
Follows the T wave and can be present normally. It is increased in hypokalaemia (see Fig. 7.22c, p. 77).

Common abnormalities
Rhythm
Causes of bradycardia
• Sinus (originating from sinoatrial node; normal P waves)—physiological (e.g. athletes), β-blockers, hypothyroidism, hypothermia.
• Complete heart block.

Causes of tachycardia
Narrow-complex tachycardia. Normal duration of QRS complex, i.e. depolarization starts in or above the AV node.
• *Supraventricular tachycardia* (Fig. 7.14).
• *Atrial tachycardia.* If the rate of supraventricular depolarization is about 150/min (one beat for every two large squares) the ventricles usually follow beat-for-beat. The P waves can sometimes be found in the preceding T wave.

If the atrial depolarization arises in or close to the AV node (*nodal* or *junctional tachycardia*) the P wave may be buried in the QRS complex.

If the rate of supraventricular depolarization is over 200/min, AV block occurs and only some (2 : 1 or 3 : 1) episodes of atrial depolarization are followed by ventricular depolarization—the ventricles cannot keep up with the atria.

At an atrial rate of 300/min (one to every small square) there is a 'saw-tooth' baseline and the rhythm is called *atrial flutter* (Fig. 7.15). The ventricular rate is then 150/min in 2 : 1 block and 100/min in 3 : 1 block.
• *Atrial fibrillation* (Fig. 7.16). Uncoordinated contraction of separate atrial muscle fibres. Unless controlled by digoxin it is usually fast (> 120/min), totally irregular without P waves, and has an irregular baseline.

Broad-complex tachycardia. Wide and abnormal QRS complex, i.e. depolarization, starts above the AV node with abnormal conduction below it (*supraventricular tachycardia with aberrant ventricular conduction*) or depolarization starts below the AV node (*ventricular tachycardia*).
• *Ventricular tachycardia* (Fig. 7.17). P waves are absent or dissociated from QRS complexes; the QRS complexes vary in shape and are often very broad. It can be difficult to distinguish from supraventricular tachycardia with aberrant conduction. The diagnosis is favoured by the presence of a known cardiac abnormality (ischaemic heart disease or cardiomyopathy). Supraventricular tachycardia is usually terminated by a rapid intravenous injection of 3 mg adenosine, whereas ventricular tachycardia is not.
• *Ventricular fibrillation* (Fig. 7.18). Very rapid irregular ventricular activation causes a 'saw-

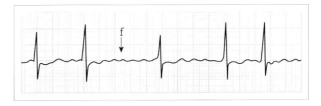

Fig. 7.16 Atrial fibrillation.

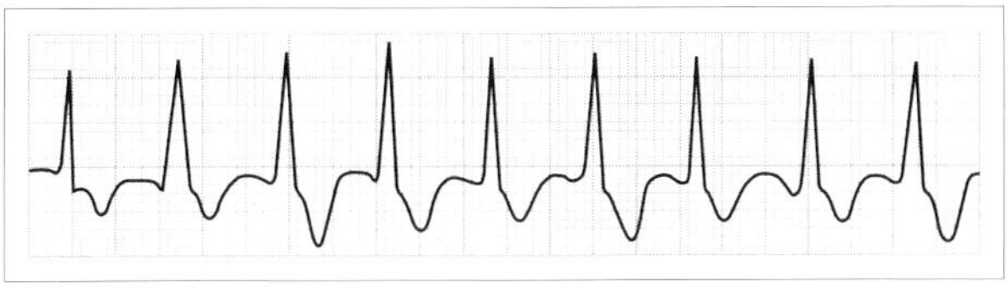

Fig. 7.17 Ventricular tachycardia with slightly irregular ventricular QRS complexes and variable T waves because of dissociated superimposed P waves.

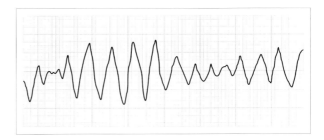

Fig. 7.18 Ventricular fibrillation. This is often seen in cardiac arrest and may be irreversible. It may sometimes alternate with ventricular tachycardia (and sinus rhythm).

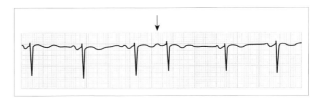

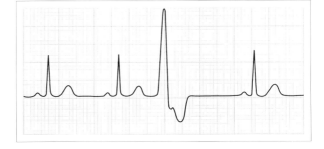

Fig. 7.19 Atrial extrasystole.

Fig. 7.20 Ventricular ectopic beat. A bizarre ventricular QRS complex. These are more ominous if multifocal, i.e. QRS of varying shape.

tooth' appearance. It is associated with no mechanical output resulting in cardiac arrest.

Occasional *extrasystoles* (ectopic or extra beats which do not fit in the otherwise regular rhythm) occur normally. The QRS complex may be normal (atrial (Fig. 7.19) or supraventricular) or wide (ventricular (Fig. 7.20) or supraventricular with aberrant conduction).

ECG patterns in common clinical conditions

Myocardial infarction (see p. 255 for definition)
A characteristic pattern of ECG changes evolves as follows.
• First few minutes—peaked T waves.
• First few hours—ST segment elevation, inversion of T waves.

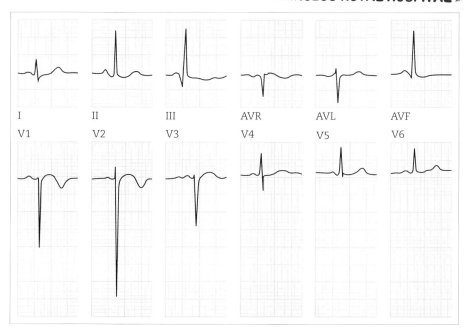

Fig. 7.21 Acute pulmonary embolism with S1, Q3, T3 pattern, a mean frontal QRS axis towards the right (+90°) and right ventricular (RV) strain pattern in leads V1–3.

• After the first few hours Q waves develop.
• After a few days the ST segment returns to normal (persistent elevation raises the possibility of left ventricular aneurysm).
• The T waves may eventually become upright but Q waves persist indefinitely.
• Rhythm abnormalities are common.
• Bundle branch block may occur at any stage, making further interpretation of the site, timing or extent of an infarct impossible.

Pulmonary embolism (Fig. 7.21)
• Tachycardia and transient arrhythmias (particularly AF).
• Right axis deviation.
• Right ventricular strain pattern—dominant R wave and inverted T waves in V1–4.
• RBBB.
• Occasionally S1, Q3, T3 pattern (S wave in lead I, Q and inverted T in III).

Ventricular hypertrophy
Large R waves occur over the appropriate ventricle in the chest leads (V1–2 for right and V5–6 for left). There tend to be large negative S waves in reciprocal leads (e.g. large S in V1 in left ventricular hypertrophy). If the sum of the S in V1 plus the R in V5 is greater than 35 mm, left ventricular hypertrophy is present on voltage criteria.

Digoxin
Sagging (reverse tick) ST segments, T wave inversion.

Metabolic abnormalities
Hyperkalaemia (Fig. 7.22a). Flattened P wave, broad QRS complex, peaked T wave.

Hypokalaemia (Fig. 7.22c). Prolonged PR, depressed ST, flattened T wave and prominent U wave.

Hypocalcaemia (Fig. 7.23). Prolonged QT interval.

Fascicular block
There are three fascicles to the bundle of His: right, left anterior and left posterior. Block of one (unifascicular block) produces the following patterns.

Fig. 7.22 (a) Hyperkalaemia; (b) normal; and (c) hypokalaemia. The T-wave amplitude varies directly with the serum potassium and the U wave inversely (it is often normally present in V3–4). In hyperkalaemia the P waves become smaller and the QRS complex widens into the ST segment. In hypokalaemia the PR interval lengthens and the ST segment becomes depressed.

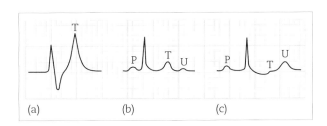

Fig. 7.23 Hypocalcaemia. Normal complexes apart from a prolonged QT_c (QT interval corrected for heart rate). Rate 95/min, QT 0.40, QT_c 0.50.

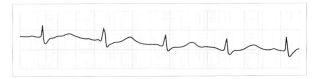

1 Right: RBBB.
2 Left anterior: left anterior hemiblock, left axis deviation.
3 Left posterior: left posterior hemiblock, right axis deviation.

Sinoatrial disease (sick sinus syndrome)
This is a chronic disorder often associated with ischaemic heart disease in which sinus bradycardia and/or episodic sinus arrest can alternate with episodes of rapid supraventricular arrhythmia. Symptoms include dizziness, syncope, palpitations and dyspnoea. Permanent pacing may be necessary. Diagnosis is most easily made using 24-h ambulatory ECG monitoring.

Exercise testing

The most widely used method is the treadmill test using the Bruce protocol. The speed and incline gradually increase at 3-min intervals to a maximum at stage seven when the patient is walking at 9.7 km/h at a gradient of 22%. The ECG, heart rate, blood pressure, symptoms and maximal workload are recorded during the test. The ECG signal is often averaged by computer to reduce noise caused by movement. ST segment depression of > 1 mm (0.1 mV) is usually regarded as a positive test, but many other parameters can signify cardiac disease. These include inability to achieve maximum heart rate or workload, inappropriate response in blood pressure (normal response is a small rise) and symptoms of angina.

Chest X-ray

The standard view is a PA (X-rays passing posterior to anterior with the patient's chest against the film), in inspiration. The X-rays are diverging from the source and magnify structures furthest from the film (e.g. vertebrae). An anteroposterior (AP) view (taken if the patient is too ill to stand) magnifies the heart. Lateral views are used largely for localization of lesions visible on the PA film.

The maximum diameter of the heart on a PA film is normally less than half the maximum diameter of the thoracic cage (cardiothoracic ratio less than 0.5). Enlargement of the heart occurs with cardiac dilatation (heart failure, valvular disease, prolonged hypertension) or the presence of a pericardial effusion.

Left atrial enlargement (mitral stenosis) causes:
• prominence of the left atrial appendage (upper left heart border);
• double contour adjacent to the right heart border; and
• elevation of the left main bronchus.

Enlargement of other chambers is difficult to distinguish radiologically.

Main vessels. Look for aortic dilatation (hypertension, aortic valve disease, aneurysm) which causes a prominent aortic shadow to the right of the mediastinum. Enlargement of the pulmonary artery (right-to-left shunts, pulmonary hypertension) produces a prominent bulge on the left border of the mediastinum. Look for valvular calcification (rheumatic valve disease). Pericardial calcification usually indicates old tuberculosis.

Check the density and texture of the lung markings, including the apices (the only markings visible in normal lungs are blood vessels). Pulmonary venous hypertension causes prominence and dilatation of the upper-lobe pulmonary vessels. Pulmonary oedema causes mottling of the lung fields, areas of consolidation and fluid collections which become visible as pleural effusions or fluid in interlobar fissures or interlobular septa (Kerley B lines).

Echocardiography

Ultrasound beams scanned rapidly across the heart record two-dimensional images of the anatomy and motion of the heart. The motion of individual cardiac structures can be recorded in detail by M-mode cardiography, which records echo signals in one particular direction of the beam over time. Relatively stationary structures generate straight lines, whereas moving structures (e.g. valves) generate undulating lines. Continuous-wave Doppler quantifies blood velocity and pressure gradients across valves. In combination two-dimensional, M-mode and Doppler echocardiography defines ventricular function, myocardial and valvular disease, congenital malformations and pericardial effusion. Transoesophageal echocardiography using a probe introduced into the oesophagus visualizes cardiac structures, including left atrial appendage, prosthetic valves, intracardiac tumours and vegetations of infective endocarditis, and intrathoracic structures, including the thoracic aorta and paracardiac tumours.

Ventricular function is assessed from changes in cavity size or wall motion, and ejection fraction from stroke volume (end-diastolic minus end-systolic volume) divided by end-diastolic volume. Normal ejection fraction is > 60%. Disturbances of wall motion (usually due to ischaemia) are assessed subjectively in different regions of the ventricle.

Radionuclide studies

Technetium. (^{99}Tc)-sestamibi-labelled red cells are used to assess myocardial perfusion and left ventricular function by gated radionuclide ventriculography (multiple uptake gated acquisition, MUGA). The ECG is used to gate the scan into different periods of the cardiac cycle. Myocardial disease tends to cause dilatation of the heart, and reduced ejection fraction, which may fall on exercise—a poor prognostic sign. Regional abnormalities of the ventricular muscle are recorded as areas of akinesia and hypokinesia. This is usually evidence of myocardial ischaemia or infarction. Regional paradoxical movement suggests an aneurysm.

Thallium. (^{201}Tl) behaves like potassium and is distributed through heart muscle in proportion to coronary blood flow. Uptake is decreased in areas of ischaemia or infarction. On exercise there may be areas of decreased perfusion which reverse after rest, indicating areas of reversible ischaemia.

Swan–Gantz catheterization

Right atrial pressure measured using a CVP line gives a poor indication of circulating intravascular volume in the presence of cardiac disease. A pulmonary artery flotation catheter (e.g. Swan–Gantz catheter) can be used to assess left atrial pressure. A light flexible catheter with a balloon on the end is introduced through a central vein into the right side of the heart. The balloon, inflated with air, 'floats' into the pulmonary artery and eventually wedges in a small pulmonary artery, where it registers a pressure similar to left atrial pressure (pulmonary capillary wedge pressure, PCWP).

Normal (systolic/diastolic) cardiac pressures are: right atrial pressure 7/3 mmHg; right ventricular pressure 15–25/3–7; pulmonary arterial pressure 25/10; mean PCWP 6–12 mmHg.

Essential Background
Information

Neurology

Headache and giddiness constitute the most commonly presenting neurological symptoms. Faints, dizzy turns and blackouts are common and may originate from the cardiovascular system, e.g. aortic stenosis, dysrhythmias such as complete heart block and sick sinus syndrome (p. 77), hypotensive drugs and cerebral emboli. Cerebrovascular accidents are the most common cause for hospital admission.

Physiology

Neurotransmitters

Amino acids. L-*glutamate* is the most important excitatory neurotransmitter in fast relay pathways of the motor and sensory systems. These include corticospinal, spinothalamic, lemniscal, somatosensory and specialized sensory (visual, auditory) pathways. It is also important in memory and learning. It acts through various receptors (e.g. the *N*-methyl-D-aspartate receptor) to open ion channels. Inactivation is through reuptake.

γ-aminobutyric acid (GABA) is found in inhibitory interneurons throughout the central nervous system (CNS). $GABA_A$ receptors act through chloride channels to stabilize membrane potentials. Activation of $GABA_A$ receptors is potentiated by benzodiazepines and barbiturates. $GABA_B$ receptors are G protein-linked. Inactivation of GABA is through reuptake.

Pharmacology

• *Benzodiazepines* are thought to exert their effect by potentiating the effects of endogenous GABA.

• *Barbiturates* have similar effects, but at high dosage they mimic the effects of GABA. Thus their action does not rely on endogenous GABA, and they can cause more profound CNS depression.

• *Gabapentin* is structurally similar to GABA, although its action may be independent of the GABA system.

• *Lamotrigine* probably acts through inhibition of excitatory amino-acid release.

• *Vigabatrin* (γ-vinyl GABA) inactivates the enzyme GABA-transaminase (GABA-T).

Monoamines

The catecholamines *dopamine*, *noradrenaline (norepinephrine)* and *adrenaline (epinephrine)* are synthesized from L-tyrosine (Fig. 8.1).

Dopamine in brainstem neurons, particularly within the substantia nigra, is important for motor control. In the hypothalamus its principal neuroendocrine function is the inhibition of prolactin synthesis. Dopaminergic neurons in the mesolimbic system are thought to control emotions. Dopamine interacts with a number of receptors, including the D_1- and D_2-receptors, which are abundant in the corpus striatum.

Noradrenaline (norepinephrine)- and *adrenaline (epinephrine)*-containing neurons originate in the pons and medulla oblongata, and connect with the limbic system, hypothalamus and spinal cord. In the peripheral nervous system, noradrenaline (norepinephrine) is the principal neurotransmitter in postganglionic sympathetic fibres. Adrenaline (epinephrine) is also released into the circulation as a hormone from the adrenal medulla. Noradrenaline (norepinephrine) and adrenaline (epinephrine) interact with α_1-, α_2- and β-adrenergic receptors in the brain and spinal cord. α_1- and β-receptors mediate the sympathetic effects of noradrenaline (norepinephrine).

SYNTHESIS OF CATECHOLAMINES

$$\text{L-tyrosine} \xrightarrow[\text{hydroxylase}]{\text{Tyrosine}} \text{Dopa} \xrightarrow[\text{decarboxylase}]{\text{Dopa}} \text{Dopamine} \xrightarrow[\text{β-hydroxylase}]{\text{Dopamine}} \underset{\text{(norepinephrine)}}{\text{Noradrenaline}} \xrightarrow[\text{N-methyltransferase}]{\text{Phenylethanolamine-}} \underset{\text{(epinephrine)}}{\text{Adrenaline}}$$

Fig. 8.1 Synthesis of catecholamines.

Inactivation of catecholamines is through reuptake, and enzymatic breakdown by monoamine oxidases and catechol-*O*-methyl-transferase (COMT). Dopamine is catabolized to homovanillic acid. In the brain adrenaline (epinephrine) and noradrenaline (nore-pinephrine) are catabolized to 3-methoxy-4-hydroxy-phenylethyleneglycol, whereas in the peripheral nervous system the principal metabolite is vanillylmandelic acid.

Serotonin (5-hydroxytryptamine; 5-HT) is synthesized from L-tryptophan in neurons arising in the brainstem raphe nuclei which project throughout the brain and spinal cord. It is also present in the myenteric plexus, and circulates as a hormone. The four main receptor sub-types (5-HT$_1$, 5-HT$_2$, 5-HT$_3$, 5-HT$_4$) are differentially distributed throughout the brain and spinal cord. 5-HT$_1$ receptors can be subdivided into 5-HT$_{1A-1E}$. 5-HT$_{1D}$-receptors are abundant in cerebral vessels where they mediate vasoconstriction. Inactivation of serotonin is through reuptake or metabolization by monoamine oxidase to 5-hydroxyindoleacetic acid.

Histamine is synthesized from L-histidine in hypothalamic neurons which innervate various parts of the brain and spinal cord. It is also stored in and released by mast cells and basophils. Histamine interacts with H$_1$-, H$_2$- and H$_3$-receptors. Cerebral H$_1$-receptors are important in controlling arousal. Reuptake of histamine does not occur. Inactivation is through metabolism by histamine-*N*-methyltransferase and monoamine oxidase to methylimidazoleacetic acid.

Pharmacology

Drugs that antagonize the effects of adrenaline (epinephrine) and noradrenaline (norepineph-rine) generally have sedative effects, whereas dopamine antagonists cause drug-induced parkinsonism.

Major tranquillizers (e.g. *phenothiazines*) are thought to exert their effects by antagonizing the effects of dopamine in the cerebral cortex and limbic system.

Monoamine oxidase inhibitors increase all cerebral catecholamines by reducing their metabolism. *Tricyclic antidepressants* potentiate the action of brain amines by preventing reuptake at nerve terminals. However, their delayed action suggests that other mechanisms are involved in their antidepressant activity.

Antiparkinsonian drugs potentiate the effects of dopamine. *Levodopa* is the treatment of choice. It is given with a dopa-decarboxylase inhibitor (e.g. carbidopa or benserazide) to prevent the peripheral effects of dopamine. *Selegiline* is a *monoamine oxidase B inhibitor* which can be used in severe parkinsonism. *Bromocriptine* is a *dopamine receptor agonist*. Dopamine deficiency results in a relative excess of acetylcholine, and *antimuscarinic agents* (e.g. *trihexyphenidyl (benhexol)*) are sometimes effective in mild parkinsonism. Dopamine agonists reduce prolactin secretion.

Drugs that affect the actions of 5-HT are used in the treatment of migraine and depression. *Sumatriptan*, a 5-HT$_{1D}$ agonist, provides symptomatic relief from migraine by constricting cerebral blood vessels. *Pizotifen* antagonizes 5-HT$_1$- and 5-HT$_2$-receptors and is used in migraine prophylaxis. The antidepressant *mianserin* is a 5-HT-receptor antagonist.

Agents that block reuptake of 5-HT are effective in the treatment of depression. They include *fluoxetine* (Prozac), *paroxetine* (Seroxat) and *sertraline* (Lustral). The hallucinogen lysergic acid diethylamide (LSD) is a partial agonist at 5-HT$_2$-receptors.

Antihistamines are commonly used in the treatment of allergy. Drowsiness is a common problem.

Acetylcholine

Acetylcholine interacts with nicotinic receptors at the neuromuscular junction and autonomic ganglia, and with muscarinic receptors in the CNS and in postganglionic parasympathetic pathways. Inactivation is through hydrolysis by acetylcholinesterase. Cholinergic transmission is thus potentiated by anticholinesterases.

Pharmacology

Anticholinergic agents are used to inhibit peripheral effects of acetylcholine. *Atropine* acts at postganglionic (muscarinic) receptors and is used in the treatment of bradycardia and as a premedication to dry secretions. *Hyoscine* is structurally related to atropine, but differs by causing CNS depression and amnesia. Drugs that block the actions of acetylcholine at the neuromuscular junction are used as muscle relaxants in anaesthesia. They act by either competition (*non-depolarizing agents*, e.g. *pancuronium*, *tubocurarine*) or by depolarization (e.g. *suxamethonium*). Competitive muscle relaxants can be reversed by *anticholinesterases* (e.g. *edrophonium*, *neostigmine*). Anticholinesterases are also used in the treatment of myasthenia gravis.

In the eye *cholinergic agents* (e.g. the alkaloid *pilocarpine* or *anticholinesterases*) cause pupillary constriction, whereas *antimuscarinic agents* can be used to dilate the pupil (e.g. *homatropine*, *tropicamide*).

Neuropeptides

Neuropeptides occur throughout the central and peripheral nervous systems. Many act as hormones and have vasoactive actions (e.g. vasopressin, somatostatin) or gastrointestinal effects (e.g. vasoactive intestinal polypeptide, cholecystokinin). They are particularly important in regulating hypothalamic function (e.g. hypothalamic-releasing hormones), pain perception (e.g. substance P, endorphins) and autonomic pathways (e.g. neuropeptide Y).

Anatomy

- Internal capsule (Fig. 8.2).
- Arterial supply (Fig. 8.3).

Headache

Headache is one of the most common of all presenting symptoms. The aim is to exclude treatable underlying intra- or extracranial disease and to make a definitive diagnosis (e.g. migraine). Patients with headache and facial pain may not give histories that fit conveniently into any well-recognized category. They should be seen at intervals to determine:

- symptoms of increasing anxiety or depression;
- symptoms of changing pain patterns; and
- developing abnormal clinical signs.

In the absence of these, treatment is with reassurance and simple analgesics.

Tension headache

A severe continuous pressure is characteristically felt bilaterally over the vertex, occiput or eyes. It may be band-like or non-specific and of variable intensity. It is most common in middle-aged women but may occur at any age or in either sex in association with stress or depression (ask about family, work, money and for symptoms of depression). The headache may be described with considerable drama and standard analgesics are invariably ineffective. Occasionally, it may be symptomatic of worry about a brain tumour and relieved by definite reassurance and thorough normal physical examination.

Postconcussion headache

This has many features of tension headache but is usually associated with dizziness (not vertigo) and loss of concentration. There is often a history of inadequate recovery following the head injury, and of impending litigation.

CORONAL SECTION THROUGH THE THIRD VENTRICLE

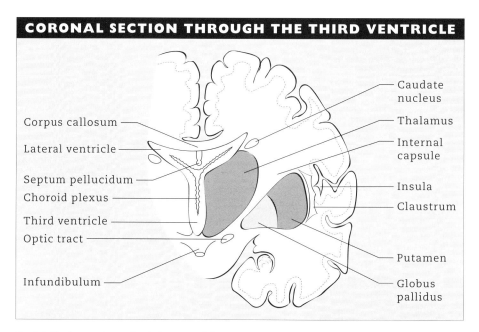

Caudate nucleus

Thalamus

Internal capsule

Insula

Claustrum

Putamen

Globus pallidus

Corpus callosum

Lateral ventricle

Septum pellucidum

Choroid plexus

Third ventricle

Optic tract

Infundibulum

Fig. 8.2 The internal capsule, thalamus and third ventricle in coronal section.

THE LEFT CEREBRAL HEMISPHERE

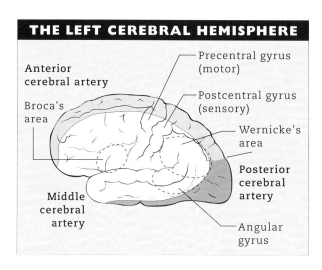

Anterior cerebral artery

Broca's area

Middle cerebral artery

Precentral gyrus (motor)

Postcentral gyrus (sensory)

Wernicke's area

Posterior cerebral artery

Angular gyrus

Fig. 8.3 Surface anatomy of the left cerebral hemisphere with the areas supplied by each cerebral artery. Light grey shading: anterior cerebral artery; dark grey shading: posterior cerebral artery; white area: middle cerebral artery.

Raised intracranial pressure

This is most often brought about by intracranial tumour, haematoma or abscess. The pain is worse on waking in the morning after lying down and is associated with vomiting. It improves 1–2 h after rising and is exacerbated by coughing, sneezing or straining. Visual deterioration may not occur despite papilloedema. The pain usually responds to standard analgesics. NB (for teetotallers) Alcoholic hangovers also cause early-morning headaches.

Patients whose histories do not fit into one of these categories usually have either an obvious diagnosis (meningitis, subarachnoid haemorrhage, sinusitis, otitis media) or a less obvious local cause (teeth, cervical spine, skull, orbits). Benign hypertension, defects in visual acuity, glaucoma and ocular muscle imbalance seldom present as headache.

Preliminary investigation of headache

Most hospital physicians, when seeing the patient referred from a family practitioner, would request:

- full blood count, including erythrocyte sedimentation rate (ESR; to exclude temporal arteritis in the over-50s);
- chest X-ray for bronchial carcinoma;
- computed tomography (CT) or magnetic resonance imaging (MRI) scan should be performed to exclude a space-occupying lesion where clinically indicated, especially in the presence of:

  (a) frontal headache on waking with nausea, i.e. symptoms suggestive of raised intracranial pressure

  (b) occipital headache of sudden onset (subarachnoid haemorrage)

  (c) abnormal and, in particular, progressive neurological signs including confusional dementia.

Unilateral facial pain

Migraine

Migraine is episodic and affects approximately 10% of the population. It usually begins around puberty and continues intermittently to middle age. It is more common in females than males (3 : 1) and there is often a family history. There may have been episodes of unexplained nausea and/or abdominal pain in childhood. It may be associated with periods and the contraceptive pill, with various foods (especially chocolate, cheese and red wine) and emotions (anger, tension, excitement). A characteristic attack starts with a sense of ill health and is followed by a visual aura (shimmering lights, fortification spectra, scotomas) usually in the field opposite to the side of the succeeding headache. The throbbing unilateral headache is associated with anorexia, nausea, vomiting, photophobia and withdrawal. There may be transient hemiparesis or sensory symptoms. It is very rarely associated with organic disease and CT scan with contrast or MRI is only indicated if of late onset (over 45 years) or to exclude arteriovenous malformation if abnormal physical signs persist or progress.

Management of the acute attack

Precipitating causes, including emotional factors and the menstrual cycle (including oral contraceptives), should be identified and removed—a patient's diary of symptoms and diet (chocolate, cheese, alcohol) may help—and simple analgesia taken early (aspirin, non-steroidal anti-inflammatory drugs (NSAIDs), paracetamol). Metoclopramide or domperidone may be given with them to reduce nausea. If attacks are frequent, interfere with work and social life, and do not respond to simple analgesia, use a 5-HT$_1$ agonist such as sumatriptan (oral, nasal or subcutaneous), preferably at the onset of the prodrome. The use of ergot alkaloids is limited by side-effects and habituation. Treat prophylactically if the patient has more than two attacks a month, with pizotifen, β-blockade or tricylic antidepressants. Very occasionally, sodium valproate, methysergide, lithium, calcium-channel blockers or even steroids need to be used by specialist neurologists.

Cluster headaches

(migrainous neuralgia)

These are related to migraine. Attacks, more common in males, occur in clusters every 1–2 years and consist of very severe unilateral pain around an eye occurring 1–10 times daily lasting 10 min–3 h, often at night (coinciding with the first phase of rapid eye movement (REM) sleep) for a period of 1–3 months. The eye becomes red and waters and the nostril of the same side blocked up and runny. It often responds to treatment for migraine as above.

Neuralgias

Neuralgias are intermittent, but brief, severe,

lancinating pains occurring along the distribution of a nerve.

Trigeminal neuralgia (tic douloureux)
This occurs almost exclusively in the elderly. In a patient under 50 years old it may be symptomatic of multiple sclerosis. The agonizing, knife-like pain is confined to the distribution of the trigeminal nerve on one side, most commonly the maxillary or mandibular divisions. It lasts only 1 or 2 s and is usually triggered from a place on the lips or the side of the nose or by chewing, eating, speaking or touching the face, or by blowing wind. It tends to get worse with age but may be specifically relieved by carbamazepine (Tegretol) or gabapentin. A small aberrant vessel overlying the nerve as it leaves the brainstem can be the cause. Dissection or cryotherapy of this completely relieves the symptoms. A patient may need thermocoagulation or section of the sensory root of the 5th nerve. Tumour can be a rare cause that can be excluded by CT/MRI scan. Suicide is a definite risk.

Glossopharyngeal neuralgia
Precipitated by swallowing, which produces pain in the pharynx.

Auriculotemporal neuralgia
Precipitated by swallowing, and may be treated by correcting dental malocclusion.

Postherpetic neuralgia
Occurs in patients with a history of herpes zoster infection (shingles) and the scars of the healed disease are usually obvious. Amitriptyline, gabapentin or topical capsaicin may help, but the pain may be almost impossible to relieve.

Giant cell arteritis

In giant cell arteritis the pain varies from scalp soreness to severe and intractable (p. 127).

Atypical facial pain

This refers to episodic aching in the jaw and cheek, lasting several hours and usually occurring in young to middle-aged women who are frequently depressed. It is often bilateral. It may respond to antidepressants or antihistamines.

Unilateral pain

Local pathologies involving the eyes, sinuses, teeth or ears may give unilateral pain, as may tumours involving the 5th nerve (cerebellopontine angle tumours). Pain from herpes zoster may occur before the rash appears.

Stroke

Stroke affects about 1 in 600 patients per year, and approximately 5% of the population over 65 will suffer from stroke. Approximately 85% are ischaemic (thrombosis or embolism), 10% are caused by intracerebral haemorrhage and 5% by subarachnoid haemorrhage. Stroke accounts for up to 12% of all deaths in industrialized countries.

Risk factors include smoking, hypertension, hyperlipidaemia, atrial fibrillation, ischaemic heart disease, valvular heart disease and diabetes.

In stroke units 5–13% of cases have a non-vascular lesion (tumour, subdural haematoma, postictal paresis, migraine, intracranial infection, metabolic disturbance, hysteria).

Investigations to confirm the diagnosis
The distinction between cerebral haemorrhage and infarction cannot be made on the basis of clinical or cerebrospinal fluid (CSF) findings, but requires CT/MRI scanning. All patients with acute stroke should undergo scanning as soon as possible. On CT a low-density area appears within a few hours of a cerebral infarct, whereas a high-density area appears immediately after a bleed. Brainstem, cerebellar and small cortical infarcts are often not visible. MRI is more sensitive for detecting ischaemic stroke, but is more expensive, takes longer to perform, and requires more cooperation from the patient.

Investigations to establish the aetiology
Less common causes of stroke should be considered, particularly in young patients and those without risk factors.

The following investigations are usually performed:
• full blood count (FBC), ESR, coagulation and

thrombophilia screens, urea and electrolytes, glucose, lipids, syphilis serology;
- electrocardiogram (ECG) and cardiac enzymes;
- chest X-ray;
- CT/MRI of head;
- echocardiography to detect cardiac source of embolus (25–30% of ischaemic strokes are caused by cardioembolism); and
- duplex imaging of the extracranial carotid and vertebral arteries provides information on arterial occlusion or source of emboli.

Other investigations which may be indicated include serum protein electrophoresis, auto-antibody screen (for anticardiolipin antibody, antinuclear antibody, antineutrophil cytoplasm antibody), protein C, S and antithrombin III levels, sickle test, blood cultures, urine for homocystinuria.

Cerebral angiography may be helpful in detecting cerebral vasculitis.

Management

Give general care to maintain comfort and an adequate airway. Ensure swallowing is safe, and keep the patient hydrated and nourished. Swallowing should be assessed (watch the patient trying to drink), and if there is difficulty, fluids should be given by nasogastric tube or intravenously. If thrombosis is demonstrated, give aspirin. The roles of thrombolysis and anticoagulation are not yet determined.

Aspirin, 300 mg o.d., should be given as soon as the diagnosis of ischaemic stroke is confirmed. The International and Chinese Acute Stroke Trials showed that aspirin started within 48 h of onset prevents death or disability, mainly by reducing early recurrence. Alteplase (recombinant tissue plasminogen activator, rtPA) may improve outcome if given within the first 3 h of stroke.

Aspirin and warfarin are equally effective in the secondary prevention of non-cardiogenic ischaemic stroke. See Trials Box 8.1.

Prevention and treatment of complications

- *Cardiovascular*. Treat cardiac arrhythmias and hypertension. Most physicians do not treat high blood pressure in the early stages for fear of lowering cerebral blood flow and exacerbating ischaemia. Urgent treatment is required if hypertensive encephalopathy or hypertensive cardiac or renal failure is suspected. Long-term aspirin is indicated in most patients for secondary prevention.
- *Chest infections* account for 20–40% of deaths. Aspiration is common and treatment with antibiotics and physiotherapy should be started if the diagnosis is suspected.
- *Deep venous thrombosis* occurs in 50% of patients, and may be difficult to diagnose in a paralysed leg. Graduated compression stockings can be used for prophylaxis.
- *Hypertension* may be previously undiagnosed or inadequately treated.
- *Pressure sores* are common in bed-ridden patients. Avoidance requires careful positioning and regular turning.
- *Urinary infections* are associated with catheterization.
- *Seizures* occur in 5% of patients, and may require treatment with anticonvulsants (p. 92).
- *Hyperglycaemia* in non-diabetic patients suffering an acute stroke results from increased cortisol, catecholamine and glucagon levels. Insulin may be required temporarily.
- *Hyponatraemia* may result from excessive use of intravenous dextrose. In 10% of patients it is caused by inappropriate antidiuretic hormone secretion, which usually resolves spontaneously.

Recovery and rehabilitation require an integrated approach between physicians, nurses, physiotherapist, speech therapist, occupational therapist and social worker.

Lateral medullary syndrome
(see Fig. 1.2, p. 4)
This is the most common brainstem vascular syndrome and presents acutely with vertigo, vomiting and ipsilateral facial pain. Dysphagia and dysarthria may occur. The following features may be present.

Ipsilateral
- Palatal paralysis.
- Horner syndrome.
- Spinothalamic sensory loss in the face.
- Cerebellar signs in the limbs.

TRIALS BOX 8.1

The **British Aneurysm Nimodipine Trial** compared placebo with nimodipine 60 mg 4-hourly, started within 96 h of subarachnoid haemorrhage and continued for 21 days, in 554 patients. Nimodipine improved outcome and reduced the incidence of cerebral infarction. *Br Med J* 1989; **298**: 636–642.

In the **Multicentre Acute Stroke Trial—Europe (MAST-E)**, streptokinase increased mortality compared with placebo when given in the first 6 h after an ischaemic stroke. *N Engl J Med* 1996; **335**: 145–150.

The **International Stroke Trial (IST)** studied the effect of aspirin, subcutaneous heparin, both, or neither in 19 435 patients with acute ischaemic stroke. Heparin did not offer a clinical advantage, but aspirin 300 mg/day reduced death or non-fatal recurrent stroke. *Lancet* 1997; **349**: 1569–1581.

The **Chinese Acute Stroke Trial (CAST)** studied 21 016 patients in a randomized placebo-controlled trial. Aspirin 160 mg/day started within 48 h of suspected acute ischaemic stroke reduced mortality and non-fatal stroke. *Lancet* 1997; **349**: 1641–1649.

A combined analysis of 40 000 randomized patients from the **Chinese Acute Stroke Trial** and the **International Stroke Trial** concluded that early aspirin is of benefit for a wide range of patients, and its prompt use should be routinely considered for all patients with suspected acute ischemic stroke, mainly to reduce the risk of early recurrence. *Stroke* 2000; **31**: 1240–1249.

Intracerebral haemorrhage after intravenous tissue plasminogen activator (t-PA) therapy for ischemic stroke performed subgroup analyses of data from a randomized, double-blind, placebo-controlled trial of intravenous t-PA administered to stroke patients within 3 h of onset. They concluded that despite a higher rate of intracerebral hemorrhage, patients with severe strokes or oedema or mass effect on the baseline-CT are reasonable candidates for t-PA, if it is administered within 3 h of onset. *Stroke* 1997; **28**: 2109–2118.

The **Alteplase Thrombolysis for Acute Non-interventional Therapy in Ischemic Stroke (ATLANTIS) trial** evaluated the clinical outcomes of 61 patients enrolled in the ATLANTIS study who were randomized to receive intravenous t-PA or placebo within 3 h of symptom onset. The data supported recommendations to administer intravenous t-PA to eligible ischaemic stroke patients who can be treated within 3 h of symptom onset. *Stroke* 2002; **33**: 493–496.

A **Cochrane review of low-molecular-weight heparins or heparinoids versus standard unfractionated heparin for acute ischaemic stroke (Cochrane Review)** concluded that low-molecular weight heparin or heparinoid appear to decrease the occurrence of deep vein thrombosis compared to standard unfractionated heparin, but there are too few data to provide reliable information on their effect on other important outcomes, including death and intracranial haemorrhage. *Cochrane Database Syst Rev* 2001; **4**: CD000119.

Mohr et al. compared the effect of warfarin (INR 1.4 to 2.8) and aspirin (325 mg/day) on recurrent ischaemic stroke or death in 2206 patients with a prior non-cardioembolic ischaemic stroke. There was no difference between aspirin and warfarin in prevention of recurrent ischaemic stroke or death, or the rate of major haemorrhage. *N Engl J Med* 2001; **345**: 1444–1451.

Contralateral

- Spinothalamic loss in the body.

Extracerebral haemorrhage

EXTRADURAL

This results from traumatic damage to the middle meningeal artery as it passes upwards on the inside of the temporal bone. Classically, momentary loss of consciousness is followed by apparent recovery and death 1–7 days later.

Not every fracture of the temporal bone results in middle meningeal haemorrhage but suspicion alone warrants CT scan of the head and admission of the patient to observe conscious level. Should signs of local haemorrhage ensue, burr holes are performed, the clot is removed and the vessel tied.

SUBDURAL

This occurs most frequently in the elderly,

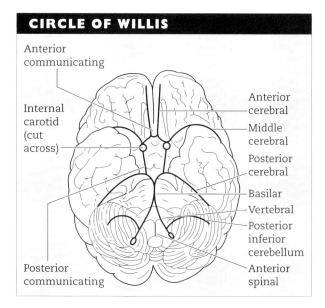

CIRCLE OF WILLIS

Anterior communicating

Internal carotid (cut across)

Anterior cerebral

Middle cerebral

Posterior cerebral

Basilar

Vertebral

Posterior inferior cerebellum

Posterior communicating

Anterior spinal

Fig. 8.4 Cerebral arteries: basal view.

alcoholics and children. It often follows trauma. A small venous haemorrhage occurs and the clot slowly enlarges in size, absorbing fluid osmotically from the CSF.

Clinical presentation
The symptoms may develop over a period of weeks to months. Headache, confusion and progressive loss of conscious level occur with fluctuation of consciousness. The other signs are of a one-sided intracranial mass with contralateral weakness and hemiplegia, possibly with signs of raised intracranial pressure (falling pulse rate, rising blood pressure, papilloedema).

Management
CT scan may show the haematoma and removal may give full recovery, irrespective of the patient's age. Subdural haematomas may be bilateral.

Subarachnoid haemorrhage
Subarachnoid haemorrhage presents with abrupt onset of severe generalized headache. There may be loss of consciousness, vomiting or seizures. Meningeal irritation causes neck stiffness and photophobia. This follows rupture of a berry aneurysm of the circle of Willis (Fig. 8.4). Focal neurological signs suggest local

compression (e.g. 3rd-nerve palsy caused by posterior communicating artery aneurysm) or associated intracerebral haematoma. Rising blood pressure, falling pulse and papilloedema indicate raised intracranial pressure.

Many patients give a history of previous similar but milder episodes, possibly caused by smaller leaks.

Diagnosis
Unenhanced CT scan shows intracranial blood in over 90% of cases and reveals any associated haematoma. It may indicate the site of a leaking aneurysm, and any associated hydrocephalus. If CT scan is unavailable, or intracranial blood is not seen but clinical suspicion is high, lumbar puncture is performed to examine CSF for uniform bloodstaining and xanthochromia. Lumbar puncture can precipitate coning, and should not be performed if signs suggest raised intracranial pressure or cerebral or cerebellar haemorrhage.

Complications
Some 25% of patients die on the first day, and a further 25% die in the first month.

Hydrocephalus occurs in 20% of patients, and may require ventricular drainage. It results from obstruction to CSF flow by blood.

Delayed *ischaemic* brain damage caused by cerebral vasospasm presents with deteriorating conscious level or focal neurological signs. Death and severe neurological deficits because of vasospasm were reduced by 66% compared with placebo by prophylactic treatment with the calcium antagonist nimodipine. It should be prescribed as soon as the diagnosis is established. Sudden deterioration suggests *rebleeding*, which can be confirmed by repeat CT scan. *Haematoma*, if compressing, requires evacuation.

Transient ischaemic attacks

Transient ischaemic attacks (TIAs) are focal brain or retinal deficits that resolve within 24 h. Most clear within 1 h. The risk of stroke or myocardial infarction following TIA is approximately 5% within 1 month, 12% during the first year and 25% over 5 years.

The most common cause is platelet emboli from large atheroscerotic arteries supplying the brain. Ten per cent of people with ischaemic strokes have previously had a TIA. Rarely, cerebral vasculitis, hypercoagulable states and arterial dissection present as TIAs. Non-vascular causes that may mimic TIA include seizures, migraine, tumour, subdural haematoma and hypoglycaemia.

• Carotid artery TIAs affect the cortex and produce ischaemia to the ipsilateral eye or brain, resulting in blurring of vision, or contralateral weakness or sensory disturbance.

• Vertebrobasilar TIAs affect the brainstem and cause dizziness, ataxia, vertigo, dysarthria, diplopia, and unilateral or bilateral weakness and numbness in the limbs.

Management
Reduction of risk factors
• Control hypertension.
• Stop smoking.
• Treat underlying heart disease (arrhythmias, valvular heart disease, coronary artery disease and heart failure).

Improving diabetic control, treating hyperlipidaemia and reducing excessive alcohol intake are all advisable, although the effect of

---

TRIALS BOX 8.2

The **Canadian Cooperative Study Group** compared placebo with aspirin 1300 mg/day, sulphinpyrazone 800 mg/day, or aspirin and sulphinpyrazone in combination in 585 patients with transient ischaemic attack (TIA) or minor stroke. Aspirin significantly reduced the risk of stroke in men but not women, possibly because fewer women were enrolled. Sulphinpyrazone provided no benefit either alone or in combination with aspirin. N Engl J Med 1978; **299**: 53–59.

The **UK-TIA aspirin trial** compared placebo with two doses of aspirin (300 and 1200 mg/day) in 2435 patients with TIA or minor stroke. Aspirin reduced the risk of the combined end-points of stroke, myocardial infarction and death. There was no significant difference between the two doses of aspirin but gastrointestinal symptoms were more common with the higher dose. J Neurol Neurosurg Psychiatry 1991; **54**: 1044–1054.

The **Dutch TIA trial** compared carbaspirin calcium at a dosage of 30 mg/day with 283 mg/day in 3131 patients with TIA or minor stroke. Both doses were equally effective in reducing the risk of stroke, but the 30-mg dose caused fewer gastrointestinal problems. N Engl J Med 1991; **325**: 1261–1266.

The **Swedish aspirin low-dose trial** compared placebo with aspirin 75 mg/day in 1360 patients with TIA or minor stroke. Low-dose aspirin reduced the risk of stroke or death compared with placebo. Lancet 1991; **338**: 1345–1349.

The **Antiplatelet Trialists' Collaboration** performed a meta-analysis of 145 randomized trials involving nearly 100 000 patients with coronary cerebral or peripheral vascular disease. They found a 23% reduction in non-fatal stroke, non-fatal myocardial infarction and vascular death in patients with a history of stroke or TIA. There was no evidence that any antiplatelet drug, alone or in combination, was more effective than medium-dose aspirin (75–325 mg/day). Higher doses of aspirin were as effective but caused more unwanted effects. Br Med J 1994; **308**: 81–106.

TRIALS BOX 8.3

The **North American Symptomatic Carotid Endarterectomy Trial (NASCET)** studied 659 patients with TIA or minor stroke and 70–99% with carotid artery stenosis. Endarterectomy reduced the risk of non-fatal and fatal stroke. NASCET is continuing for patients with 30–69% stenosis. *N Engl J Med* 1991; **325**: 445–453.

The **European Carotid Surgery Trial (ECST)** studied 2518 patients with mild (0–29%), moderate (30–69%) or severe (70–99%) stenosis. Surgery reduced the risk of stroke or death in patients with severe stenosis, but medical treatment was better than surgery in patients with mild stenosis. *Lancet* 1991; **337**: 1235–1243.

The **European Carotid Surgery Trialists' Collaborative Group** investigated the risk of stroke in the distribution of asymptomatic carotid artery stenosis in 2295 patients. The risk of stroke over 3 years was 2.1%, and neither screening nor endarterectomy for asymptomatic lesions was felt to be justified. *Lancet* 1995; **345**: 209–212.

The **North American Symptomatic Carotid Endarterectomy Trial Collaborators** assessed the benefit of carotid endarterectomy in patients with symptomatic moderate stenosis, defined as stenosis of less than 70%. Endarterectomy in patients with symptomatic moderate carotid stenosis of 50–69% yielded only a moderate reduction in the risk of stroke.

They concluded that decisions about treatment for patients in this category must take into account recognized risk factors, and exceptional surgical skill is obligatory if carotid endarterectomy is to be performed. Patients with stenosis of < 50% did not benefit from surgery. Patients with severe stenosis (≥ 70%) had a durable benefit from endarterectomy at 8 years of follow-up. *N Engl J Med* 1998; **339**: 1415–1425.

The **North American Symptomatic Carotid Endarterectomy Trial Collaborators** studied patients with unilateral symptomatic carotid-artery stenosis and asymptomatic contralateral stenosis from 1988 to 1997. Among 1604 patients with stenosis of < 60% of the luminal diameter, the risk of a first stroke was 1.6% annually, as compared with 3.2% annually among 216 patients with 60–99% stenosis. In the group with 60–99% stenosis, the 5-year risk of stroke in the territory of a large artery was 9.9%, that of lacunar stroke was 6.0% and that of cardioembolic stroke 2.1%. The collaborators concluded that the risk of stroke among patients with asymptomatic carotid-artery stenosis is relatively low. Forty-five per cent of strokes in patients with asymptomatic stenosis of 60–99% were attributable to lacunes or cardioembolism, suggesting that the absolute benefit associated with endarterectomy may be overestimated. *N Engl J Med* 2000; **342**: 1693–1700.

each on reducing stroke risk is unclear. Mild to moderate alcohol consumption reduces the risk of coronary artery disease, and may have a mild protective effect on stroke risk.

Medical treatment
Aspirin reduces the risk of stroke or myocardial infarction or vascular death in patients with TIA by 25% (see Trials Box 8.3). Aspirin in a dosage of 75–300 mg/day (with or without dipyridamole) is as effective as or better than any other agent or combination of agents. Clopidogrel can be used in those who are aspirin intolerant. In the absence of risk factors for cardioembolism (atrial fibrillation, valvular disease, prosthetic heart valves, myocardial

infarction within the last 3 months) there are no conclusive data to support the use of oral anticoagulants. However, in those who do fulfil these criteria, and in whom haemorrhage has been excluded by imaging, full anticoagulation is indicated from 2 weeks poststroke (Royal College of Physicians. *National Clinical Guidelines for Stroke*. 2000).

Surgical treatment
The indications for carotid endarterectomy in patients with TIA depend on many factors, including the severity of the stenosis and the surgical morbidity and mortality at the centre involved. In centres with a low surgical morbidity and mortality (< 6%) surgery is of

GLASGOW COMA SCALE

Category	Score
Eye opening	
None	1
To pain	2
To speech	3
Spontaneous	4
Best verbal response	
None	1
Incomprehensible	2
Inappropriate	3
Confused	4
Oriented	5
Best motor response	
None	1
Extending	2
Flexing	3
Localizing	4
Obeying	5

Patients are scored for each of the three categories. The sum of the three scores gives a measure of their overall conscious level, the range being from 3 (completely unresponsive) to 14 (fully conscious).

Table 8.1 Glasgow Coma Scale.

proven value in patients with a stenosis of > 70% and a history of TIA.

Glasgow Coma Scale

Conscious level may be charted using the Glasgow Coma Scale (Table 8.1).

Brain death (two independent medical opinions are required)

The three main criteria essential to this medicolegal diagnosis are the following.
1 A known untreatable cause, such as cardiac arrest, intracerebral haemorrhage or severe trauma. Patients with hypothermia or drug overdose are not acceptable.

2 Absent cortical function: deep coma, as shown by absent response to any stimulus (other than spinal reflexes).
3 Absent brainstem function. This is demonstrated by:
   (a) fixed dilated pupils;
   (b) absent corneal, gag and cough reflexes;
   (c) absent eye movements and no movement on rolling the head (i.e. the normal 'doll's eye movements', in which the eyes lag behind head movement, are absent);
   (d) absent caloric responses. Ice-cold water into an external auditory meatus causes eye movements towards the stimulated ear in normal people; and
   (e) lack of spontaneous respiration.

Epilepsy

Epilepsy is a clinical diagnosis. It results from a paroxysmal electrical discharge in the cerebral neurons that results in a wide variety of clinical patterns. Epilepsy is an expression of brain dysfunction and the diagnosis makes it imperative to search for the cause, although two-thirds of all cases are idiopathic, i.e. of undetermined cause. Most commonly there is a continuing tendency to experience episodes of altered movement, sensory phenomena and odd behaviour, usually with altered consciousness. A single unprovoked episode is insufficient to make a diagnosis of epilepsy. Patients with established epilepsy tend to have stereotypical attacks.

Many patients who present following a 'fit' have only had an episode of unconsciousness. It is important to consider and exclude other conditions that are commonly confused with epilepsy.

Classification
Partial seizures—seizures that start locally
Partial seizures have a single focus (origin) of activity. This may be scar tissue following trauma, a stroke or a tumour. Either:
• *simple partial seizures*—no impairment of consciousness. Symptoms may be illusional, olfactory, psychic, cognitive, aphasic, sensory or motor (Jacksonian); or

• *complex partial seizures*—in which consciousness is impaired. These are chiefly 'temporal lobe seizures' which may start with an aura and include automatisms or other psychological phenomena (see below).
NB Partial seizures (secondarily generalized) may proceed to generalized seizures.

Generalized seizures—in which there is no evidence of a focal onset
Generalized seizures in which there is widespread activity affecting both cerebral hemispheres. They include:
• childhood absence seizures (petit mal);
• myoclonic epilepsy—sudden convulsive movements of the limbs and trunk, usually in children; and
• tonic–clonic (grand mal) seizures (see below). Also tonic (spasm) and clonic (jerking) seizures; atonic or akinetic seizures.
    Many seizure patterns remain unclassified.

Aetiology
Usually no cause is identified and the epilepsy is termed idiopathic. This includes patients who have suffered intrauterine, perinatal or neonatal insults. There may be a strong family history, suggesting genetic susceptibility, particularly with petit mal seizures.
    Seizures may be secondary to cerebral disorders, metabolic disorders and drug intake.

Cerebral disorders
• Cerebral tumour or arteriovenous malformation.
• Post-tramatic—a sequel to severe head injury or birth injury.
• Cerebrovascular disease.
• Infection—encephalitis, bacterial meningitis, cerebral abscess, toxoplasmosis (the most common intracranial lesion in acquired immunodeficiency syndrome (AIDS)), cysticercosis, syphilis. Falciparum malaria should be considered in travellers (examine blood film).
• Inflammatory lesions—systemic lupus erythematosus (SLE), vasculitis, multiple sclerosis.
• Degenerative—Alzheimer disease, Huntington chorea.

Metabolic disorders
• Hypoglycaemia.
• Hypocalcaemia or hypomagnesaemia.
• Renal or hepatic failure.
• Hyponatraemia.

Drugs (particularly following overdose)
• Alcohol: severe intoxication, rapid withdrawal by habitual heavy drinker, or following head injury while intoxicated.
• Amphetamines, tricyclic antidepressants, phenothiazines.

Provocation of seizures
Many aetiological factors (e.g. drug overdose, hypoglycaemia) can provoke seizures in patients not usually prone to epilepsy. In known epileptics, seizures can be provoked by sleep deprivation, stress, alcohol and, occasionally, stimuli such as television or disco lighting. In women seizures may increase in frequency around the time of menstruation.

Differential diagnosis
It is important to consider other causes of loss of consciousness, including:
• syncope: vasovagal fainting attacks; postmicturition and cough syncope;
• cerebrovascular disease: TIAs, carotid artery stenosis, vertebrobasilar ischaemia;
• low cardiac output: cardiac arrhythmia (Stokes–Adams attacks in heart block, sinoatrial disease); aortic stenosis; cardiomyopathy;
• metabolic: hypoglycaemia;
• postural hypotension may be caused by hypotensive or sedative drugs, particularly in the elderly; and
• psychiatric: conversion hysteria, malingering.
    An account of the fit from a witness is invaluable.
    In the differential diagnosis from faints, epileptics are stiff and not floppy in the fall, usually have staring open eyes rather than half-closed, have no memory of the fall and take over 30 s to recover.
    Drop attacks occur only past middle age, usually in women in whom there is no loss of consciousness but there is a sense of surprise about the lack of external cause.

A hysterical episode is exacerbated by witnesses, is associated with coarse dramatic movement rather than neat jerking, and clenched flickering eyelids with the eye rolled up (if the lids can be prised apart). Recovery is rapid with full mental alertness ('What happened, where am I?') and no neurological signs.

Clinical features

Generalized, tonic–clonic seizures (grand mal)
In over 50% of cases a fit is preceded by an *aura*. This is followed by loss of consciousness and the *tonic* phase, which usually lasts up to 30 s. Cyanosis may occur as the respiratory muscles are also tonically contracted. The *clonic* phase follows in all limbs. Micturition and tongue biting (and biting of any fingers unwisely inserted into the mouth to pull the tongue forwards) which is followed by sleep, lasting for 1–3 h. During sleep, the corneal and limb reflexes may be absent and the plantar responses upgoing.

The patient should be protected from injury during the acute phase. Intravenous diazepam, given as an emulsion to reduce thrombophlebitis (Diazemuls 5 mg for 2–4 min), will control most fits. Alternatively, rectal solutions, 2.5–20 mg, are well absorbed. Status epilepticus may require continued diazepam or a clomethiazole or phenytoin infusion with close attention to breathing. General anaesthesia with muscle relaxants and artificial ventilation are sometimes needed to suppress abnormal cerebral electrical activity.

Absence seizures (petit mal)
This presents in childhood (4–10 years old) and is characterized by brief (10–15 s) moments of absence without warning and with immediate recovery. The electroencephalogram (EEG) shows typical spike-and-wave complexes at 3 s. It virtually never continues beyond puberty, but about 5% of children will develop adult grand mal seizures.

Temporal lobe epilepsy
This is characterized by temporary disturbances of the content of consciousness. Hallucinations may occur (e.g. *déjà-vu* phenomena), as may visual disturbance such as macropsia and micropsia. Unreasoning fear and depersonalization may be present. Olfactory or gustatory auras may be the only symptom and are related to abnormal foci in the uncinate lobe. Automatism may follow the aura. Patients perform a complex movement pattern, repeated with each attack (psychomotor epilepsy).

Jacksonian (focal) epilepsy
Epileptic activity originates in one part of the precentral motor cortex. Fits begin in one part of the body (e.g. the thumb) and may proceed to involve that side of the body and then the whole body. Subsequent paresis of the affected limb may last up to 3 days (Todd paralysis). Sensory epilepsy is a parallel condition originating in the sensory cortex.

Investigation
The object is to detect treatable underlying brain disease and to exclude the factors that may be provoking the attacks.

A full history and clinical examination are taken to exclude other causes of loss of consciousness (see above).

Check blood for evidence of *alcohol* (blood levels, mean corpuscular volume, γ-glutamyl transferase), *hypoglycaemia* or *hypocalcaemia*.

All patients should have a *chest X-ray*.

An *EEG* may be helpful by demonstrating the type of epilepsy, site of an epileptic focus (slow-wave activity may suggest the presence of a tumour) and guide drug therapy. A diagnosis of epilepsy cannot be made from an EEG alone—epilepsy is a clinical diagnosis, not an electrical one. Of the general population, 10–15% have an abnormal EEG.

If there is a possibility of a transient cardiac arrhythmia as a cause of fits, *24-h ambulatory ECG* monitoring should be performed.

Brain CT scan to exclude focal brain disease. It is of particular value in late-onset epilepsy, partial seizures and in patients with generalized epilepsy where the EEG discloses a focal abnormality, particularly if this is accompanied by slow waves.

Management

A single fit rarely requires treatment. Any underlying cause should be identified and patients should be advised not to drive and to inform the licensing authority (p. 96).

Antiepileptic treatment should be reserved for those who have two or more seizures within a year. It is essential that the diagnosis is confirmed before starting treatment.

About 200 000 people in the UK are taking antiepileptic drugs. The aim is to prevent seizures without causing adverse effects. The initial choice depends on the type of epilepsy, and the risk of unwanted effects, and the likelihood of compliance. Seizure control with minimal adverse effects can be achieved using a single agent in about 80% of patients.

Established antiepileptic therapies

Carbamazepine is often regarded as the drug of first choice for simple and complex partial seizures, and for tonic–clonic seizures. Side-effects include gastrointestinal disturbances, dizziness, hepatitis and skin rashes (5–10%). It induces its own metabolism, so increased dosage may be needed to achieve therapeutic levels—optimum response occurs at plasma concentration of 4–12 mg/l (20–50 µmol/l). It is ineffective in absence seizures, which may be exacerbated.

Sodium valproate can be effective in controlling simple and complex partial seizures and all forms of generalized seizures, including tonic–clonic seizures, myoclonic seizures, atonic and tonic seizures and absence attacks. Because of its widespread use, some recommend it as the drug of choice for new-onset epilepsy.

TRIAL BOX 8.4

The **Medical Research Council Antiepileptic Drug Withdrawal Study Group** randomized 1013 patients to continuation or slow withdrawal of treatment. A total of 78% of those still on treatment and 59% of those in whom it had been withdrawn were seizure-free after 2 years. *Lancet* 1991; **337**: 1175–1180.

Unwanted effects include weight gain (one of the most common reasons for non-compliance), hair loss and tremor. Hepatotoxicity, thrombocytopenia and pancreatitis (check amylase if abdominal pain) are rare adverse effects. Plasma concentrations are unhelpful in monitoring efficacy.

Phenytoin is effective in both partial and tonic–clonic seizures, but a narrow therapeutic index and adverse effects limit its usefulness. Cosmetic changes (gum hypertrophy, hirsutism, coarsening of facial features) are particularly undesirable in adolescents. Optimum plasma concentrations are 10–20 mg/l (40–80 µmol/l).

Phenobarbital is effective in partial and generalized seizures, but causes sedation in adults and behavioural changes and hyperkinesia in children. It is usually reserved for patients who are intolerant of other therapies.

Ethosuximide is the drug of choice for simple absence seizures. It may also be used in myoclonic seizures. It can cause sedation, but skin rashes, liver changes and haematological disorders are rare. Optimum plasma concentration is 40–100 mg/l (300–700 µmol/l).

Benzodiazepines are useful for the treatment of status epilepticus, but sedation and tolerance limit their usefulness in chronic treatment. *Clobazam* is a 1,5 benzodiazepine (differing in structure from other compounds, such as diazepam and clonazepam which are 1,4 benzodiazepines). It may cause less sedation and psychomotor impairment, but tolerance is still a problem. *Clonazepam* is occasionally used in tonic–clonic or partial seizures.

Newer antiepileptic drugs form useful adjunctive therapy in uncontrolled epilepsy.

Gabapentin is structurally similar to the inhibitory neurotransmitter GABA, although it does not appear to interact with the GABA system. It is effective as an adjunctive treatment of partial seizures, with or without secondary generalization. Side-effects are uncommon, although somnolence, dizziness and ataxia can occur.

Lamotrigine probably acts through inhibition of excitatory amino acid release. It is used as adjunctive treatment in partial or tonic–clonic seizures. It is generally well tolerated, although headache, dizziness, ataxia and gastrointestinal disturbance can occur.

Vigabatrin (γ-vinyl GABA) inactivates the enzyme (GABA-T). It is used, usually as monotherapy, in partial or tonic–clonic seizures which are not controlled by other antiepileptics. Sedation, depression, weight gain and gastrointestinal symptoms limit its usefulness in some patients.

Epilepsy and pregnancy

Maternal epilepsy is associated with an increased risk of fetal malformation, which increases further if the mother is taking antiepileptics. Common anomalies include fingernail hypoplasia, facial deformities such as low-set eyebrows, broad nasal bridge, irregular teeth and low-set ears. More serious abnormalities, including cleft lip and palate, congenital heart disease and spina bifida, are less common. The incidence of neural tube defects is particularly common with sodium valproate (1.5%) and carbamazepine (1%). The newer antiepileptics (gabapentin, lamotrigine and vigabatrin) are not licensed for use in pregnancy, although there is no evidence to date that they are teratogenic in humans.

Epileptic women who wish to become pregnant should receive advice about the risk of congenital abnormality, and also about the need to continue treatment. The lowest dosage of a single agent should be used wherever possible. Folic acid, 5 mg daily, should be given before and for 12 weeks after conception. Screening for neural tube defects (α-fetoprotein levels and second trimester ultrasound) should be performed if sodium valproate or carbamazepine is used.

Most antiepileptics are excreted in breast milk, but concentrations are usually low and not harmful to the infant.
NB Carbamazepine, phenytoin and phenobarbital all induce hepatic microsomal enzymes and increase metabolism of oestrogens and progestagens, making oral contraception unreliable. Sodium valproate and the newer add-on agents (gabapentin, lamotrigine and vigabatrin) do not affect the efficacy of oral contraceptives.

Prognosis in epilepsy

Six years after diagnosis, 40% of patients will have been fit-free for 5 years. Relatively poor prognoses are associated with combinations of grand mal with other seizures, traumatic epilepsy, clustering of episodes, physical signs and mental retardation. Attempts to withdraw treatment in patients who are symptom-free should be considered on an individual basis.

Advice to the patient with epilepsy

There are no rules, but it is sensible to avoid heights, ladders, unsupervised swimming and cycling for 2 years from the last episode. Fires should be guarded and children should not be left in the bath unattended. Patients with epilepsy are unable to perform certain occupations (e.g. the armed forces, jobs involving driving), but epilepsy should not be a bar to most occupations.

Epilepsy and driving

From the guide to UK medical standards of fitness to drive.

Group 1 entitlement (cars and motorcycles)
First epileptic seizure/solitary fit
One year off driving with medical review before restarting.

Patients suffering from epilepsy
To be granted a licence patients should have been free from epileptic attacks for 2 years, or have had an epileptic attack while asleep more than 3 years previously and no epileptic attacks while awake but only while asleep since that attack.

If epileptic medication is withdrawn, the Driver and Vehicle Licensing Authority (DVLA) advises patients not to drive during withdrawal, and for 6 months after cessation of therapy. If an epileptic attack occurs the above criteria then apply.

Provoked seizures are dealt with by the DVLA on an individual basis.

A single loss of consciousness for which no cause is found requires cessation of driving for 1 year. Multiple episodes are treated as for epilepsy (i.e. at least 2 years off driving).

Stroke
At least 1 month off driving after the event. When clinical recovery is fully satisfactory, driving may restart.

Narcolepsy

This rare condition usually starts in late puberty. The onset is sudden, with episodes of irresistible and inappropriate sleep usually without fatigue, although often in sleep-provoking circumstances such as medical lectures. It is associated with cataplexy—attacks of sudden, brief muscle atonia often causing falls but without loss of consciousness precipitated by strong emotions such as laughter (also in medical lectures?). There may be abnormal mental states while passing between awake and asleep: sleep paralysis like cataplexy, and presleep, 'hypnagogic' hallucinations like vivid dreams. These are disorders in which REM sleep is present in the waking state. They are strongly associated with human leucocyte antigen (HLA) DR2. Narcolepsy may respond to amphetamines, and cataplexy to clomipramine.

Multiple sclerosis

A demyelinating disease characterized by episodes of neurological deficit appearing irregularly throughout the CNS both in anatomical site and time. Prevalence is 50–80 in 100 000 with a slight preponderance in females. First episodes usually occur in young adulthood, with a peak at around 30 years.

Aetiology
Current evidence suggests an acquired auto-immunity against myelin proteins. This is determined in part by genetic susceptibility as evidenced by:

• racial variation;
• clustering in families, and excess concordance in monozygotic vs. dizygotic twins; and
• HLA associations—in particular between multiple sclerosis in white patients and HLA DR15, DQ6, Dw2.

Geographical variations, with a high prevalence in temperate climates, emphasize the importance of environmental factors. Individuals who migrate before the age of 15 acquire the risk of the country to which they have migrated.

Experimental autoimmune encephalomyelitis (EAE) has provided a model for studying multiple sclerosis. EAE is a T-cell-mediated disease that is produced by immunizing animals with myelin basic proteins.

Pathology
Patches of demyelination occur in discrete areas (plaques) in the white matter of the brain and spinal cord, especially in:
• optic nerves—the most common initial site;
• brainstem;
• cerebellar peduncles; and
• dorsal and pyramidal (lateral) tracts.

Oedema around acute lesions contributes to the neurological deficit. Function typically improves as oedema resolves. Later, scarring gives rise to the characteristic white plaque.

Clinical presentation
Plaques can occur at any site, so presentation is extremely variable. Symptoms include visual disturbance, clumsiness, weakness, numbness, tremor, cognitive impairment, bowel or bladder disturbance and sexual dysfunction.

Typical features
• *Visual disturbance*—almost all patients have visual loss or diplopia at some stage. Between 30 and 70% of patients with isolated optic neuritis subsequently develop multiple sclerosis. Recovery from optic neuritis is characterized by optic atrophy or temporal pallor of the disc.
• *Upper motor neuron deficit* with weakness, as a paraparesis, hemiparesis or monoparesis.

• *Sensory deficit* with paraesthesia and pro-prioceptive loss in a limb or half of the body.
• *Cerebellar signs* with intention tremor, nystagmus, vertigo and dysarthria.
• *Bladder dysfunction* is common, and is occa-sionally the presenting complaint. Initially there is urgency and frequency, followed by incontin-ence. Constipation is the usual *bowel disturbance*, but urgency of defecation can occur. *Erectile impotence* and *ejaculatory failure* are common.
• *Cognitive impairment*—IQ and language skills often remain until late in the disease. However, memory, learning and the ability to deal with abstract concepts often deteriorate in chronic forms.

Chronic progressive forms are characterized by evidence of optic atrophy, cerebellar lesions and spastic paraparesis, frequently with posterior column loss. There is dementia with altered mood—both depression and euphoria occur.

Symptoms are commonly made worse by exertion and heat (patients may be able to get into a hot bath but not out of it).

Diagnosis

Clinically the diagnosis is made on the basis of at least two characteristic episodes of neuro-logical dysfunction.

Visually evoked potentials (VEP) test the integrity of the visual pathways. Demyelination causes an abnormality (usually delay) in occipi-tal EEG tracings in response to a stimulus such as a chessboard pattern presented to the eyes. Abnormalities are present in 95% of patients with multiple sclerosis but it is not specific. Sensory and auditory evoked potentials may also show delay.

Lumbar puncture reveals a raised CSF protein (up to 1 g/l) in 50% of patients. The most useful test in CSF is immunoelectrophoresis, which shows an increased proportion of immunoglobulin G (IgG) in 60% and oligoclonal bands in 90%.

MRI is the imaging procedure of choice for the diagnosis of multiple sclerosis. Plaques of demyelination appear as bright lesions, which are especially numerous in the periventricular area. Clinically silent lesions are frequently revealed. Refinements such as fluid attenu-ation inversion recovery (FLAIR) MRI can be used to suppress the signal from CSF and detect lesion in the spinal cord.

Prognosis

The average duration of life from onset of symptoms is 20–30 years. Overall, 80% experi-ence steadily progressive disability, 15% follow a relatively benign course and 5% die in 5 years. There may be a long latent period (15–30 years) after an episode of optic neuritis before further neurological symptoms occur. Patients whose disease onset is sensory rather than motor tend to have a better prognosis. Poor prognostic factors are older age of onset, early cerebellar involvement and loss of mental acuity.

Management

Physiotherapy, rehabilitation, pharmacological treatment, surgery and psychological support all have a role. Support for the family should be provided. Interferon-β (1a and 1b) is of benefit in relapsing/remitting and progressive disease (see Trials).

Visual loss. High-dose intravenous steroids accelerate visual recovery in isolated optic neuritis (see Trials), and delays the onset of further neurological signs.

Weakness. Physiotherapy and rehabilitation are important. Several studies have shown a bene-fit from aminopyridines, which promote nerve conduction by blocking potassium channels in excitatory nerve membranes.

Spasticity. This responds to stretching exer-cises, alone or in combination with antispas-modic agents such as benzodiazepines or baclofen. Baclofen is a GABA analogue that binds to GABA receptors in the dorsal horn of the spinal cord. Dantrolene sodium acts directly on skeletal muscle to reduce spasm. Intractable spasticity may require tendono-tomy or neurectomy.

Bladder dysfunction. Antimuscarinic agents (e.g. oxybutynin, flavoxate) increase bladder capacity by diminishing unstable detrusor contractions.

TRIALS BOX 8.5

The **IFN-β Multiple Sclerosis Study Group** compared β-interferon (IFN-β) and placebo in a double-blind multicentre study of 372 ambulatory patients with relapsing–remitting multiple sclerosis. IFN-β was effective in reducing relapses over a 3-year period, but did not significantly affect disability. *Neurology* 1993; **48**: 655–661.

The **Optic Neuritis Study Group** compared intravenous steroids (methylprednisolone 250 mg q.d.s. for 3 days followed by oral prednisone for 11 days), oral steroids and placebo in 457 patients with optic neuritis. Intravenous steroids accelerated visual recovery from optic neuritis, and delayed subsequent development of multiple sclerosis over a 2-year period. By 4 years the rate of developing multiple sclerosis was similar in all three treatment groups. *N Engl J Med* 1993; **329**: 1764–1769.

The **Multiple Sclerosis Collaborative Research Group (MSCRG)** randomized 301 patients with relapsing multiple sclerosis into a double-blinded, placebo-controlled, trial of interferon β-1a. Interferon β-1a had a significant beneficial impact in relapsing multiple sclerosis patients by reducing the accumulation of permanent physical disability, exacerbation frequency, and disease activity measured by gadolinium-enhanced lesions on brain magnetic resonance images. *Ann Neurol* 1996; **39**: 285–294.

The **European Study Group** on interferon β-1b in secondary progressive multiple sclerosis compared interferon-β (358 patients) and placebo (360 patients) in the treatment of patients who are in the secondary progressive phase of multiple sclerosis. Treatment with interferon β-1b delayed sustained neurological deterioration in patients with secondary progressive multiple sclerosis. *Lancet* 1998; **352**: 1491–1497.

The **Prevention of Relapses and Disability by Interferon β-1a Subcutaneously in Multiple Sclerosis (PRISMS) Study Group** undertook a double-blind, placebo-controlled study in relapsing/remitting multiple sclerosis to investigate the effects of subcutaneous interferon β-1a in 560 patients. Subcutaneous interferon β-1a was an effective treatment for relapsing/remitting multiple sclerosis in terms of relapse rate, defined disability, and all MRI outcome measures in a dose-related manner, and it was well tolerated. *Lancet* 1998; **352**: 1498–1504.

PRISMS-4 reported the long-term efficacy of interferon β-1a in relapsing multiple sclerosis. Clinical and MRI benefit continued for up to 4 years, with evidence of dose response. Outcomes were consistently better for patients treated for 4 years than for patients in crossover groups. Efficacy decreased with neutralizing antibody formation. *Neurology* 2001; **56**: 1628–1636.

α-Adrenoceptor blockers (e.g. prazosin, terazosin) relax smooth muscle and may also be of benefit. Antidiuretic hormone (vasopressin), and its synthetic analogue desmopressin, have been used to control disabling nocturia. Self-catheterization enables some patients to remain free from a permanent indwelling catheter.

Sexual dysfunction. Counselling should be provided. Oral sildenafil or intracavernosal injection of papaverine may be of value in erectile impotence.

Psychological support. This is essential. Patients often remain surprisingly euphoric, but not infrequently there is marked depression.

Motor neuron disease

This disease involves progressive degeneration of:
- anterior horn cells in the spinal cord;
- cells of the lower cranial motor nuclei; and
- neurons of the motor cortex with secondary degeneration of the pyramidal tracts.

Clinical presentation

Motor neuron disease (MND) usually presents between the ages of 50 and 70 years, slightly more frequently in men than women (1.5 : 1), with the clinical features of one of the above groups but usually progresses to produce features of the other two as well. It is rare in all its forms: UK prevalence is 5 in 100 000 of the population (incidence: 1.5 in 100 000). About 20% of people with familial MND have mutations in the copper-zinc superoxide dismutase (*SOD1*) gene.

It is characterized by:
- muscular weakness and fasciculation; and
- absence of sensory signs.

There are three classical forms of clinical presentation.

1 Lower motor neuron weakness, with wasting and fasciculation of the small muscles of the hand. This is followed by wasting of the upper and lower limb muscles. This lower motor neuron wasting and fasciculation is termed *progressive muscular atrophy*.

2 Lower motor neuron weakness, fasciculation and wasting of the tongue and pharynx producing dysarthria, dysphagia, choking and nasal regurgitation (*progressive bulbar palsy*).

3 Upper motor neuron spastic weakness starting in the legs, and later spreading to the arms (*amyotrophic lateral sclerosis*—a term sometimes used for motor neuron disease as a whole, particularly in the USA).

Any combination of the above three groups can occur. In most cases upper and lower motor neuron lesions are combined at the time of presentation.

Fasciculation of some limb musculature is a hallmark of this disease. Lower limb lesions are usually of upper motor neuron type, and the upper limb lesions of lower motor neuron type. The limbs may demonstrate marked muscular wasting but still have exaggerated reflexes. The abdominal reflexes are usually preserved until late in the disease. Pseudobulbar palsy may occur but is very uncommon. The bladder is not affected.

Management

Physiotherapy, rehabilitation, psychological and family support are important. Terminal care including help with ventilation and swallowing may be required late in the disease. The physician should be prepared to discuss issues of physician-assisted suicide and euthanasia. Riluzole might slow the rate of disease progression in the amyotrophic lateral sclerosis form of the disease.

Parkinson's disease and extrapyramidal disorders

Parkinson's disease
James Parkinson, 1755–1824, London.
Prevalence: 1–1.5 in 1000 in the UK (1 in 200 in those over 70 years).

Aetiology of parkinsonism
Idiopathic Parkinson's disease (paralysis agitans)
This is of slow onset and inexorably progressive. It presents in the 50–60-year age group and in males more often than females. It results from deficiency of dopamine in the substantia nigra and relative excess of acetylcholine stimulation in the corpus striatum as a consequence. Dopamine granules are reduced in the cells of the substantia nigra. It is asymmetrical, particularly at first, and may be familial.

Atherosclerosis
This is often associated with other manifestations of vascular disease (stroke, dementia, ischaemic heart disease, intermittent claudication and hypertension). There tends to be less tremor and more festination than in idiopathic parkinsonism.

Drugs
Neuroleptics, e.g. chlorpromazine and, less commonly, reserpine, may produce parkinsonism. The high doses used in psychiatry make it relatively common in schizophrenics. Dystonic movements—facial grimacing, involuntary movements of the tongue and oculogyric crises—are more common than in idiopathic parkinsonism, and are usually symmetrical. Tremor is less common.

NB Acute extrapyramidal syndromes with grinding teeth and masseter spasm may result from phenothiazines used as sedatives (e.g. perphenazine) and other dopa antagonists such as metoclopramide. They respond rapidly to intravenous procyclidine.

Poisoning

Rarely, Parkinson-like disorders may result from poisoning with heavy metals e.g. manganese and copper (NB Wilson disease, p. 102) and after carbon monoxide poisoning.

Postencephalitic

Parkinsonism occurred following outbreaks of encephalitis lethargica (between 1917 and 1925) and still occurs sporadically.

Punch-drunk syndrome

This is caused by brain damage in boxers.

Clinical presentation

This disturbance of voluntary motor function is characterized by the triad of *rigidity*, *tremor* and *bradykinesia* (slow movements) plus postural abnormalities. Vague muscle ache and clumsiness with physical and mental fatigue may be seen, in retrospect, to have been early evidence.

The classical picture of parkinsonism is of immobile flexion at all joints (neck, trunk, shoulders, elbows, wrists and metacarpophalangeal joints) except the interphalangeal. Even in the early case, on walking the arms do not swing fully and later in the disease the gait is stuttering and shuffling and the patient may show festination. He or she is slow and unstable on the turn and may freeze. The face is expressionless and unblinking, and speech slurred and monotonous. In the long-standing case, other symptoms are commonly present:
• difficulty in initiating movement (starting to walk, rising from a chair or turning in bed);
• poor balance with a tendency to fall because of slow correcting movements;
• small handwriting;
• seborrhoea, especially of the face;
• rarely, increased salivation (which, with dysphagia, may give rise to drooling); and
• a soft unintelligible voice (dysarthria).
Constipation and urinary frequency occur, sometimes with incontinence.

Oculogyric crises (forced upwards deviation of the eyes) occur characteristically in drug-induced and postencephalitic parkinsonism.

These patients may also have symptoms of the side-effects of treatment (see below).

The tremor (4–6/s) is usually most obvious in the hands ('pill-rolling'), improved by voluntary movement and made worse by anxiety. Titubation refers to tremor involving the head. Repeated movements, such as tapping with the fingers, although regular in rate and amplitude (unlike those with cerebellar disorders), are reduced in both amplitude and speed. The rigidity may be lead-pipe or, with the tremor superimposed, cogwheel. The patient may demonstrate a glabellar tap sign—the patient continues to blink when the mid-forehead between the eyebrows is repeatedly tapped. False positives are fairly common. Parkinsonism is usually asymmetrical. Patients are frequently, and understandably, depressed. Dementia with confusion and hallucination may supervene later.

Management

The object is to reduce each of the symptoms—rigidity, tremor and bradykinesia. This debilitating chronic illness requires not only specific drug therapy but also expert supportive physiotherapy, occupational and speech therapy.

Two major groups of drugs are used in parkinsonism: dopaminergic and the antimuscarinic.

Dopaminergic drugs

Levodopa is a precursor of dopamine and replenishes the depleted striatal dopamine. It is the drug of choice for idiopathic parkinsonism and is effective in 75% of patients; excellent in 20%, particularly in those with bradykinesia, less so in those with tremor. It is not used in drug-induced parkinsonism. It is not given alone because the side-effects of levodopa (anorexia, nausea and vomiting) are reduced by concomitant administration of an extracerebral dopa-decarboxylase inhibitor. It is therefore usually given as co-beneldopa (with benserazide as Madopar) or co-careldopa (with carbidopa as Sinemet). Late side-effects of levodopa include the sudden unpredictable swings of the on/off syndrome, peak-dose dyskinesias (often

welcomed), early-morning akinesia and end-of-dose deterioration. This is managed by increasing the dose frequency (but not the total daily dosage) of the levodopa preparation using a slow-release preparation, and adding one of the following drugs.
• The monoamine oxidase B inhibitor, *selegiline*, slows the disposal of dopamine.
• The dopamine agonists stimulate the remaining dopamine receptors (D_1, D_2 and D_3). They include the *ergot derivatives*, bromocriptine, cabergoline, lisuride and pergolide. *Ropinirole* is a D_2-, and *pramipexole* is a D_2- and D_3-receptor agonist.
• *Entacapone* is a COMT (p. 82) inhibitor that potentiates levodopa.
• *Apomorphine* is a potent D_1- and D_2-receptor stimulant, given by subcutaneous injection.

These drugs can be of value in those patients who cannot tolerate levodopa, as well as in those in whom control is unsatisfactory. They tend to be ineffective in those who are not primarily improved by levodopa. The chief indication therefore is for late failure of levodopa. The most common side-effect is nausea, which can be controlled by domperidone. Hallucinatory psychosis and dementia may develop.

Antimuscarinic drugs
Standard atropine-like drugs can be used first in mild disease and patients intolerant of dopa, e.g. trihexyphenidyl (benzhexol; Artane 2 mg b.d. increasing to 5 mg b.d.), orphenadrine (Disipal), benztropine (Cogentin) and procyclidine. They have more effect on tremor. Side-effects include blurred vision, dry mouth, tachycardia, urinary retention, constipation and glaucoma. There may be confusion and loss of concentration, especially in the elderly. Benztropine and procyclidine may be given parenterally in emergencies and with dysphagia.

Stereotactic thalamotomy is used only for intractable symptoms of rigidity and tremor in the non-dominant limbs on the contralateral side.

Depression is easy to overlook in parkinsonism because of reduced emotional expression. It should be treated with a tricyclic antidepressant but not with monoamine oxidase inhibitors because the combination with levodopa may induce acute hypertension.

Neurodegenerative diseases
A number of these have parkinsonism as a component.
1 Alzheimer's disease with gross early cognitive impairment.
2 The 'Parkinson-plus' syndromes:
   (a) Steele–Richardson syndrome with failure of voluntary gaze (see below);
   (b) Shy–Drager syndrome with autonomic failure and postural hypotension; and
   (c) multisystem atrophy with cerebellar and pyramidal involvement.

Steele–Richardson syndrome
(a progressive supranuclear palsy)
This is a very rare condition that affects males more than females (2 : 1) in late middle age. It is a degenerative condition of the upper brainstem akin to Parkinson's disease and often confused with it in the early stages. It may start with no more than an expressionless facies with axial rigidity and a tendency to extension rather than the flexion of parkinsonism. There may be lead-pipe rigidity and cogwheeling. Characteristically, voluntary vertical eye movements become progressively more fixed, and then lateral and convergence movements. Pseudobulbar palsy leads to dysphagia, dysarthria and emotional lability. Falls are common. As with parkinsonism, there may be dementia. Response to antiparkinson therapy is poor.

Hepatolenticular degeneration
(Wilson disease)
Aetiology
This is an autosomal recessive disorder where the primary defect is a failure to excrete copper into the bile. Accumulation of hepatic copper inhibits the formation of caeruloplasmin, the copper-binding serum protein. When the storage capacity of the hepatocytes is exceeded, copper is released into the blood and is deposited in the:
• *liver*—producing cirrhosis, hepatosplenomegaly and jaundice;

- *basal ganglia*—producing choreoathetosis (p. 24);
- *cerebrum*—producing dementia and emotional lability;
- *eyes*—producing Kayser–Fleischer rings (a green–gold 'fuzz') around the cornea, and cataract in the lens;
- *renal tubules* (rarely)—producing the effects of heavy metal poisoning and renal tubular acidosis (aminoaciduria, phosphaturia, glycosuria and hypercalciuria);
- *bones*—producing osteoporosis and osteoarthritis; and
- *red cells*—producing haemolytic anaemia.

The cerebral type is more common than the hepatic type.

Management
- Low dietary copper intake.
- D-penicillamine (1–2 g/day for 6 months–2 years followed by maintenance treatment)—a chelating agent to increase 24-h urinary copper excretion.

The prognosis for improvement is very good. Siblings should be examined and screened for low serum copper and caeruloplasmin plus increased 24-h urinary copper output.

Chorea
This term describes jerky, explosive, involuntary movements, usually of the face and/or arms, which appear pseudopurposive unless very marked. They may interfere with voluntary movements of limbs and with speech, eating and respiration. They cease during sleep.

Chorea may follow a stroke or kernicterus. It may occur in pregnancy (chorea gravidarum) and with the oral contraceptive, and may be congenital.

HUNTINGTON'S CHOREA
George Sumner Huntington, 1851–1916, America.

This is a Mendelian dominant disorder on the short arm of chromosome 4 and there is usually a family history (p. 120). GABA and acetylcholine are reduced in the substantia nigra and globus pallidus. The symptoms usually start between 30 and 45 years of age. The chorea is distal initially and involves the legs (with ataxia), arms (with clumsiness) and face. The movements are rapid and jerky. Epilepsy occurs. The chorea may respond to tetrabenazine, which depletes nerve endings of dopamine. Mental changes develop gradually, usually without insight, and progress to dementia and death in about 10–15 years (p. 120).

SYDENHAM'S CHOREA
Thomas Sydenham, 1624–1689, England.

A child of 5–15 years, female more often than male, is described as restless, clumsy or fidgety. There is proximal chorea of the arms and, less so, legs, and grimacing. It is associated with rheumatic fever and usually recovers completely in 2–3 months. It must be differentiated from a nervous tic. Like rheumatic fever, it is very rare now in the UK.

Cerebral tumours

They are rare, with a UK incidence of 1 in 20 000. They may be primary (20%), or secondary (80%) from bronchus, breasts, kidney, colon, ovary, prostate or thyroid.

Primary tumours originate from:
- *supporting tissues* such as gliomas (50%; or astrocytomas), oligodendrogliomas and ependymomas (both benign);
- *meninges* producing meningiomas (25%);
- *blood vessels*—angiomas and angioblastomas; and
- *nervous tissue* (very rare).

Symptoms and signs
Caused by raised intracranial pressure
- Headache, classically throbbing bilateral frontal and early-morning, associated with nausea, vomiting and later papilloedema and increased by stooping.
- Mental confusion, change in personality, apathy, drowsiness and dementia.
- Sixth-nerve palsy results from pressure on the nerve as it crosses the petrous temporal bone (a 'false localizing sign').

Epilepsy
Occurs in 30% of tumours, particularly of the frontal or temporal lobes.

Progressive focal signs
These depend upon the site of the tumour.
• *Prefrontal.* Progressive dementia with loss of affect and social responsibility. Anosmia may be present and the grasp reflex is present in the contralateral hand.
• *Precentral.* Contralateral hemiplegia and Jacksonian epilepsy.
• *Parietal.* The chief parietal signs are falling away of the contralateral outstretched arm, astereognosis and tactile inattention. Apraxia and spatial disorientation may occur. Low-sited tumours may produce lower quadrantic homonymous hemianopia rather than complete homonymous hemianopia (or visual inattention). Dysphasia occurs with lesions in the dominant temporoparietal region.
• *Temporal lobe.* Symptoms of temporal lobe epilepsy with aphasia (if on the dominant side) and an upper quadrantic homonymous hemianopia.
• *Occipital lobe.* Lesions produce homonymous hemianopia, either complete or quandrantic, with macular sparing.

Investigation
CT or nuclear MRI scanning is the investigation of choice. Lumbar puncture can be dangerous because of the risk of coning.

Screen for primary neoplasms at the sites that most frequently metastasize to the brain (bronchus, breast and kidney).

Raised alkaline phosphatase and calcium suggest associated secondary bone deposits.

Acoustic neuroma
A neurofibroma of the acoustic (8th) nerve. It is relatively rare and is more common in neurofibromatosis (see below).

Clinical presentation
Typically, symptoms begin at 35–45 years with progressive deafness and diminished reaction on caloric testing, sometimes with tinnitus and mild vertigo. Pressure on other nerves and the brainstem of the same side at the cerebellopontine angle produce:
• 7th nerve—facial palsy;
• 5th nerve—weakness of mastication, loss of corneal reflex and facial sensory loss;
• 6th nerve—lateral rectus palsy; and
• cerebellar syndrome (ipsilateral).

Investigation
Skull radiology may reveal erosion of the internal auditory meatus and/or petrous temporal bone. CT scanning will confirm the diagnosis. CSF protein is usually considerably raised to above 1 g/l. It is a slowly enlarging tumour and by the time it presents may be large (3–6 cm in diameter). Because of this and its vascularity, it is easily seen on an enhanced CT scan.

Neurofibromatosis type 1 (von Recklinghausen's disease) is an autosomal dominant disorder characterized by multiple pigmented skin lesions (*café-au-lait* spots and freckling in the axillae) and benign and malignant tumours, including neurofibromas and optic gliomas. It is caused by a defect in neurofibromin which maps to 17q11. Neurofibromatosis type 2, caused by a deficit in merlin (**m**oezin-**e**zrin-**r**adixin-**l**ike prote**in**) typically causes acoustic neuromas, although other central and peripheral nerve tumours occur.

Benign intracranial hypertension
This mimics cerebral tumour with headaches and papilloedema. It may be caused by impaired absorption of CSF by the arachnoid villi. It is more common in obese young women and is associated with oral contraceptives and pregnancy, and may follow head injury and treatment of infection (e.g. otitis media). The blind spot can enlarge and sight may be threatened. Lumbar puncture shows normal CSF under high pressure. CSF pressure is uniform in the cerebrum, so a CT/MRI scan shows normal ventricles and sulci. The absence of pressure gradient reduces the risk of coning on lumbar puncture. It tends to recover spontaneously in a few months, but carbonic anhydrase inhibitors (e.g. acetazolamide), steroids or ventriculo-peritoneal shunting may be required.

Peripheral neuropathy

A disorder of peripheral nerves, sensory, motor or mixed, usually symmetrical and affecting distal more than proximal parts of the limbs, i.e. furthest from the nerve nucleus. By convention, isolated cranial nerve palsies and isolated and multiple peripheral nerve lesions (median, ulnar, lateral popliteal palsies and mononeuritis multiplex) are excluded.

Aetiology
In general medical practice four disorders must be considered: diabetes mellitus, carcinomatous neuropathy, vitamin B deficiency (including B_{12}), especially in alcohol excess, and drugs or chemicals. Only the first is common.

Diabetic neuropathy (see p. 157)
Apart from causing isolated cranial and peripheral nerve lesions (including mononeuritis multiplex), diabetes causes a distal, predominantly sensory neuropathy commonly affecting the distal lower limbs in a stocking distribution. Symptoms of numbness, paraesthesiae and sometimes pain in the feet are associated with loss of vibration and position sense. Characteristically the ankle reflex is lost. It can be associated with Charcot joints.

Carcinomatous neuropathy
Carcinoma may be associated with either a sensory neuropathy affecting the 'glove-and-stocking' regions or motor neuropathy in which there is muscle weakness and wasting, usually of the proximal limb muscles. The neuropathy may be mixed. If distal muscles are affected, the neuropathy may be indistinguishable from any motor neuron disease.

Vitamin B deficiency
Sensory neuropathy characterizes deficiency of vitamin B_1. Patients, often alcoholics, present with numbness ('walking on cotton wool') and paraesthesiae. Pain and soreness of the feet may be a feature. In vitamin B_{12} deficiency the peripheral neuropathy may be associated with megaloblastic anaemia (p. 301) and subacute combined degeneration of the cord (p. 114).

Drugs
Peripheral neuropathy may result from treatment for tuberculosis with isoniazid, which is pyridoxine-dependent and occurs in 'slow acetylators'. Other drugs include vincristine, vinblastine, phenytoin and nitrofurantoin.

Other rare causes
Uraemia, myxoedema, polyarteritis nodosa, heavy metal and industrial poisoning (e.g. lead, triorthocresyl phosphate), infectious disorders (leprosy, diphtheria, Guillain–Barré syndrome), amyloidosis, sarcoidosis and porphyria.

NB Investigation of patients with peripheral neuropathy is aimed at excluding underlying carcinoma and confirming the other common and treatable disorders. In about 50% of cases the aetiology remains unknown.

Brachial neuralgia
(neuralgic amyotrophy)

This may follow a presumed virus infection and presents with pain in the shoulder (C5 dermatome) and root pain down the arm with rapidly progressive weakness and wasting (usually of C5–6 innervated muscles). Sensory loss is segmental in distribution. Adjacent nerve roots may be involved. The sensory symptoms usually resolve completely but the weakness and wasting may not.

Mononeuritis multiplex

A disorder affecting two or more peripheral nerves at one time, producing symptoms of numbness, paraesthesiae and sometimes pain in their sensory distribution with associated muscle weakness and wasting. The lower limbs are more commonly affected and the neuropathy is asymmetrical. This uncommon syndrome occurs in diabetes mellitus, carcinoma, amyloidosis, polyarteritis nodosa and, less commonly, in other autoimmune diseases. Leprosy is the most common cause worldwide but the diagnosis is usually obvious.

Hereditary ataxias

These are familial disorders, usually transmitted as Mendelian dominant traits. Pathological changes of degeneration are present in one or more of the optic nerves, cerebellum, olives and long ascending tracts of the spinal cord. Each family presents its own particular variants. All are rare.

Friedreich's ataxia
Pathology
Degeneration is maximal in the dorsal and lateral (pyramidal) columns of the cord and the spinocerebellar tracts. It is autosomal recessive.

Clinical presentation
Cerebellar ataxia is noted at 5–15 years affecting first the lower and then upper limbs. Pes cavus and spinal scoliosis may be present. Pyramidal tract involvement produces upper motor neuron lesions of the legs, and dorsal column involvement sensory changes and absent ankle jerks. Arrhythmias and heart failure are common resulting from cardiomyopathy. There may be optic atrophy. Mild dementia occurs late in the disease and patients tend to die from cardiac disease in their 40s.

Cerebellar degenerations

This group of hereditary ataxias affects primarily the cerebellum and the cerebellar connections of the brainstem. All are rare. These disorders may present in late middle age and must be distinguished from:
- tumours of the posterior fossa;
- primary degeneration secondary to bronchial carcinomas; and
- myxoedema.

Hereditary spastic paraplegia

The pyramidal tracts are affected and the patients develop progressive spasticity. The onset occurs from childhood to middle age. The disorder, when first seen, must be distinguished from cord compression (which may require emergency decompression) and mul-

tiple sclerosis in the elderly. Dantrolene sodium or baclofen are used to reduce spasticity.

Meningitis

Aetiology
The bacterial and viral causes are listed in Table 8.2. The following points should be considered.
- Tuberculosis meningitis is easily missed and should be considered in the differential diagnosis of all cases of viral meningitis.
- Cerebral tumours, lymphomatous infiltration, abscesses and venous sinus thrombosis may produce a lymphocytosis and raised protein in the CSF.
- Neck stiffness and headache without more severe signs may follow a small subarachnoid haemorrhage.
- Diabetics may be precipitated into coma by meningitis.
- The confident diagnosis of meningism may mean failure to diagnose meningitis.
- If in doubt, lumbar puncture must be performed.
- Pneumococcal meningitis is often secondary to underlying pneumococcal infection in the lung, sinuses or ear.

Clinical features
These are of:
- infection;
- meningism (± mild encephalitic features); and
- raised intracranial pressure.

Meningococcal meningitis

The meningitis is part of a septicaemia. The meningococcus is carried in the nasopharynx often asymptomatically (carriers) and tends to produce epidemics of infection, chiefly in children and young adults. These occur in conditions of overcrowding and in closed communities. After a short incubation period of 1–3 days the disease begins abruptly with fever, headache, nausea, vomiting and neck stiffness. Mental confusion and coma may follow. There may be a characteristic rash with widespread irregular petechiae of variable size.

CAUSES OF MENINGITIS

Organism	Special clinical features	Cerebrospinal fluid	Microbiology	Antibiotic of choice
Common causes				
Meningococcus	Purpuric rash Septicaemic shock	Polymorphs: $0.5–2.0 \times 10^9/l$ Protein: 1–3 g/l Glucose: very low	Gram-negative intracellular diplococci Positive blood culture Positive CSF immuno- electrophoresis	Penicillin or cefotaxime
Pneumococcus	Cranial nerve damage Otitis media Lobar pneumonia High mortality (10–20%)	Polymorphs: $0.5–2.0 \times 10^9/l$ Protein: 1–3 g/l Glucose: very low	Gram-positive diplococci Positive blood culture Positive CSF immuno- electrophoresis	Penicillin or cefotaxime
Haemophilus influenzae	Most common in children under 5 years	Polymorphs: $0.5–2.0 \times 10^9/l$ Protein: 1–3 g/l Glucose: very low	Gram-negative bacilli	Cefotaxime or chloramphenicol
Coxsackievirus and echovirus	Paralysis (very rare)	Lymphocytes: $0.05–0.5 \times 10^9/l$ Protein: 0.5–1 g/l Glucose: normal	Positive throat swab Positive stool culture Serum antibody: rising titre	None
Mumps vlrus		Lymphocytes: $0.05–0.5 \times 10^9/l$ Protein: 0.5–1 g/l Glucose: normal	Positive throat swab Positive stool culture Serum antibody: rising titre	None
Rare causes				
Mycobacterlum tuberculosis	Subacute onset Altered personality Strokes Cranial nerve lesions Fits in children Pyrexia of unknown origin	Lymphocytes $0.1–0.6 \times 10^9/l$ Protein: 1–6 g/l Glucose: low, < 1.4 mmol/l	Acid- and alcohol- fast bacilli Ziehl–Neelsen staining and fluorescence microscopy	See p. 248
Leptosptra ictero- haemorrhaglae (Weil disease)	Follows exposure to rat urine (sewers) Associated hepatitis and nephritis High peripheral white blood cell count: $10–20 \times 10^9/l$	Lymphocytes: $0.2–0.3 \times 10^9/l$ Protein: raised by 0.5–1.5 g/l Glucose: normal	Serum antibody: rising titre	Penicillin
Lyme disease	Associated with cranial nerve lesions (unilateral or bilateral seventh nerve and asymmetrical arthalgia and erythema chronicum migrans	Immunofluorescent antibody tested		Tetracycline
Poliovirus	Meningitis (common) Asymmetrical paralysis (rare) Polio incidence increasing with decrease in immunization	Lymphocytes: $0.05–0.5 \times 10^9/l$ Protein: 0.5–1 g/l Glucose: normal	Positive throat swab Positive stool culture Serum antibody: rising titre	None

NB Other rare causes: acquired immunodeficiency syndrome (AIDS), herpes simplex virus, arbovirus, *Staphylococcus*, *Listeria*, *Pseudomonas*, *Cryptococcus* in immunosuppressed; *Escherichia coli*, streptococci and *Listeria* in neonates.

Table 8.2 Bacterial and viral causes of meningitis.

There is risk of cardiorespiratory collapse and disseminated intravascular coagulation (p. 310).

Vaccines are available against groups A and C; most cases in the UK are group B. Travellers to at-risk areas should be immunized.

Lumbar puncture
The CSF is purulent and shows a raised protein to about 1–3 g/l, 500–2000 polymorphs/mm^3 and a low or almost absent sugar. Intracellular and extracellular Gram-negative diplococci are present. The organism can also be isolated in blood culture.

Treatment
Drug of choice
Benzylpencillin 2–4 g infusion, 6-hourly.

Second-line treatment (when the patient is allergic to penicillins)
Cefotaxime (1–2 g, 8-hourly) or chloramphenicol (20 mg/kg body weight, 6-hourly).

Supportive therapy with fluids, inotropes and clotting factors may be needed.

In hospital patients should be isolated for 24 h from the onset of treatment, and close family contacts should be given rifampicin.

If meningococcal disease is suspected general practitioners should give parenteral benzyl penicillin (or cefotaxime if penicillin allergic) before urgent transportation to hospital.

Pneumococcal meningitis
Infection may be secondary to pneumococcal pneumonia or it may spread from infected sinuses or ears or through fractures of the base of the skull. It is more common in paediatric and geriatric practice, and after splenectomy. Symptoms develop rapidly, sometimes within hours, and fever, headache, nausea and vomiting may quickly proceed to coma.

Lumbar puncture
The CSF is purulent with a raised protein, high polymorph count and low sugar. Gram-positive diplococci are present. Blood culture is often positive (as it is in pneumococcal pneumonia).

Treatment
Drug of choice
Benzylpenicillin, as for meningococcal meningitis providing the organism is sensitive. The dosage can be reduced after about 3–4 days provided the fever has fallen and there is clinical improvement. Treatment should continue for 10 days.

Second-line treatment
Cefotaxime or chloramphenicol, as for meningococcal meningitis.

Pneumococcal meningitis is extremely serious and especially so if the patient is in coma before therapy is started. The overall mortality is high (20–30%).

Haemophilus influenzae meningitis
This usually occurs in children under 5 years old because after that age they develop specific antibodies. It may be insidious in onset with a longer incubation period than in the meningitides described above (5 days). It usually follows an influenzal type of illness and presents with fever, nausea and vomiting.

Lumbar puncture
The CSF is purulent with a high protein and polymorph count and low sugar. Gram-negative bacilli can be seen, and grown on culture.

Treatment
Drugs of choice
Cefotaxime 1–2 g, 8-hourly; chloramphenicol 3–5 g/day (children 50–100 mg/kg/day for 10 days, although a lower dosage is required in the neonate) is an alternative.

The overall mortality is 5–10%.

Intrathecal penicillin therapy
There is no evidence to support the use of intrathecal benzylpenicillin therapy through the lumbar puncture needle on finding a purulent CSF.

Acute bacterial meningitis of unknown cause
This problem occurs when a purulent CSF is

obtained from a patient with meningitis but no organisms are seen with Gram staining. This is most frequently caused by preadmission antibiotic therapy. There is no time to wait for the results of culture and antibiotics must be started immediately.

• Cefotaxime is the drug of choice.
• Chloramphenicol with penicillin is an alternative.

Tuberculous meningitis (see also Tuberculosis, pp. 247 and 334)

This may present as acute meningitis but, more commonly, as an insidious illness with fever, weight loss and progressive signs of confusion and cerebral irritation leading to mental deterioration and finally coma.

The CSF looks opalescent and by investigation resembles viral meningitis but the glucose is very low.

Three of four drugs (rifampicin, isoniazid with pyridoxine, ethambutol and pyrazinamide) should be given initially and the dosage of isoniazid doubled. If streptomycin is used, blood levels must be monitored to prevent ototoxicity. (There is no place for intrathecal streptomycin.)

Viral meningitis

A large number of viruses have been implicated, including enteroviruses (coxsackie A and B, echoviruses, polioviruses), herpesviruses (herpes simplex virus-1, (HSV-1), HSV-2, Epstein–Barr virus, varicella zoster virus), mumps, measles and adenoviruses. The CSF is clear with normal or raised protein content, and normal glucose. Mononuclear cells may be seen, but there are no organisms. The symptoms of headache and meningism are self-limiting.

Herpes simplex encephalitis

Encephalitis implies infection of the brain parenchyma. The most common cause is HSV. Most episodes are thought to result from reactivation of latent virus. It occurs in otherwise healthy individuals, but is most common in the immunosuppressed. A brief prodrome of headache, fever and malaise is followed by

severe CNS dysfunction, with focal signs, seizures and coma.

CT shows low-density lesions with ring enhancement and EEG may show focal abnormalities. Lesions are most common in the temporal lobes. CSF findings are similar to those in viral meningitis. Identification of HSV in CSF by polymerase chain reaction, rising titres to HSV and/or brain biopsy may all aid diagnosis, but treatment with acyclovir 10 mg/kg t.d.s. i.v. should be started if the diagnosis is strongly suspected.

Intracranial abscess

The primary source of the infection is usually chronic middle-ear infection (50%), the paranasal sinuses or the lungs. There may be a history of head trauma or neurosurgery. The clinical presentation is usually that of a space-occupying lesion (headache, nausea, vomiting and papilloedema, with or without focal signs) plus the evidence of the primary infection. A CT scan defines the lesion. Lumbar puncture is potentially dangerous because of the risk of coning. Neurosurgical advice should be sought concerning the optimum time for aspiration and/or open drainage. Mixed infections occur in 50%. Blood cultures and aspiration of any other infected sites help to identify the organisms.

Initial treatment is with intravenous cefotaxime with metronidazole to cover *Staphylococcus*, *Streptococcus* and anaerobes until sensitivities are known. Even with modern management the mortality is 30%. Of those who survive, one-third develop epilepsy and many physicians give anticonvulsants to all survivors.

Guillain–Barré syndrome

This is characterized by 'ascending paralysis' with sub-acute weakness and reduced tendon reflexes, usually without sensory loss. Most commonly, there is an inflammatory demyelinating polyradiculoneuropathy affecting predominantly motor nerves.

Aetiology

About three-quarters of patients give a history of an infectious illness preceding the onset of weakness by 1–2 weeks. *Campylobacter jejuni* or *cytomegalovirus* (CMV) have occurred in up to 50%. Antibodies to ganglioside GM1 are found in 20–30% of patients. A particular strain of *C. jejuni* (Penner serogroup 19), which has been implicated in pathogenesis, contains β-*N*-acetylglucosamine residues homologous to the terminal carbohydrate residue of ganglioside GM1.

There is a strong association between antibodies to ganglioside GQ1b and the Miller–Fisher syndrome (see below).

Clinical features

Typically, presentation starts with paraesthesia in the toes, rapidly (hours) followed by flaccid paralysis of the lower limbs that ascends to involve the arms and sometimes the facial muscles, the muscles of the palate and pharynx (causing dysphagia) and the external ocular muscles. Less commonly, the disease affects the upper limbs or the cranial nerves alone, or proximal more than distal muscles, and sensory symptoms are usually minimal or absent.

Paralysis is of lower motor neuron type with flaccidity and early loss of tendon reflexes. Maximal disability occurs at 3–4 weeks.

The major complications are:
- respiratory failure from weakness of respiratory muscles (in one-quarter of patients);
- autonomic involvement causing lability of blood pressure and arrhythmias; and
- venous thrombosis with pulmonary embolism.

The *Miller–Fisher syndrome* is characterized by brainstem features of ataxia and ophthalmoplegia plus areflexia. There is no significant limb weakness.

Investigation

Lumbar puncture characteristically reveals a very high CSF protein (3–10 g/l) with no, or very few, white cells.

Differential diagnosis

Poliomyelitis is excluded by a known history of immunization, the presence of sensory symptoms, the symmetrical pattern of paralysis and the CSF findings (in polio the protein is lower and the white cell count raised).

Transverse myelitis usually causes sphincter disturbance, and is characterized by the presence of a sensory level.

The rapid speed of onset can suggest *brainstem stroke*, and in some cases myalgia is a prominent feature, raising the possibility of *muscle* or *joint disease*.

Management

The most important aspect of treatment is the prevention of complications. Complete recovery occurs over several months in 80–90% of patients.

In all cases careful nursing with physiotherapy is required, usually in an intensive treatment unit (ITU), to prevent pressure sores, chest infection and contractures, and to maintain morale.

Anticoagulants, passive movements of the legs and graduated compression stockings may reduce the risk of deep venous thrombosis and death from pulmonary embolism.

Careful fluid balance and nutrition is necessary if dysphagia occurs.

Vital capacity should be monitored frequently if paralysis ascends to involve the respiratory muscles. Intubation with ventilation may be necessary. Shoulder adduction (C6, 7, 8) is a good clinical test of intercostal muscle function. Early tracheostomy is required in patients with respiratory failure because muscle activity takes weeks or months to recover.

Temporary cardiac pacing may be required for persistent bradycardia (< 50 b.p.m.).

Plasma exchange is of benefit, but intravenous immunoglobulin is as effective as, or slightly better than, plasma exchange (see Trials Box 8.6). Several trials have shown that steroids alone have no beneficial effect.

Poliomyelitis

Poliovirus is one of the enteroviruses (with echovirus and Coxsackievirus) and a picorna (*pico* = small; *rna* = RNA) virus. The incidence

TRIALS BOX 8.6

Guillain–Barré Syndrome Trial Study Group compared intravenous methylprednisolone 500 mg/day for 5 days with placebo in 242 patients. Treatment was started within 15 days of onset of neurological symptoms. No beneficial effect of steroids was observed. *Lancet* 1993; **341**: 586–590.

The **French Cooperative Group in Plasma Exchange in Guillain–Barré Syndrome** studied the effect of four plasma exchanges with fresh frozen plasma or albumin replacement in 220 patients in a randomized controlled trial. Plasma exchange improved both short-term and 1-year functional status. Fresh frozen plasma showed no additional benefit compared with albumin. *Ann Neurol* 1992; **32**: 94–97.

The **Dutch Guillain–Barré Study Group** compared intravenous immunoglobulin with plasma exchange using a replacement fluid that did not contain immunoglobulin in 150 patients who were unable to walk independently. Treatment was started within 14 days of onset of neurological symptoms. Treatment with intravenous immunoglobulin was at least as effective as, and in some respects superior to, plasma exchange. *N Engl J Med* 1992; **326**: 1123–1129.

The **Plasma Exchange/Sandoglobulin Guillain–Barré Syndrome Trial Group** compared plasma exchange, intravenous immunoglobulin and combined plasma exchange and intravenous immunoglobulin started within 14 days of onset of neurological symptoms in 383 patients who had difficulty walking. Plasma exchange and intravenous immunoglobulin had equivalent efficacy, and the combination did not confer a significant advantage. *Lancet* 1997; **349**: 225–230.

in the UK has fallen dramatically since immunization began in 1957, but polio remains endemic in the tropics.

Immunization
Sabin vaccine is live attenuated poliovirus types 1, 2 and 3 given as a drop orally.

Clinical features
In areas without an immunization scheme, infection with poliovirus is common but the serious features of acute meningitis and muscle paralysis are rare.

About 90–95% of infected patients have mild upper respiratory or gastrointestinal symptoms that settle completely. The rest have a more severe early infection with fever, sore throat, diarrhoea or constipation and muscle pains. This *minor illness* usually settles but 1–2% of patients go on to develop a *major illness* 5–10 days later with features of acute viral meningitis. A small number of patients who have acute poliovirus meningitis develop flaccid lower motor neuron muscle paralysis with loss of reflexes as a result of damage to the anterior horn cells. This may be preceded by muscular pain. The legs are most commonly affected and

paralysis may spread to involve the arms and the medulla oblongata and lower pons, causing a bulbar palsy.

Respiratory failure is a result of paralysis of the respiratory muscles and may be further complicated by aspiration pneumonia following the dysphagia and inability to cough caused by bulbar palsy.

There are no sensory neurological changes.

Diagnosis
CSF is the same as other forms of virus meningitis with raised protein (50–100 g/dl), increased cells, initially polymorphs, followed by lymphocytes 50–400/mm^3. The glucose is normal.

The virus can be grown from throat, stool and CSF and paired sera will show a rising titre.

Paralytic poliomyelitis (all motor) must be distinguished from the Guillain–Barré syndrome (mixed motor and sensory).

Management
Patients should be isolated and contacts immunized. Artificial ventilation is required for respiratory failure—the most common cause of death. Careful nursing is necessary in all

paralysed patients to prevent sores, combined with monitoring of fluid and electrolyte balance. Physiotherapy and progressive rehabilitation are started after the fever has settled.

Full muscle recovery is rare if limbs are paralysed. Patients with isolated bulbar palsy usually recover completely but those with paralysis of the respiratory muscles rarely do, and may require continued artificial ventilation.

Syphilis of the nervous system

Tertiary syphilis of the CNS never develops in a syphilitic patient who has received early and correct treatment. All forms are now rarely seen in the industrialized world except as chronic cases with residual symptoms and signs, but it remains common worldwide. Tertiary syphilis may be divided into four groups:
1 meningovascular disease, occurring 3–4 years after primary infection;
2 tabes dorsalis, occurring 10–35 years after primary infection;
3 general paralysis of the insane, occurring 10–35 years after primary infection; and
4 localized gumma.

The first three produce symptoms by a combination of primary neuronal degeneration and/or arterial lesions.

Meningovascular syphilis
This affects both the cerebrum and the spine (*meningo*, producing fibrosis of the meninges and nipping of nerves; *vascular*, producing endarteritis and ischaemic necrosis). Headache is a common presenting symptom.

Cerebrum. Syphilitic leptomeningitis produces fibrosis and thickening of the meninges with nipping and paralysis of cranial nerves. The 2nd, 3rd and 4th nerves are most frequently involved.

Vascular endarteritis. Produces ischaemic necrosis. Hemiplegia may result. Syphilitic endarteritis is one cause of isolated cranial nerve lesions.

Spinal meningovascular syphilis. Meningeal thickening involves posterior spinal roots to produce pain and anterior roots to cause muscle wasting.

Endarteritis. May produce ischaemic necrosis, and transverse myelitis and paraplegia.

Tabes dorsalis
The signs result from degeneration of the dorsal columns and nerve roots.

Clinical presentation
Lightning pains because of dorsal nerve root involvement characterize the disease. There are severe paroxysmal stabbing pains (crises) that occur in the limbs, chest or abdomen. Paraesthesiae may also occur. Ataxia follows degeneration of the dorsal columns of the spinal cord. The gait is wide-based and stamping because position sense is lost.

Examination
The facies is characteristic. Ptosis is present and the forehead wrinkled because of overactivity of the frontalis muscle. Argyll Robertson pupils are small, irregular pupils that do not react to light, but constrict with accommodation. There may be optic atrophy. Cutaneous sensation is diminished typically over the nose (tabetic mask), sternum, ulnar border of the arm and outer borders of the legs and feet. Vibration and position sense are lost early in the disease. Deep pain sensation (pressure on testicles or Achilles tendon) may also be lost. Charcot neuropathic joints are grossly disorganized from painless arthritis (also rarely seen in diabetes mellitus and syringomyelia when there is loss of pain sensation). Absence of visceral sensation results in overfilling of the bladder. The reflexes are diminished or absent in the legs. The plantar responses are flexor in pure tabes dorsalis. Romberg's sign (increased unsteadiness on closing the eyes) is present and is evidence of loss of position sense.

General paralysis of the insane (GPI)
This is a late manifestation of systemic syphilis.

Pathologically, the meninges are thickened, particularly in the parietal and frontal regions. Primary cortical degeneration produces a small brain with dilatated and enlarged ventricles. The dorsal columns degenerate.

Clinical presentation
The pathological changes are associated with marked mental impairment. This may produce loss of memory and concentration with associated anxiety and/or depression. Later, insight is lost and the patient may become euphoric with delusions of grandeur and loss of emotional response. Epilepsy occurs in 50% of cases.

Examination
Euphoria may be present. The face is vacant and memory lost. Argyll Robertson pupils are present. The tongue demonstrates a 'trombone' tremor. Dorsal column involvement produces limb ataxia from loss of position sensation. Upper motor neuron lesions occur in the legs with increased reflexes and upgoing plantar responses.

NB In taboparesis there is a combination of the lower limb upper motor neuron signs of general paralysis of the insane and the signs of dorsal root degeneration from tabes dorsalis. This produces a combination of absent knee reflexes with upgoing plantar responses.

FTAA and TPHA tests
The TPHA and FTAA tests are the most specific tests available for diagnosis. They may remain positive for years after adequate treatment.

Management
Penicillin by injection is the drug of choice for active syphilitic infection. Improvement, stabilization or deterioration may occur in any one case despite adequate penicillin therapy.

The Herxheimer reaction is an acute hypersensitivity reaction and results from toxins produced by spirochaetes killed on the first contact with penicillin. Death has been reported and some authorities give steroids during the first days of penicillin therapy.

Disorders of spinal cord

Syringomyelia
A longitudinal cyst in the cervical cord and/or brainstem (syringobulbia) occurs just anterior to the central canal and spreads, usually asymmetrically, to each side. It may be caused by outflow obstruction of the fourth ventricle from a congenital anomaly such as the Arnold–Chiari malformation (also associated with spina bifida). It starts in young adults and is usually very slowly progressive over 20–30 years. It is very rare.

Damage to the cord (see Figs 1.6 and 1.7, pp. 14 and 15) occurs as follows.
• At the root level of the lesion:
   (a) in the decussating fibres of the lateral spinothalamic tracts (pain and temperature) since they cross anteriorly (NB fibres of the posterior column enter posteriorly and are not involved—hence the dissociated sensory loss); and
   (b) the cells in the anterior horn where the lower motor neuron starts.
• Distant from the lesion in the upper motor neuron in the pyramidal tracts.

The classical case of syringomyelia therefore presents with:
• painless injury to the hands (sensory C6, 7, 8); and
• weakness and wasting in the small muscles of the hands (T1).

Examination may reveal more extensive dissociated sensory loss in the cervical segments, and upper motor neuron signs in the legs. These are usually asymmetrical. All signs and symptoms are ipsilateral to the lesion. Charcot joints may occur in the upper limbs. Surgical decompression and aspiration of cysts should be considered.

Syringobulbia
In brainstem syringomyelia the descending root of the trigeminal nerve (pain and temperature) may be involved from the first division downward and a Horner's syndrome from involvement of the cervical sympathetic tract. The motor nuclei of the lower cranial

nerves may be involved in syringobulbia and there may be a rotatory nystagmus from involvement in vestibular and cerebellar connections.

Subacute combined degeneration of the cord

The neurological consequences of vitamin B_{12} deficiency include subacute combined degeneration of the cord, signs of peripheral neuropathy and, very rarely, dementia and optic atrophy.

Combined degeneration refers to the combined demyelination of both pyramidal (lateral columns) and posterior (dorsal) columns, the signs and symptoms being predominantly in the legs. It is now rare.

Clinical presentation

Sensory peripheral neuropathy with numbness and paraesthesia in the feet are the usual presenting symptoms. Less commonly, the disease presents as a spastic paraparesis. The signs are of:
• posterior column loss (vibration and position senses, with positive Rombergism);
• upper motor neuron lesion (weakness, hypertonia and hyperreflexia, with absent abdominal reflexes and upgoing toes); and
• peripheral neuropathy (absence of all the jerks, reduced touch sense and deep tenderness of the calves).

Investigation

Rarely, there is no anaemia or macrocytosis in the peripheral blood film. The following are indicated:
• serum B_{12} and folate levels;
• marrow histology for megaloblastic change; and
• parietal cell and intrinsic factor antibodies.
These are the only tests of value if the patient has been given vitamin B_{12} injections.

Management

Vitamin B_{12} (hydroxocobalamin 1 mg, repeated five times at 2-day intervals and then 1 mg every 3 months for life).

Prognosis

Neurological symptoms and signs usually improve to some degree. However, they may remain unchanged or, rarely, continue to progress. Sensory abnormalities resolve more completely than motor, the peripheral neuropathy more than the myelopathy.

Peroneal muscular atrophy

(Charcot–Marie–Tooth)
This condition is often confused with the muscle dystrophies. It is rare and genetic counselling is advisable.

Pathology

It is usually transmitted as an autosomal dominant trait, but in some families is recessive or sex-linked. It may be classified into two groups of hereditary motor and sensory neuropathy affecting the peripheral nerves:
• type I with thickened peripheral nerves as a result of repeated demyelination and remyelination (ulnar at elbow, and common peroneal at the neck of the fibula); and
• type II as a result of axonal degeneration, without thickening.

Clinical presentation

It presents about the age of 20 years with wasting and weakness of all the distal lower limb muscles and pes cavus. Later, the upper limbs may be affected. The wasting stops at midthigh, producing an inverted champagne-bottle appearance, and at the elbows. Fasciculation and sensory loss are sometimes present, and reflexes depressed. The disease usually arrests spontaneously and life expectancy is normal. Contractions may produce talipes equinovarus.

Cord compression

This is a neurosurgical emergency.

Aetiology

Disorders of vertebrae (extradural)
These constitute 45% of cases:
• cervical spondylosis;
• collapsed vertebral body (usually secondary to carcinoma, myeloma or, rarely, osteoporosis);

- prolapsed intervertebral disc; and
- rarely, tuberculosis, abscesses, Paget disease, reticuloses, angiomas, cervical and lumbar stenosis.

Meningeal disorders (intradural)
Also constitute 45% of cases:
- neurofibromas (dumb-bell tumours); and
- meningiomas (usually thoracic and more common in women).

Disorders of spinal cord (intramedullary)
These constitute 5–10% of cases:
- gliomas; and
- ependymomas.

Clinical presentation

Patients present with a spastic paraparesis: there is upper motor neuron weakness in the legs, loss of sphincter control (an ominous sign) and loss of abdominal reflexes if the lesion is in or above the thoracic cord. The level of the sensory loss indicates the level of the neurological lesion, which may, however, be up to two roots higher. Remember that, compared with the vertebral column, the cord is about one segment short in the lower cervical region, two segments short in the upper thoracic region, and three to five segments short in the lower thoracic region. The sacral segments and end of the cord lie opposite the L1 vertebra. Remember also that the cervical spine has seven vertebrae and the cervical spinal cord eight segments.

It is important to consider the possibility of cord compression in all cases of spastic paresis. Cord compression is a neurosurgical emergency, particularly if of recent onset and rapid progression. Decompression must be performed as early as possible if recovery is to occur.
NB The tumours that commonly metastasize to bone arise in bronchus, breast, prostate, thyroid and kidney.

Investigation

- MRI scan to show the cord.
- Chest X-ray for carcinoma of the bronchus.
- Lumbar puncture for spinal block and raised protein.
- Myelography to delineate the level and character of obstructing tissues. This investigation may increase the severity of transverse myelitis and should therefore be performed only if scanning is not available and after receiving expert advice.

Differential diagnosis

Other causes of spastic paraparesis are:
- Multiple sclerosis. Demyelination may cause isolated slow progressive paraparesis in the middle-aged.
- Subacute combined degeneration of the cord.
- Transverse myelitis.
- Anterior spinal artery thrombosis.
- Motor neuron disease.
- Parasagittal cranial meningioma.

Cervical spondylosis

Over 70% of the adult population in the UK have X-ray changes of osteoarthritis of the joints of the cervical spine. The most frequent and obvious abnormality is the presence of osteophytes. These radiological changes are unrelated to the presence or severity of symptoms.

Clinical features

Most patients are symptom-free. Pain in the neck, associated with and precipitated by movements of the neck, is the most common symptom. Occasionally, compression of the cervical nerve roots causes root pain, paraesthesiae, numbness and sometimes segmental weakness with muscle wasting (even with fasciculation). Rarely, narrowing of the cervical canal with compression of the spinal cord or occlusion of the spinal cord vessels (spinal stenosis) produces brisk reflexes in the arms and upper motor neuron damage affecting the legs.
NB Lumbar spinal canal stenosis may produce weakness of the legs and sometimes pain in the calves on walking (intermittent claudication). It must be distinguished from femoral artery

stenosis, the most common cause of inter-mittent claudication (or limping).

Disorders of muscles

Myasthenia gravis

This is a very rare disorder of muscle weakness resulting from failure of neuromuscular trans-mission. There is a reduction in the number of functioning postsynaptic acetylcholine recep-tors (AChR) and a high titre of specific anti-AChR antibodies has been shown in most cases. Thymoma is associated in 10% of cases and thymus abnormalities in 75%. Excessive muscular fatigability may also occur in poly-myositis and SLE, and there is an increased incidence of myasthenia gravis in thyrotoxico-sis. The Lambert–Eaton myasthenic syndrome associated with carcinoma is clinically different (see below).

Clinical presentation

Painless muscular weakness is produced by repetitive or sustained contraction. It is usually most marked in the face and eyes producing a symmetrical ptosis and diplopia. Weakness of speech and swallowing may occur. The prox-imal muscles are more often affected than the distal, and the upper limb muscles more than the lower. There is no wasting and tendon reflexes are preserved.

Prognosis

The disorder may never progress beyond ophthalmoplegia and periods of remission up to 3 years occur. Death may be rapid if the respiratory muscles are involved. Thymectomy usually improves the outlook unless a thy-moma is present.

Diagnosis

Edrophonium (Tensilon) 10 mg intravenously with cardiac monitor (in case of brady-cardia/asystole) reduces the weakness of affected muscles for 3–4 min. The anterior mediastinum should be searched with chest X-rays and MRI/CT scan for thymoma. AChR IgG antibodies are present in 90% of cases.

Very rarely, mitochondrial muscle diseases may mimic myasthenia.

Treatment

Therapy is achieved with long-acting anti-cholinesterases orally, such as neostigmine or pyridostigmine (Mestinon), preferably by increasing the dosage slowly until measured muscular strength is optimal. Overdosage may give depolarization block with weakness. Thymectomy at any age appears to increase the percentage of patients in remission. An alternate-day regimen of steroids (between 10 and 80 mg on alternate days) is of proven value and immunotherapy with azathioprine may be useful and allow a reduction in steroid dosage. Plasmapheresis has been used in intractable cases but the effect is short-lasting (days–months).

The differential diagnosis is from other causes of ptosis (p. 4), muscular dystrophies involving the face, familial hypokalaemic para-lysis and the Lambert–Eaton syndrome. In this, a disorder of acetylcholine release, the myasthenia is associated with a carcinoma, usually oat cell, of the bronchus. It differs from classical myasthenia gravis in that the eyes are less frequently affected, that proximal limb muscle weakness is common and their strength initially *increased* by repeated movement. There is no response to edrophonium but oral 3,4 diaminopyridine may help.

Myotonia

Myotonia is the inability of muscles to relax normally after contraction. This produces a reluctant release of handshake, and percus-sion contraction for instance of the thenar muscles.

DYSTROPHIA MYOTONICA

An autosomal dominant (chromosome 9) dis-order producing progressively more severe symptoms and signs with succeeding genera-tions, i.e. anticipation. It is rare.

Genetics

There is expansion of a CTG repeat in the 3′ untranslated region of the myotonin protein kinase gene (genetic locus 19q13). Trinucleo-tide repeat is a novel form of genetic mutation in which there is expansion of a sequence of DNA that contains a series of repeated nucleotide triplets (p. 120).

Clinical presentation
Both males and females are affected with usual onset at 15–40 years. UK incidence is 1 in 20 000. The classical case demonstrates the following.
• Abnormal facies—with frontal balding, pto-sis, a smooth expressionless forehead, cataracts and a lateral smile or sneer.
• Wasting of the facial muscles, sternomas-toids, shoulder girdle and quadriceps.
• The forearms and legs are involved and reflexes lost. There is no fasciculation.
• Myotonia which increases with cold, fatigue and excitement and may reduce with repeated activity.
• Testicular or ovarian atrophy with impot-ence and sterility.
• Mental deficiency.
NB The heart may be involved (e.g. heart block) and diabetes mellitus may develop. Phenytoin may reduce myotonia.

MYOTONIA CONGENITA
This is a hereditary disorder, transmitted as a Mendelian dominant trait, which affects both sexes equally, and first presents in childhood. There is no muscle wasting and no long-term effects. It is very rare. The myotonias should not be confused with two disorders of chil-dren: amyotonia congenita and progressive spinomuscular atrophy.

AMYOTONIA CONGENITA
A congenital disorder producing weakness and hypotonia which is first noticed in children at the head-lifting stage. The muscle disturbance becomes less severe as the children grow older, although contractures may produce scoliosis.

PROGRESSIVE SPINOMUSCULAR ATROPHY (WERDNIG–HOFFMANN)
A hereditary disorder involving progressive degeneration of the anterior spinal horn cells starting in the first year of life and producing weakness, muscle wasting and fasciculation, and death within 6 months.

Muscular dystrophies
Each family produces its own pattern of disease but some forms are more common than others. They are all rare. Genetic counselling is advised. There is no effective treatment. Chromosome studies may define the carrier state.

PSEUDOHYPERTROPHIC (DUCHENNE)
A sex-linked recessive disorder affecting males with a prevalence of 3 in 100 000 and incidence of 25 in 100 000 male births. The age of onset is 5–10 years with symptoms of difficulty in climbing stairs, or even walking, and the use of Gowers' manoeuvre to rise from the floor. On examination the posture is lordotic and the gait waddling because of weakness of the muscles of the pelvic girdle and proximal lower limb. The calves are hypertrophied but weak and the creatine phosphokinase level is raised. The electromyogram (EMG) and muscle biospy are characteristic. In later stages muscle contracture of the legs may produce talipes equinovarus and muscle weakness may spread to the upper limbs, although not to the face. The child dies in the early teens, usually from chest infection or cardiomyopathy. Becker dystrophy is a mild form.

Genetics
The cytoskeletal protein dystrophin (genetic locus Xp) is either abnormal or absent. In Becker muscular dystrophy a milder form of muscular dystrophy is caused by mutations of the dystrophin gene, resulting in partially func-tional dystrophin protein that is reduced in amount or size.

FACIOSCAPULOHUMERAL (LANDOUZY–DÉJÉRINE)
Transmitted as an autosomal dominant trait and affects both sexes equally. The onset is at puberty with progressive wasting in the upper

limb-girdle and face. The disorder may abort spontaneously or progress to the muscles of the trunk and lower limbs. Individuals usually live to a normal age.

LIMB-GIRDLE (ERB)

Transmitted as an autosomal recessive trait and affects both sexes equally. It presents at 20–40 years. It involves the muscles of the shoulders and pelvic girdles and is slowly progressive, with death usually in middle age.

Other forms may affect the muscles of the face and eyes (oculomuscular dystrophy) or the distal limb muscles (Gower muscular dystrophy). They are very rare.

Dementia

Dementia means a loss of mind which can present with both behavioural and psychological symptoms. The earliest feature is loss of memory for recent events. There is a global disruption of personality with the gradual development of abnormal behaviour, loss of intellect, mood changes often without insight, blunting of emotions and cognitive impairment with failure to learn. Eventually, there is a reduction in self-care, restless wandering and incontinence. In patients under 65 years of age it is usually termed presenile dementia, although this distinction is not fundamental.

The most common causes are Alzheimer's disease, vascular (multi-infarct) dementia and frontotemporal dementia, but treatable disorders, especially the sedative effect of drugs, must always be excluded.

Causes of dementia
Degenerative
- Alzheimer's disease.
- Huntington disease.
- Frontotemporal dementia (Pick disease)
- Steele–Richardson syndrome.
- Spinocerebellar degeneration (including Friedreich ataxia).
- Parkinson's disease (sometimes).
- Multiple sclerosis.

Vascular
- Multi-infarct dementia.
- Cerebral vasculitis (rare).

Toxic
- Poisoning with carbon monoxide, lead.
- Alcoholism.

Drug-induced
- Usually overmedication with sedatives.

Traumatic
- Head injury.
- Subdural haematomas.
- Boxers ('punch drunk').

Malignancy
- Primary cerebral tumour (meningiomas may grow very slowly).
- Posterior fossa tumour with hydrocephalus.
- Metastases.

Metabolic
- Uraemia.
- Hepatic encephalopathy.
- Hypothyroidism (myxoedema madness).
- Wilson disease.
- B_{12} deficiency.

Infection
- AIDS.
- Herpes simplex encephalitis.
- Cerebral syphilis.
- Progressive multifocal leukoencephalopathy.
- Subacute sclerosing panencephalitis.
- Creutzfeldt–Jakob disease.

Pseudodementia
- In depression.

Investigation
Investigation is aimed at establishing the diagnosis and excluding treatable causes. Patients should have:
- psychometric evaluation to establish the diagnosis and assess severity;
- FBC and ESR;
- urea and electrolytes, glucose, calcium;
- liver function tests;

- thyroid function studies;
- serological tests for syphilis;
- vitamin B$_{12}$;
- chest X-ray (for bronchial carcinoma); and
- CT/MRI scan of the head is advisable in all patients, and essential in younger patients, to exclude tumour, hydrocephalus and subdural haematoma.
- In selected patients, serological tests and examination of CSF to exclude toxicity or infection.

Alzheimer's disease

Alois Alzheimer, 1864–1915, Poland.

Alzheimer's disease affects about 10% of people over the age of 65, and between 25 and 40% of those over 85. About 50% of cases of severe dementia are caused by Alzheimer's disease (most of the remaining cases are caused by multi-infarct dementia, alone or in combination with Alzheimer's disease).

Pathology

Two characteristic features are found in the brain of patients with Alzheimer's disease:

1 *Senile plaques* consist of extracellular deposits of β-amyloid, a peptide formed by cleavage of β-amyloid precursor protein (genetic locus 21q21–22). Abnormal deposits of β-amyloid are also found in blood vessels.

2 *Neurofibrillary tangles* are dense bundles of abnormal fibres in the cytoplasm of neurons which contain an altered form of the microtubule-associated protein, τ. Neither senile plaques nor neurofibrillary tangles are specific to Alzheimer's disease. They occur in other chronic cerebral conditions and can be found in elderly patients without dementia.

The brain amines, 5-HT, noradrenaline (norepinephrine) and GABA, are all reduced at postmortem.

Aetiology

Risk factors are:

- increasing age;
- head trauma;
- Down syndrome (trisomy 21); and
- genetic susceptibility.

A family history can be obtained in 30–50% of cases. Rare familial forms in which young-onset Alzheimer's disease is inherited in an autosomal dominant pattern show linkage to chromosome 21 and, in some cases, chromosome 14. Associations between sporadic and familial late-onset Alzheimer's disease and polymorphisms of the apolipoprotein E gene on chromosome 19 have been reported.

In Down syndrome an extra chromosome 21 (trisomy 21) results in the typical facial appearance (flat face, slanting eyes, small low-set ears) and simian crease (single palmar crease), together with mental retardation and an increased incidence of congenital heart disease (p. 280).

Clinical features

Loss of memory for recent events is the usual presenting feature. Insight may be preserved in the early stages and depression is common. Later, more marked memory disturbance is accompanied by impaired motor abilities, often with extrapyramidal features. Disturbed sleep pattern, loss of sphincter control and personality change all contribute to the progressive social disintegration.

Management

It is important to exclude treatable causes of dementia. Management is largely supportive, towards both patient and family—97% of carers have emotional difficulty. Treatment of depression may be effective in the early stages. Acetylcholinesterase-inhibiting drugs, such as donepezil and galantamine, can slow cognitive decline (see Trials Box 8.7). They have cholinergic side-effects.

Multi-infarct dementia

In dementia resulting from cerebrovascular disease the onset may be abrupt with a step-wise progression, and other focal neurological signs may be present. Predisposing factors (e.g. smoking, hypertension, hyperlipidaemia, diabetes) and other evidence of vascular disease are often present. Postmortem studies have shown that pathological changes associated

---

TRIALS BOX 8.7

Tacrine (a cholinesterase inhibitor) in high doses (160 mg/day) had a beneficial effect on Alzheimer's disease, assessed by both clinical impression and neuropsychological test scores, in a 30-week randomized placebo controlled trial. *J Am Med Assoc* 1994; **271**: 985–991.

However, the usefulness of tacrine may be limited by side-effects, including hepatotoxicity. *J Am Med Assoc* 1994; **271**: 992–998.

The **Donepezil Study Group** evaluated the efficacy and safety of donepezil in patients with mild to moderately severe Alzheimer's disease. Patients treated with donepezil showed dose-related improvements in the Alzheimer's disease assessment scores. Donepezil was not associated with any hepatotoxicity, as observed with acridine-based cholinesterase inhibitors. *Dementia* 1996; **7**: 293–303.

The **Alzheimer's Disease Cooperative Study** conducted a double-blind, placebo-controlled, trial of selegiline, α-tocopherol, or both in

patients with patients with moderately severe impairment from Alzheimer's disease treatment with selegiline or α-tocopherol slowed the progression of disease. *N Engl J Med* 1997; **336**: 1216–1222.

Feldman *et al*. investigated the efficacy and safety of donepezil in 290 patients with moderate to severe Alzheimer's disease. The results suggested that the benefits of donepezil extend into more advanced stages of Alzheimer's disease than those previously investigated, with very good tolerability. *Neurology* 2001; **57**: 613–620.

Tariot *et al*. performed a 24-week, randomized, double-blind, placebo-controlled study of the efficacy and safety of donepezil in 208 patients with Alzheimer's disease in the nursing home setting. Patients treated with donepezil maintained or improved in cognition and overall dementia severity in contrast to placebo-treated patients who declined during the 6-month treatment period. *J Am Geriatr Soc* 2001; **49**: 1590–1599.

---

with vascular lesions and Alzheimer's disease often coexist.

Frontotemporal dementia
(Pick disease)

Frontotemporal dementia may account for up to 25% of presenile dementia caused by cerebral atrophy. It occurs predominantly between the ages of 45 and 65 years. Half are inherited (autosomal dominant, chromosome 17, long arm). There is focal cortical atrophy with astrocytosis and intraneural inclusion bodies (Pick bodies) in surviving pyramidal cells. Disinhibition (including violence), apathy, and poverty of speech with relatively preserved spatial skills and memory help to distinguish the disease clinically from Alzheimer's disease.

Creutzfeldt–Jakob disease (CJD)

Creutzfeldt–Jakob disease usually presents in late middle age with dementia which progresses to death within months. Spongiform changes are found in the brain at postmortem. The

agents of this and other transmissible spongiform encephalopathies, such as scrapie and bovine spongiform encephalopathy (BSE), are prion proteins that are resistant to inactivation by heat or chemicals.

Huntington's disease (see also p. 103)

Progressive dementia and involuntary movements (chorea) develop in middle age. Inheritance is autosomal dominant, although the disease is late and variable in its presentation. Death usually occurs 10–15 years after the onset of symptoms.

Disease-related gene

The Huntington's disease gene (chromosome 4p16) contains an expanded CAG trinucleotide repeat. *Trinucleotide repeat* is a genetic mutation in which there is expansion of a sequence of DNA that contains a series of repeated nucleotide triplets. The repetitive sequence is present in the gene of normal individuals, but is expanded up to 1000-fold in the gene of affected patients. The length of the trinucleotide repetitive sequence tends to increase as the gene passes from parent to offspring, providing an explanation for anticipation, the phenomenon by which the disease gets progressively more severe through successive generations.

The Huntington's disease gene encodes a novel protein of currently unknown function.

Management
Tetrabenazine may help the chorea by depleting nerve endings of dopamine. Extrapyramidal dysfunction and depression are common side-effects. Identification of the genetic mutation has increased the precision of genetic testing. However, presymptomatic testing for Huntington disease must be approached with great care because of the implications of a positive test for the patient and family.

Normal-pressure hydrocephalus
Enlargement of all of the ventricles is associated with dementia, usually with pyramidal signs in the limbs, an ataxic gait and urinary incontinence. CSF pressure is normal, but continuous monitoring may reveal intermittent periods of raised pressure. Some patients respond to ventriculoperitoneal shunting.

Rheumatic Disease

Musculoskeletal strains are very common and the cause of most referrals in general practice (sports injuries and back pain). Osteoarthritis affects most people who live past middle age.

Non-organ-specific autoimmune disorders, such as systemic lupus erythematosus (SLE) and systemic vasculitis, remain uncommon, but should come to mind in the clinical situations of:
• pyrexia of unknown origin, malaise and weight loss;
• multisystem disease; and
• renal disorders.

The following named diseases describe more common clinical pictures. Lesions chiefly affect skin, glomeruli, joints, serous membranes and blood vessels.

Systemic lupus erythematosus

SLE commonly presents in women aged 20–40 years (90%) and is exacerbated by sunlight and infection. In the UK the prevalence (per 100 000) is 36 for white women, 90 for Asian women, and 200–500 for Afro-Caribbean women. It is uncommon in Africans in Africa.

Clinical presentation
The early features are fever (75% of cases), arthralgia and general ill health, with exhaustion and weight loss. It can mimic rheumatoid arthritis, subacute bacterial endocarditis, and may produce the nephrotic syndrome. Only one-third develops the typical butterfly rash on the face. One or more of the following systems may be involved.

Joints (90% of cases)
A migratory, usually asymmetrical polyarthralgia, not unlike rheumatoid arthritis but very rarely (5%) erosive or deforming, affects the fingers, wrists, elbows, shoulders, knees and ankles. Avascular necrosis may follow prolonged steroid therapy. Myalgia is common.

TRIALS BOX 9.1

Subcommittee for Systemic Lupus Erythematosus Criteria of the American Rheumatism Association Diagnostic and Therapeutic Criteria Committee 1982 revised criteria for the classification of SLE. *Arthritis Rheum* 1982, **25**: 1271–1277.

The subcommittee proposed a diagnosis of SLE if four of the following 11 criteria are present, serially or simultaneously, during any interval of observation:
1 malar rash
2 discoid rash
3 photosensitivity
4 oral ulcers
5 arthritis
6 serositis (pleuritis, pericarditis)
7 renal disorder
8 neurological disorder (seizures or psychosis)
9 haematological disorder (haemolytic anaemia, leucopenia, thrombocytopenia)
10 immunological disorder
11 antinuclear antibody.

R. Leonard has suggested the following mnemonic for remembering the diagnostic criteria—SLE: A RASH POINts MD. Arthritis Renal disease ANA Serositis Haematological disorders Photosensitivity Oral ulcers Immunological disorder Neurological disorders Malar rash Discoid rash.
Ann Rheum Dis 2001; **60**: 638.

Skin (80%)

Non-specific erythema, photosensitivity, alopecia and malar (butterfly) rash (30%) are the most common features. Oral and mucosal ulceration is not uncommon (30%).

Nail fold infarcts may occur (10%). Follicles are blocked, and telangiectases present. It may involve the ears, neck, chest and upper limbs. Raynaud's phenomenon is present in 10%.

Kidneys (100% in some studies)

Renal involvement is common and associated with a worse prognosis. Clinical presentation is with almost any manifestation of renal disease, including hypertension, haematuria, proteinuria, nephrotic syndrome, acute renal failure and end-stage renal disease (p. 193).

Nervous system (50% at presentation)

The most common abnormalities are headache and peripheral neuropathy. Cranial nerve abnormalities, strokes, psychoses and depression also occur. Central nervous system abnormalities are associated with a poorer prognosis. Rarely, epilepsy is the presenting feature. Symptoms mostly result from ischaemia caused by vasculitis, coagulopathy, embolism, dissection and premature atherosclerosis.

Lungs (50%)

Pleurisy, occasionally with effusion, is relatively common. Patchy consolidation and plate-like areas of collapse, and/or diffuse reticulonodular shadowing on chest X-ray may be seen. 'Shrinking lungs', usually best seen on X-ray, is uncommon but characteristic. Lupus pneumonitis, which may be haemorrhagic, is rare but often fatal.

Cardiovascular system (40%)

Pericarditis is sometimes the first indication of SLE. Raynaud's phenomenon (10%, p. 290), cardiac failure of cardiomyopathy and non-bacterial endocarditis of mitral (Libman–Sacks) and aortic valves all may occur. Hypertension is usually associated with renal involvment.

Blood

The erythrocyte sedimentation rate is raised in active disease, and often leads to first suspicion of disease. Thrombocytopenia with purpura may be the first indication of SLE. The antiphospholipid syndrome, with intravascular coagulation, may be present (see below). Normochromic, normocytic anaemia of chronic disease occurs in over 70%. About 10% also have haemolytic anaemia (with reticulocytosis and hyperbilirubinaemia) and leucopenia may occur. There may be splenomegaly.

Lymphatic system

Generalized lymphadenopathy (50%) with or without hepatosplenomegaly (15%) may occur.

Ocular

Sjögren syndrome may be present (p. 135).

Endocrine

Dysthyroidism, usually hypothyroidism, rarely occurs.

Investigation

Routine tests show a normal or low white blood cell count (WBC)—particularly lymphocytes—and a normal or mildly elevated C-reactive protein (CRP). Both are high in systemic vasculitis. The erythrocyte sedimentation rate (ESR) and immunoglobulin levels are raised. Antibodies against double-stranded DNA (dsDNA) are found in up to 90% of those with active disease. Low serum complement, particularly the C3 and C4 fractions, occurs, especially in lupus nephritis. Antiphospholipid antibodies (p. 124) and anti-bodies to extractable nuclear antigens (anti-Ro, anti-La, anti-Sm and anti-RNP) are present.

Disease activity is assessed by titres of dsDNA and by low complement levels and increased ESR. The development of infection may be shown by rises in both WBC and CRP.

Management

General measures include avoidance of sunlight, warm socks and gloves for Raynaud's syndrome and antibiotics for intercurrent infection.

Non-steroidal anti-inflammatory drugs may be sufficient to relieve joint symptoms.

Antimalarials (e.g. hydroxychloroquine) are used when skin and joint disease predominate. They can cause lens opacities, which are not serious clinically (and resolve on stopping it), and retinal degeneration, which is rare but irreversible. Skin involvement can be helped by sunscreen preparations and by topical steroids.

Systemic steroids may be required when non-steroidal anti-inflammatory drugs and anti-malarials are insufficient to control symptoms, often in combination with *cytotoxic immuno-suppressants* (azathioprine, cyclophosphamide, methotrexate). Steroids in combination with monthly pulsed intravenous cyclophosphamide have been used to induce remission in renal lupus.

Prognosis

The history is of episodic relapses and remissions lasting months to years. Five-year survival is over 95% unless there is renal involvement. Death usually results from active generalized disease, sepsis or cardiovascular disease.

Antiphospholipid syndrome

Although first described in SLE, most patients with the antiphospholipid syndrome do not meet the criteria for SLE. It is characterized by venous (deep vein thrombosis (DVT) and pulmonary embolism) or arterial (transient ischaemic attack (TIA) stroke, migraine) thromboses, and the presence of antiphospholipid antibodies that typically bind to charged phospholipids (present in cell membranes), the classical example used in assays being cardiolipin. These antibodies bind to phospholipids used in coagulation tests, paradoxically causing

---

TRIAL BOX 9.2

Khamashta *et al.* retrospectively studied 147 patients with the antiphospholipid syndrome and a history of thrombosis. Treatment with high-intensity warfarin (international normalized ratio (INR) > 3) with or without low-dose aspirin was more effective in preventing thrombosis than treatment with low-intensity warfarin (INR < 3) with or without low-dose aspirin, or treatment with aspirin alone. *N Engl J Med* 1995; **322**: 993–997.

---

an anticoagulant effect *in vitro* (hence the term lupus anticoagulant). Other important features of the syndrome are thrombocytopenia and recurrent spontaneous abortion, usually in the second or third trimester. Babies born to mothers with anti-Ro (SS-A) and/or anti-La (SS-B) are at risk of severe bradycardia heart block. Histologically there is a thrombus without inflammation of the vessel wall. Life-long anticoagulation is usually required.

Systemic vasculitis

Inflammation of small and medium-sized blood vessels occurs in a number of generalized inflammatory diseases (see also p. 201). It can present as the primary feature of a disease (e.g. microscopic polyarteritis and Wegener's granulomatosis) or as a secondary feature of conditions such as rheumatoid arthritis (p. 130) or SLE (p. 122). The cause is unknown, although flare-up of disease is often associated with infection. Many organs can be affected; common sites are skin, lungs, kidney, joints, eyes and nervous system.

Clinical features

- Malaise, fever, rashes, uveitis, arthritis.
- Dyspnoea, cough, haemoptysis (from pulmonary haemorrhage).
- Haematuria, renal failure (glomerulonephritis).
- Psychiatric disturbance.
- Epilepsy, strokes, peripheral neuropathy.

Vasculitis may be classified according to the size of vessel involved, or the presence of serological markers. Antineutrophil cytoplasm antibodies (ANCAs) recognize cytoplasmic components (usually proteases) of neutrophils. The pattern of staining seen by immunofluorescence and the target antigen vary. Diffuse cytoplasmic staining (classical or cANCA) is seen with antibodies against proteinase 3 and is associated with Wegener's granulomatosis. Perinuclear staining (pANCA) occurs with antibodies against myeloperoxidase which occur in microscopic polyarteritis nodosa.

A number of different disease patterns are recognized.

Polyarteritis nodosa

Polyarteritis nodosa is characterized by necrotizing inflammation of small- and medium-sized arteries, leading to the formation of small aneurysms. Clinical presentation is usually with organ infarction in the presence of a systemic illness. Some cases are associated with hepatitis B virus (HBV).

• Malaise, fever, weight loss, arthralgia, myalgia.
• Hypertension (sometimes malignant) occurs almost invariably at some stage, and in 50% at presentation.
• Renal disease—over half of cases have an abnormal urinary sediment, but renal impairment is less common and usually mild.
• Nervous system (over 50%). Mononeuritis multiplex or polyneuritis. Occasionally stroke.
• Skin (25%)—tender subcutaneous nodules. Punched-out lesions occur around the ankles.
• Arteritic lesions around the nail bed and splinter haemorrhages can mimic bacterial endocarditis (particularly if combined with fever).
• Joints (10%)—a non-deforming polyarthritis.
• Gut—infarction, haemorrhage, perforation.
• Heart—myocardial infarction, angina.
• Liver—hepatitis may be caused by HBV infection.

Investigations

There is an acute phase response with a raised ESR and CRP. Anaemia, leucocytosis, proteinuria and microscopic haematuria and are common. Biopsy of involved tissue (muscle, nerve, skin, kidney) demonstrates changes of segmental fibrinoid necrosis of the walls of medium-sized arteries and arterioles with cellular infiltration. Arteriography shows narrowing of vessels, pruning of the peripheral vasculature and the presence of aneurysms. Aneurysms are most common in the renal and hepatic vasculature. Liver and renal function tests may be affected. ANCAs, usually pANCA, are present in only 10% of cases. HBV is sometimes positive.

Microscopic polyarteritis

In microscopic polyarteritis the necrotizing vasculitis affects predominantly small vessels (capillaries, venules, arterioles). The kidney is most commonly affected (over 90%) with development of a rapidly progressive glomerulonephritis. Fifty per cent have lung disease (haemoptysis, pleurisy, asthma). Frank pulmonary haemorrhage is rare (5%), but potentially fatal. Other features include arthralgia (50%), vasculitic or purpuric rashes (40%) and hypertension (20%).

pANCA staining is seen in 50% of patients, usually with specificity against myeloperoxidase. Microaneurysms do not occur.

Wegener's granulomatosis

In Wegener's granulomatosis tissue necrosis occurs as a result of both granulomatous inflammation and systemic vasculitis. Typically, localized granulomatous inflammation, usually in the upper or lower respiratory tract, is followed by a systemic vasculitis and glomerulonephritis.

Clinical features

Ear, nose and throat involvement is a prominent early feature (95%). Nasal stuffiness, facial pain and epistaxis are common. Saddle-nose deformity results from erosion of the nasal septum and destruction of nasal cartilage. Middle-ear disease causes pain and deafness.

Lungs (95%). Cough, dyspnoea, haemoptysis and chest pain are common. Pulmonary nodules may cavitate or progress to diffuse infiltration. About 10% develop diffuse pulmonary haemorrhage. Bronchial stenosis, ulceration and inflammation are seen at bronchoscopy.

Kidneys (90%). Proteinuria, haematuria and renal impairment result from a focal, segmental, necrotizing glomerulonephritis.

Joints and muscles (70%). Transient arthralgia and synovitis are common, but chronic arthritis is not a feature.

Eyes (30%). Scleritis, episcleritis, uveitis and conjunctivitis all occur.

Involvement of *skin* (25%), *nervous system* (15%) and *gastrointestinal tract* (10%) also occurs.

Investigations

Eighty per cent of patients with active Wegener's granulomatosis have cANCA, usually with specificity against proteinase 3. Biopsy of affected tissue shows a necrotizing vasculitis with granuloma formation.

Churg-Strauss syndrome

Churg–Strauss syndrome is a systemic vasculitis affecting extrapulmonary organs: heart (myocardial infarction); lungs (infiltrates and haemorrhage); gut (colic, diarrhoea, bleeding, perforation); peripheral nerves (mononeuritis multiplex); brain (stroke); and skin (purpura). Renal involvement (focal segmental necrotizing glomerulonephritis) tends to be mild. It occurs in those with pre-existing asthma and allergic rhinitis. There is an eosinophilia in peripheral blood and eosinophils predominate in the inflammatory infiltrates, which may be granulomatous. ANCA, usually pANCA, is present in 75%.

Hypersensitivity vasculitis

This term is often used to describe inflammation of small vessels (usually postcapillary venules) in which skin lesions predominate, with or without systemic features. Although most cases are idiopathic, it is associated with autoimmune diseases (rheumatoid arthritis, SLE), malignancy (lympho- and myeloproliferative disorders), infections (hepatitis B, human immunodeficiency virus, (HIV)) and drugs (e.g. penicillin, sulphonamides, thiazides).

Henoch-Schönlein purpura

Chapter 12, Renal, p. 200. Chapter 18, Haem, p. 310. Henoch–Schönlein purpura is a systemic vasculitis with immunoglobulin A (IgA) dominant immune deposits, usually following an upper respiratory tract infection. It is most common between the ages of 3 and 15 years, more often in males, and is rare in adults in whom the prognosis is worse. There is a palpable (vasculitic) purpuric rash typically over the buttocks and legs (100%), arthritis (75%) and abdominal pain with bloody diarrhoea (30%) in association with a glomerulonephritis (50%)

indistinguishable from IgA nephropathy (p. 200). There is a leucocytoclastic necrotizing vasculitis, with IgA present in the mesangium in nephropathy, and at the dermoepidermal junction in skin biopsies. It is usually self-limiting but with relapses especially in the elderly and those with nephritis.

Mixed connective tissue disease (MCTD)

MCTD is a rare overlap disorder and patients present with progressive weakness in the proximal limb muscles, usually more marked in the lower limbs. There are high titres of autoantibodies to ribonucleoprotein (RNP). Severe Raynaud's phenomenon may lead to amputation of digits.

MCTD merges with (and usually evolves into one of the) other auto-immune syndromes such as:

• dermatomyositis and scleroderma in which skin manifestations are an obvious feature;

• other collagen disorders, such as polymyositis, in which muscle weakness may be a marked or dominant feature;

• rheumatoid arthritis; or

• SLE.

Behçet disease

Behçet disease is of unknown aetiology, twice as common in males with a peak age of onset in the 20s. The diagnosis is chiefly clinical and based on the presence of recurrent oral ulcers plus the involvement of at least two of four criteria: involvement of any of the first three organs or a positive pathergy test.

• *Genitalia* (90%). Scrotal or labial ulceration.

• *Skin* (80%). Erythema nodosum, acneiform lesions and vasculitic lesions all occur. A papule or pustule may form after puncture of the skin with a sterile needle (pathergy reaction).

• *Eye* (40%). Relapsing anterior and posterior uveitis.

• *Joints* (50%). Non-deforming mono- or polyarthritis. Arthralgia of large joints.

• *Neurological* (10%). Usually central nervous system involvement.

• *Vascular.* Recurrent thombophlebitis in the limbs, venae cavae, etc. A migrating superficial thrombophlebitis may present with DVT (and occasionally pulmonary involvement).

The ESR is usually over 50 mm/h and there is a neutrophilia.

Treatment

Ulceration is treated with topical anti-inflammatory drugs (steroidal and non-steroidal). Low dose colchicine and thalidomide have been used in the more severe cases. Treatment of uveitis and systemic vasculitis involves a combination of high-dose corticosteroids and cytotoxic drugs (azathioprine or cyclophosphamide) to induce remission. Cyclosporin is used in unresponsive disease. Anticoagulation may be needed for thrombosis.

Large-vessel vasculitis

Giant-cell arteritis (temporal arteritis, cranial arteritis)

Clinical presentation

A disease in patients, usually over 60 years, who develop severe headache, with burning and tenderness over the scalp and tenderness over the temporal arteries, sometimes with visual blurring and jaw claudication. Systemic manifestations are common with fever, weight loss, arthralgia and a myalgia identical to polymyalgia rheumatica in 50%. The ophthalmic arteries may be involved and blindness may result. Personality changes may occur from involvement of the cerebral vessels. The coronary arteries or other vessels can be involved.

Investigation

The ESR is markedly raised (often above 90 mm/h). The alkaline phosphatase may also be raised. Diagnosis is confirmed on temporal artery biopsy that shows patchy involvement of the arterial wall with areas of necrosis, large mononuclear cell infiltration and giant cells. As arterial involvement may be patchy, a negative biopsy does not exclude the diagnosis.

Management

Steroids in high doses (prednisolone 40–60 mg/day) are given urgently to suppress symptoms (this usually occurs within 2 days) and to prevent blindness. Treatment is given for 2–3 years or more, gradually reducing the dosage while monitoring symptoms and the ESR.

Takayasu arteritis

Takayasu arteritis is a granulomatous arteritis affecting the aorta and its major branches, and sometimes the pulmonary arteries. It is most common in young women. Systemic features (fever, arthralgia, myalgia, anaemia) usually precede the ischaemia/pulselessness that usually affects the upper limbs. Bruits may be audible over the aorta, carotids and subclavian vessels. The diagnosis is usually confirmed by angiography, which shows diffuse narrowing of the aorta and main arteries. The ESR and CRP are elevated, with anaemia and leucocytosis. Treatment is with high-dose corticosteroids (60–80 mg/day), with gradual reduction guided by inflammatory markers.

Polymyalgia rheumatica

Clinical presentation

Occurs in patients usually over 60 years old and is more common in women. Patients present with muscle pain, stiffness and occasionally tenderness, usually in the shoulder girdle and neck, but sometimes in the pelvic region. Symptoms are worse on waking. There is little, if any, weakness or wasting. The associated findings are headache, lassitude, depression and weight loss. It may be associated with giant-cell arteritis. The ESR is usually very high (> 70 mm/h and, rarely, < 30 mm/h).

Management

Steroids (10–20 mg/day prednisolone) are required urgently to relieve symptoms and prevent development of associated giant-cell arteritis. The response is characteristically rapid. The dosage is often reduced to a very low level, while monitoring symptoms and the ESR, which should be kept within normal limits. Treatment should be continued for 1–2 years.

Dermatomyositis

Dermatomyositis mainly affects women of 40–50 years. About 20% of all cases are associated with underlying malignancy (bronchus, breast, stomach, ovary) and in men presenting over the age of 50 years, over 60% have carcinoma, usually of the bronchus. An acute form occurs in children and is often fatal.

Clinical presentation
The onset may be acute or chronic. Skin and muscle changes occur in any order, or together, sometimes with 2–3 months separating their appearance. General ill health and fever are common.

Skin involvement (60%)
• Classically purple heliotrope (a lilac-blue flower) colour occurs around the eyes. The remainder of the face may be involved.
• Violet, oedematous lesions over the small joints of the hands with telangiectasia.
• Arteritic lesions around the nails.
• There may be generalized telangiectasia, especially of the face, chest and arms.
• The rash is photosensitive.

Muscle involvement
Tenderness and weakness of muscles occur, commonly of the shoulder and proximal muscles of the upper limb, and if this predominates the disease closely resembles polymyositis (p. 000). Dysphagia is common. Muscle wasting and fibrosis with fixed joint deformity may occur in chronic disease.

Other systems
• Lungs with plate-like areas of collapse and diffuse fibrosis.
• Heart with cardiomyopathy and cardiac failure.
• Sicca syndrome (p. 135).

Investigation
Investigation of myositis (p. 129).

Management
Steroids are given in high doses (e.g. prednisolone 60–80 mg/day) in the acute stages but are relatively ineffective in the chronic cases. Immunosuppression with azathioprine may be given if there is an inadequate response within 2 months.

Prognosis
Depends upon the underlying neoplasm if present. The disease may progress rapidly but exacerbations and remissions are the rule and continue for 10–20 years until respiratory or cardiac failure occurs.

Polymyositis and allied disorders

Clinical presentation
The disorder presents at any age, but is more common in patients over 30 years with muscle pain and tenderness with progressive weakness (50% of cases). Proximal muscles are affected more than distal ones, and patients may first notice difficulty climbing or standing from a sitting position, and difficulty lifting objects above their heads. Neck muscles are frequently involved (60%) but the facial and ocular muscles rarely (cf. myasthenia gravis). Dysphagia is common (50%) and involvement of the respiratory muscles may be severe and endanger life. Arthralgia occurs in about 25% of cases. Raynaud's phenomenon is common in the young (30%) and may proceed to scleroderma. Skin rashes are common (60%) and range from diffuse erythema to the manifestations of dermatomyositis (see above).

Prognosis
This is variable but generally worse in older patients. The disease may remit spontaneously, particularly in the young (under 30 years), but may recur and/or progress to a more diffuse systemic collagen disorder (30–50 years). In patients over 50 years the prognosis depends on the underlying carcinoma if present. The overall mortality of untreated cases is about 50%.

Differential diagnosis

The differentiation is from other causes of proximal myopathy (p. 22). *Trichinella spiralis* infection of muscles and statins may produce an acute myositis syndrome.

NB Polymyalgia rheumatica usually presents with pain and stiffness. Wasting is not a characteristic feature (p. 127). All these conditions are rare.

Investigation

Muscle biopsy

This shows muscle fibre necrosis and inflammatory cell infiltration.

Serum aldolase and creatine phosphokinase

In polymyositis, the level of these enzymes is markedly elevated, gives a measure of active muscle destruction and should decline rapidly on corticosteroids coincident with improvement in muscle strength. There may be high titres to nuclear antigens, and the antinuclear factor (ANF) may be positive. Autoantibody Jo-1 is present in 25% of patients with polymyositis—more so in those with fibrosing alveolitis.

These enzymes are also greatly elevated in the muscular dystrophies during the most active stage of muscle degeneration (in the second and third decades of life).

Electromyography

In the muscular dystrophies, evidence of decrease in active muscle is shown by the presence of short-duration, low-amplitude polyphasic action potentials. Polymyositis produces a similar picture but also with evidence of spontaneous fibrillation, possibly evidence of muscular irritability. Spontaneous fibrillation is characteristic of degenerated muscle undergoing active degeneration, and is associated with evidence of a decrease in the number of motor units on voluntary movement. Electromyograph (EMG) findings often do not fit neatly into the above patterns, as the distribution of muscle involvement is patchy and as the EMG recording depends upon the particular region of muscle sampled.

Treatment

Corticosteroids (prednisolone 40–60 mg/day) are given initially and the dosage reduced gradually, depending upon the patient's clinical state and the serum creatine phosphokinase level. This is high during active disease but falls rapidly if therapy is successful. Steroid therapy is usually needed for 1–3 years before being gradually withdrawn. Azathioprine is usually given as well and allows a reduction in steroid dosage. Physiotherapy is usually very helpful.

Scleroderma (systemic sclerosis)

Scleroderma is a rare disease mainly of middle-aged people, more commonly female. There is excessive deposition of collagen and other matrix proteins in organs, including the skin. There is progressive fibrosis with later atrophy of the skin structures (*scleroderma* literally means *hard skin*). There is vasomotor instability (usually manifest as Raynaud's phenomenon), and blood vessels also show proliferative intimal lesions leading to ischaemia.

Clinical presentation

The following systems may be involved.

General

Lassitude, fever and weight loss.

Skin (75%)

Raynaud's phenomenon with sclerodactyly and telangiectasia. In the early stages there is non-pitting oedema of the skin of the hands and feet, later involving the face, neck and trunk. Abnormal nail fold capillaries are characteristic. The skin becomes smooth, waxy and tight and finally thin, atrophic and pigmented in 50%. Skin ulcers develop in 40%. Vitiligo may occur. Changes are maximal over the hands, ankles and face, producing a typical mask-like face. Subcutaneous calcification may be present (10%). The *sicca syndrome* (p. 135) develops in 5%. *Morphoea* is a localized indurated sclerodermatous lesion usually on the trunk, neck or extremities. It is benign and only rarely proceeds to systemic sclerosis.

Lungs

Diffuse interstitial fibrosis progressing to respiratory failure occurs later. Aspiration pneumonitis from oesophageal dysfunction.

Oesophagus and intestine

Reduced motility can occur in any part of the gastrointestinal tract. Dysphagia is common (65%). Steatorrhoea and malabsorption are rare. Barium studies may reveal deformity and diminished peristalsis in the oesophagus, and dilatation of the second part of the duodenum.

Locomotor system

Polymyositis. Polyarthralgia later proceeds to a rheumatoid picture.

Heart

Pericardial effusion, cardiomyopathy and heart failure are rare.

Kidney

Progressive renal failure is usually associated with hypertension. Angiotensin-converting enzyme (ACE) inhibitors are useful in reducing blood pressure and preventing renal damage.

CREST syndrome

This is a syndrome that includes **c**alcinosis cutis, **R**aynaud's phenomenon, o**e**sophageal immobility, **s**clerodactyly and **t**elangiectasia.

Investigation

There is no specific test. The ESR is often raised and antinuclear antibodies are present in 60%. Anticentromere antibodies tend to be found in patients with diffuse cutaneous systemic sclerosis associated with extensive visceral involvement. Antitopoisomerase antibodies (Scl-70) occur in patients with a more limited cutaneous disease, in whom involvement of other organs is a much later event.

Management

No treatment has been proven to alter the course of the disease. Most therapies are symptomatic. Antacid therapy and sleeping upright may assist in preventing oesophageal reflux. Physiotherapy may help stiff fingers and joints and maintain muscle activity. Vasodilatators, calcium-channel blockers and electrically heated gloves may reduce the symptoms of Raynaud's phenomenon. Nonsteroidal anti-inflammatory drugs may be used for arthralgia (with caution if there is renal involvement). D-penicillamine has been used in an attempt to slow the fibrosis. Steroids and other immunosuppressants are sometimes tried, but have not been shown to be effective.

Rheumatoid arthritis

Women are more frequently affected than men (3 : 1). It is usually insidious in onset but may be an acute or a chronic relapsing disease marked by ill health and chronic joint deformity. The dominant clinical feature is a chronic synovitis. However, the name 'rheumatoid disease' is more appropriate because tissues other than the joints are frequently affected. The overall picture is of a systemic disease with the brunt of the disease falling upon the joints. The extra-articular manifestations are very important in determining both the morbidity and mortality of the disease. There is often a family history.

Clinical features
Musculoskeletal

The small joints of the hands and feet are the most commonly affected, usually symmetrically, but in addition other large synovial joints (hips, knees, elbows) are often involved. The onset may be gradual with progressive pain, early-morning stiffness and swelling of joints. The acute onset is associated with fever and general constitutional illness. Examination shows the following.

• Tenderness and diminished movement of involved joints with characteristic fusiform soft-tissue swelling of the metacarpophalangeal and interphalangeal joints of the hands. The wrists are commonly involved. The terminal interphalangeal joints of the fingers are spared—unlike psoriatic arthropathy. The metatarsophalangeal joints of the feet may also be tender on pressure. Chronic disease produces fixed deformities and ulnar deviation at the metacarpophalangeal joints.

• Wasting of the small muscles of the hand is common and results from a combination of disuse atrophy, vasculitis and peripheral neuropathy. Wasting occurs in the muscle around any affected joint.

• Inflammation of the soft tissues surrounding inflamed joints causes swelling, tenosynovitis (Achilles tendinitis, olecranon bursitis) and even tendon rupture. Localized subcutaneous nodules are present in 25%.

Joints less commonly involved are the ankles, which have relatively little synovial tissue, the costovertebral joints producing diminished chest expansion, temporomandibular joints, the cricoarytenoid joints (causing hoarseness and, rarely, acute respiratory obstruction) and the cervical spine. Laxity of the atlantoaxial joint ligaments with some erosion of the odontoid peg may result in acute or chronic cord compression and death. Atlantoaxial subluxation is present in 25% of patients, although only 7% have neurological signs. It may be necessary to X-ray the cervical spine in severe cases of rheumatoid arthritis prior to intubation for general anaesthesia.

NB In rheumatoid joints, acute solitary effusions should be aspirated and examined microscopically and bacteriologically for infection.

Lung

Lung involvement is clinically uncommon but lung function tests show changes in nearly half of all patients with rheumatoid arthritis. They tend to be more common in men than in women. It can occur before the arthritis and usually in seropositive disease. It presents as:

• isolated unilateral pleural effusion (must be differentiated from primary tuberculosis);

• rheumatoid nodules, single or multiple, which may be present throughout the lung parenchyma—commonly subpleural;

• diffuse fibronodular infiltration or fibrosing alveolitis; and

• Caplan syndrome: the presence of large (up to 5 cm) rheumatoid nodules in the lungs of coal miners with silicosis but also occurring in other pneumoconioses. They may calcify, cavitate or coalesce and may precede clinical arthritis. The patients are seropositive.

Cardiac

Pericarditis (with or without effusion) is clinically uncommon, although found at postmortem in about 30%.

Vascular

Arteritic lesions characteristically produce nail fold infarcts and minute 'splinter' necrosis in the digital pulps. (This form of vascular necrosis is characteristic of arteritic lesions seen in vasculitis, although multiple emboli in infective endocarditis may produce a similar picture.) Necrotizing arteritis may affect large vessels and give rise to digital gangrene, infarcted bowel or stroke. Chronic leg ulcers result from skin necrosis secondary to vasculitis—the ulcers are frequently on the lateral aspect of the tibia (cf. varicose ulcers). Raynaud's phenomenon (p. 290) is associated.

Neurological

• Peripheral neuropathy: this is predominantly sensory, and secondary to arteritis of the vessels.

• Neuropathy complicates therapy with gold and chloroquine.

• Mononeuritis multiplex, particularly of digital nerves, ulnar nerves and lateral popliteal nerves.

• Entrapment neuropathy, e.g. carpal tunnel syndrome and the ulnar nerve at the elbow.

• Spinal cord lesions secondary to cervical disease.

Reticuloendothelial

The spleen is enlarged in about 5% of cases, but only 1% develop leucopenia. Generalized lymphadenopathy is present in 10%.

Infection

Infection of all kinds (except urinary tract infections) and in all sites (especially joints) is much more common and should be looked for in all patients who deteriorate suddenly.

Blood

Normochromic normocytic anaemia is common and its severity relates to that of the disease. Iron deficiency may result from bleeding secondary to salicylate or other non-steroidal anti-inflammatory therapy but this is uncommon and peptic ulceration and colonic neoplasms should be excluded. The height of the ESR reflects the activity of the disease. The CRP is raised even in the absence of infection (see SLE, p. 123).

Renal

Amyloidosis, although common on biopsy, is seldom clinically important in rheumatoid disease. Proteinuria or nephrotic syndrome may complicate treatment with pencillamine and gold.

Ocular

• Keratoconjunctivitis sicca occurs in 15% of patients with rheumatoid arthritis: see Sjögren syndrome (p. 135).
• Scleritis presents as pericorneal injection with pain and tenderness in 0.6% of cases of rheumatoid arthritis. It predisposes to uveitis and glaucoma.
• Scleromalacia perforans is even less common and occurs in long-standing rheumatoid arthritis: a rheumatoid nodule in the sclera may perforate.
• Iatrogenic: lens opacities and retinal degeneration with chloroquine and cataracts from steroids.

Iatrogenic

From gold (proteinuria, nephrotic syndrome, skin rash, marrow suppression); aspirin and most non-steroidal anti-inflammatory drugs (gastric erosion); penicillamine (nephropathy), steroids (p. 148) and chloroquine (cataract, retinopathy, photosensitivity).

Investigation of inflammatory polyarthropathy

Normochromic normocytic anaemia is common. The ESR is performed to assess the activity of the disease and to monitor therapy. Perform ANF and DNA antibodies to exclude SLE. The serum uric acid helps to exclude gout, particularly if the distribution is asymmetrical. A chest X-ray helps to exclude the hypertrophic arthropathy of bronchial carcinoma and the arthropathy of acute sarcoid, which usually affects the ankles and knees. Human leucocyte antigen (HLA) B27 supports the diagnosis of Reiter disease and the arthropathy of ulcerative colitis or Crohn disease.

Rheumatoid factor

This is a circulating immunoglobulin of the IgM class which is an antibody to the patient's own IgG. It fixes complement and aids phagocytosis of immune complexes by neutrophils. It agglutinates sensitized sheep red cells (sheep cell agglutination test, SCAT) and also latex particles that have been coated with denatured γ-globulin (latex agglutination tests, e.g. F_2LP test, in which the F_2 fraction of denatured γ-globulin is used to coat the latex particles). High titres correlate with more severe arthritis with a worse prognosis, and with a higher incidence of extra-articular disease (nodules, arteritis, leg ulcers, digital gangrene, neuropathy, Felty syndrome and fibrosing alveolitis).

Rheumatoid factor is positive in:
• 50–70% of outpatients with rheumatoid arthritis (100% in patients with nodules and Sjögren syndrome);
• 15% of patients with juvenile rheumatoid arthritis (Still disease); and
• 4% of the general population, rising with age. Its presence does not necessarily indicate that rheumatoid disease will develop later.

Rheumatoid factor is usually negative in ankylosing spondylitis, Reiter syndrome, psoriatic arthropathy and colitic arthropathy.

Radiology

The joints may be normal in early rheumatoid disease. The characteristic sequence of abnormalities is:
1 soft-tissue swelling and periarticular osteoporosis;
2 narrowing of joint space and periarticular erosions;

3 subluxation and osteoarthritis occur in long-standing disease; and
4 fibrosis or bony ankylosis.

Management
The assessment of disease activity depends on both clinical and laboratory findings.
• *Mild disease* is characterized by slight joint swelling and pain, with brief morning stiffness. Haemoglobin and platelet count are normal and ESR normal or marginally elevated.
• *Active disease* has more severe symptomatology, and the laboratory findings are abnormal (haemoglobin low, platelets often high and ESR > 40 mm/h). The rheumatoid factor is more likely to be positive.

The objects of therapy are: first, symptom control of pain and stiffness, enabling the patient to maintain as near normal existence as possible; and, secondly, suppression of synovitis and systemic inflammation in more severe disease. A social assessment of occupation, of family help and home conditions is essential when planning therapy.

Rest diseased joints in splints, especially at night to reduce pain and prevent deformity.

Physiotherapy to maintain full joint movement and strengthen weak muscles. Early attention and advice regarding posture may prevent chronic deformity and degeneration of all involved joints.

Drugs used in rheumatoid arthritis can be broadly divided into those aimed at pain relief and those that suppress the disease process, sometimes known as disease modifying anti-rheumatic drugs (DMARDs).

Pain relief
Analgesics. Simple, such as paracetamol, or a compound such as co-proxamol or co-codamol.

Non-steroidal anti-inflammatory drugs. Aspirin, although inexpensive and effective, is less well-tolerated than newer non-steroidal anti-inflammatory drugs. Ibuprofen has fewer gastrointestinal side-effects than other similar drugs, but tends to be less effective. Piroxicam, ketoprofen, indometacin, naproxen and diclo-fenac have an intermediate risk of side effects, whereas azapropazone carries the highest risk. If there is gastrointestinal intolerance H_2-blockade or the prostaglandin E_1 analogue misoprostol may be added. Selective inhibitors of cyclo-oxygenase 2 (rofecoxib and celecoxib) may also improve gastrointestinal tolerance.

Disease-suppressing drugs
Corticosteroids are effective at producing symptomatic relief and suppressing disease activity, although concerns over side-effects (osteoporosis, weight gain, hypertension, diabetes, cataracts, p. 148) have limited their use. Local injection of steroids into joints (or other painful sites) may give relief.

Gold. Sodium aurothiomalate is given by intramuscular injection at a dosage of 50 mg/week until there is evidence of remission (usually after about 500 mg). If there is no response after a total of 1 g, treatment is usually stopped. In patients who respond, the dosage interval is gradually increased to monthly. Treatment may be continued for up to 5 years, although only one-half of patients remain on therapy after 2 years. Regular blood counts and urinalysis are required. Leucopenia and thrombocytopenia, or proteinuria (caused by membranous glomerulonephritis, p. 200), are usually reversible if gold is discontinued. Rashes may necessitate discontinuation of treatment.

Penicillamine has a similar action to gold. Side-effects of thrombocytopenia, proteinuria and rashes are common, but in some cases treatment can be continued at a reduced dose, or stopped and then reintroduced.

Chloroquine and hydroxychloroquine tend to be better tolerated than gold or penicillamine. Retinopathy is rare if recommended dosage is not exceeded (chloroquine 4 mg/kg/day; hydroxychloroquine 6 mg/kg/day).

Sulfasalazine is split into 5-aminosalicylic acid and sulfapyridine by bacteria in the large intestine. Its use is limited by gastrointestinal

TRIALS BOX 9.3

The **Arthritis and Rheumatism Council Low-Dose Glucocorticoid Study Group** compared prednisolone 7.5 mg/day with placebo in 128 adults with active rheumatoid arthritis of less than 2 years' duration. Over a 2-year period steroids reduced the rate of radiologically detectable disease progression. *N Engl J Med* 1995; **333**: 142–146.

The **Methotrexate–Cyclosporin Combination Study Group** compared methotrexate alone or in combination with cyclosporin in 148 patients who had previously demonstrated partial responses to methotrexate. Over a 6-month period patients receiving combination therapy demonstrated clinically important improvement, without substantial increases in side-effects. *N Engl J Med* 1995; **333**: 137–141.

Moreland et al. evaluated the safety and efficacy of a recombinant fusion protein that consists of the soluble TNF receptor linked to the Fc portion of human IgG_1 (TNFR:Fc) in a placebo controlled trial of 180 patients with refractory rheumatoid arthritis. TNFR:Fc was safe, well tolerated and associated with improvement in the inflammatory symptoms of rheumatoid arthritis. *N Engl J Med* 1997; **337**: 141–147.

Anti-Tumor Necrosis Factor Trial in Rheumatoid Arthritis with Concomitant Therapy Study Group treated 428 patients who had active rheumatoid arthritis despite methotrexate therapy with placebo or infliximab, a chimeric monoclonal antibody against TNF-α. In patients with persistently active rheumatoid arthritis despite methotrexate therapy, repeated doses of infliximab in combination with methotrexate provided clinical benefit and halted the progression of joint damage. *N Engl J Med* 2000; **343**: 1594–1602.

intolerance, rashes and haematological abnormalities. Leucopenia and thrombocytopenia usually occur in the first 3–6 months, and are reversible on cessation of treatment.

Immunosuppressant drugs (methotrexate, azathioprine, cyclophosphamide, cyclosporin A, chlorambucil) have all been used in active rheumatoid arthritis, either alone or in combination with corticosteroids or other agents to allow use of lower dosage.

Treatments which *neutralize the effects of TNF-α (infliximab,* a chimeric monoclonal antibody against TNF-α, and *etanercept* a recombinant fusion protein that consists of the soluble tumour necrosis factor (TNF) receptor linked to the Fc portion of human IgG_1 have been shown to improve symptoms, and in combination with methotrexate can halt progressive joint damage (see Trials Box 9.3).

Surgical management
Synovectomy (especially of the knee joint), realignment and repair of tendons, joint prostheses (hip, knee, fingers) and arthrodesis may be required for severe pain or deformity.

Advice of an expert in *rehabilitation* may allow a severely disabled patient to continue a tolerable and even happy existence at home. Depression should not be missed.

Diseases resembling rheumatoid arthritis (all seronegative)

Still disease
Adult-onset Still disease, like the juvenile form (p. 137), is characterized by a high spiking fever (85%), an evanescent rash (80%) and arthritis (100%), but occurs after the age of 15 years. Other features include splenomegaly (35%), pleurisy (30%), pericarditis (20%), neutrophil leucocytosis (100%), lymphadenopathy (70%) and hepatic abnormalities (85%). Roughly half go into remission off medication. Non-steroidal anti-inflammatory drugs are the treatment of choice, e.g. naproxen. Steroids are often needed in the acute phase.

The presence of five or more criteria, including at least two major, has a diagnostic sensitivity of 96.2% and specificity of 92.1%.

• *Major:* fever (> 39°C for > 1 week), arthralgia

(> 2 weeks), typical rash, leucocytosis (> 10 × 10⁹/l, with > 80% neutrophils).

• *Minor*: Sore throat, lymphadenopathy and/or splenomegaly, liver dysfunction, negative ANF and rheumatoid factor.
• *Exclude* infections, malignancies and other rheumatological disorders.

Sjögren syndrome

This is more common in women than in men (9 : 1). The major clinical features of the sicca syndrome result from reduced secretion from the lachrymal and salivary glands. It produces dry, gritty eyes and corneal ulcers (keratoconjunctivitis sicca) and a dry mouth (xerostomia) with accelerated dental caries, candidosis and dysphagia. Recurrent respiratory infections occur from diminished bronchial secretions. About 50% are associated with rheumatoid arthritis, 30% are uncomplicated and 20% associated with other autoimmune disease (mostly non-organ-specific). Rheumatoid factor is usually present, ANF frequently present (70%), anti-Ro and anti-La antibodies are often present (40–60%), and lupus erythematosus cells are seldom present (15%). In the Schirmer test, filter paper is hooked over the lower eyelid; in normal people at least 15 mm is wet in 5 min and in the sicca syndrome usually far less. Fluorescein demonstrates corneal ulceration. Labial salivary gland biopsy may show diagnostic histology. Treatment is symptomatic with artificial tears (hypromellose) and the arthritis is treated as uncomplicated rheumatoid arthritis.

Felty syndrome

Some patients with severe rheumatoid arthritis have enlarged lymph nodes, splenomegaly and hypersplenism (anaemia, leucopenia and thrombocytopenia). Removal of the spleen often reverses blood abnormalities but the underlying rheumatoid process is not affected and surgery is seldom indicated. Leg ulcers are common as a result of vasculitis. The ANF is usually positive.

Psoriatic arthritis

An arthritis similar to but distinct from rheumatoid arthritis may complicate psoriasis (p. 291). The clinical picture resembles rheumatoid arthritis and may be clinically indistinguishable from it in 30% but:
• psoriasis is present;
• joint involvement is usually asymmetrical and deforming and involves the terminal interphalangeal joints which may be the only affected joints (50%);
• pitting occurs in the nails (80%);
• subcutaneous nodules do not occur;
• sacroiliitis is more common (30%); and
• tests for rheumatoid factor are negative.

Ankylosing spondylitis
(sacroiliitis)

Clinical features

This is a disease mainly of young adult males (20–40 years; cf. rheumatoid arthritis) with a 6% familial incidence. Joint involvement affects the sacroiliac joints, causing persistent low back pain with morning stiffness. Characteristically, the pain improves on exertion and worsens with rest. The disease may involve the spine, producing pain and stiffness initially of the lumbosacral region and eventually of the thoracic and cervical spine. The hips are involved in 50% of patients. Examination reveals decreased spinal movements and loss of the normal lumbosacral curvature. 'Springing' the pelvis (i.e. pressing the iliac crests towards each other) causes sacroiliac pain.

Peripheral joints are involved in 25%, especially the knees and ankles. The ribs fuse to the vertebrae. Up to 15% may present with a peripheral arthropathy. The arthropathy differs from rheumatoid arthritis in that it is asymmetrical and affects large joints more than small joints.

Other features of ankylosing spondylitis are:
• general ill health;
• uveitis (in 25–30% of cases and up to 40% in long-standing cases);
• ulcerative colitis—more common in patients with ankylosing spondylitis and vice versa;
• aortic regurgitation as a result of aortitis; and
• respiratory failure may result from the fixed

ribcage with kyphoscoliosis, and from fibrosing alveolitis.

Investigation

Tests for rheumatoid factor are usually negative. The ESR is raised in 80%. HLA B27 is present in 96% (compared with 7% in the general population and 50% of asymptomatic relatives).

Radiology

The sacroiliac joints are irregular with widening, erosion and sclerosis on both sides of the articular margins of one or both joints. Bony ankylosis occurs late. The intervertebral ligaments calcify and finally ossify to produce a 'bamboo' spine.

Differential diagnoses

- Osteoarthritis of the spine.
- Prolapsed intervertebral disc.
- Tuberculosis which may affect only one sacroiliac joint.
  Rarely,
- psoriatic arthritis;
- Reiter disease; or
- the sacroiliitis of ulcerative colitis.

Management

Bed rest is contraindicated because it increases stiffness and ankylosis.

Careful posture with spinal muscle exercises is essential to prevent chronic deformity. Sleeping on a firm bed without pillows should help prevent fixed spinal flexion.

Analgesics. Indometacin or other non-steroidal anti-inflammatory drug is the treament of initial choice.

Sulfasalazine (500 mg starting dose to maintenance dosage of 2–3 g/day), as in rheumatoid arthritis, offers symptomatic improvement more of peripheral joints than sacroiliitis in 2–3 months, probably by altering the immune process.

Phenylbutazone 200–300 mg/day is particularly effective but, in view of its propensity to cause fatal adverse effects, is only used when alternative treatments have failed and only under expert supervision.

Prognosis

Many mild cases may never present to a physician. With expert care 70–80% will maintain complete or almost complete activity. More severe cases develop moderate to severe bony ankylosis of the spine to produce fixation of mobility and rounded kyphosis of the cervical and thoracic spine. This may impair ventilation. In severe cases extreme rigidity of the spine may occur within 3–5 years. The disease may remit at any stage but recurrent episodes may occur.

Reiter syndrome

A disease, usually of the young, affecting men three times more often than women. Patients present with a peripheral arthritis plus urethritis or cervicitis, with conjunctivitis in 30%. There is usually a history of sexual intercourse 2–4 weeks previously. It occurs in < 1% of patients with non-specific urethritis (*Chlamydia trachomatis*). The disease may, less commonly in the UK, follow bacillary (*Shigella*) dysentery.

Clinical features

- Arthritis: typically acute or subacute and usually oligoarticular and asymmetrical, affecting large joints of the lower limbs.
- Sacroiliitis occurs in 30%. Plantar fasciitis, calcaneal spurs and Achilles tendinitis may occur (20%).
- Conjunctivitis is common in the acute disease. Iritis is associated with chronic recurrent disease, particularly when associated with sacroiliitis.
- Skin lesions (20%): mouth ulcers are common. Urethritis and prostatitis are associated with superficial skin ulceration around the penile meatus (circinate balanitis).
- Pustular hyperkeratotic lesions of the soles of the feet and, less frequently, the palms of the hands (keratoderma blennorrhagica) occurs in 15%.
- Tests for rheumatoid factor are by definition negative.
- HLA B27, present in 70%, confers susceptibility to reactive arthritis with a relative risk of 30–50%.

Differential diagnosis

• Gonococcal arthritis (gonococcus is detected in urethral discharge or blood culture).
• Ankylosing spondylitis.
• Behçet disease.
• Psoriatic and rheumatoid arthritis.

Management

• The treatment of the acute stage is symptomatic.
• Rest and aspirate the inflamed joints.
• Indometacin is the drug of first choice. The urethritis may respond to tetracycline 2 g/day for 10 days.
• The majority of cases settle spontaneously within 4–10 weeks, but the disease recurs in up to 50%.

Acute generalized arthritis

Still disease—juvenile form

This is a childhood disease, usually of acute onset with fever and skin rashes. Joint pain is not an essential feature (absent in 25% at onset) and may be monarticular (30%) at the onset. Subcutaneous nodules are rare. Eye changes include chronic iridocyclitis (10%), corneal band opacity and complicated cataract. Lymphadenopathy is present in 30%, splenomegaly in 20% and simple pericarditis in 10%. One-third of patients present with a history of insidious polyarthritis as in adult rheumatoid arthritis. Tests of rheumatoid factor are usually negative (85%).

Prognosis

The majority of cases settle spontaneously with minimal or no disability. Bone growth may be retarded. In one-third the disease continues into adult life.

Acute rheumatic fever

This is an acute febrile systemic disorder affecting mainly the heart and joints following a streptococcal infection (group A, β-haemolytic), usually occurring between the ages of 5 and 15 years. The disease is now very rare in industrialized countries.

Diagnosis

The diagnosis is made when there is evidence of previous streptococcal infection plus one major and two minor, or two major criteria. (Guidelines for the diagnosis of rheumatic fever. Jones Criteria, 1992 update. Special Writing Group of the Committee on Rheumatic Fever, Endocarditis, and Kawasaki Disease of the Council on Cardiovascular Disease in the Young of the American Heart Association. *J Am Med Assoc* 1992; **268**: 2069–2073.)

In the text below, double asterisks denote major criteria, single asterisks minor criteria.

Symptoms

The disease usually presents with flitting polyarthropathy** or carditis** (40%), the former being more common in adults and the latter in children. Both may be present at the same time but carditis is uncommon over the age of 20. The involved joints may be exquisitely tender (arthralgia)*. There may be a history of streptococcal infection of the throat or skin 10–20 days previously. Rarely, children may present with chorea**—the writhing limb movements of extrapyramidal involvement.

Examination

General

The dominant features are fever* (90%) and flitting arthropathy of large joints (small joints may be affected in the elderly) which are exquisitely tender. Erythema nodosum and erythema marginatum** (5%) are more common in children. Symmetrical subcutaneous nodules** (10%) lying over bony prominences and extensor surfaces occur virtually only in children and their presence probably correlates with severe carditis.

Sign of carditis

Myocarditis: tachycardia, cardiomegaly, heart failure.
Endocarditis: any valve may be involved and cause transient murmurs. A transient mitral diastolic murmur (Carey Coombs) is the most

common. Mitral systolic and aortic murmurs also occur.

Percarditis: friction rub or small effusion.

Investigation

There is evidence of preceding group A strep-tococcal infection with a raised or rising anti-streptolysin (ASO) titre (> 200 units/ml) and haemolytic streptococci may be isolated from the throat. The WBC count is raised and a hypochromic normocytic anaemia, unre-sponsive to iron therapy, may develop. Acute phase proteins are raised* (ESR and CRP). The electrocardiogram may show first-degree heart block*. Almost any rhythm disorder may occur. Chest X-ray may demonstrate pro-gressive cardiac enlargement.

Management

• Bed rest.
• Immobilize inflamed joints.
• Acetylsalicylic acid. The oral dose is 6–12 g/day to achieve blood levels of 2.1–2.4 mmol/l (300–350 mg/l). Side-effects of nausea, tinnitus and blurring of vision may limit the dosage. The symptomatic response to salicylates is characteristic. Steroids are frequently used with salicylates but there is no evidence that either improves the prognosis.
• Penicillin G is given during the acute stages and oral phenoxymethyl penicillin (125–250 mg b.d.) continued in those with cardiac involvement for at least 5 years and preferably until 20 years of age to prevent recurrence. Erythromycin is used for patients sensitive to penicillin.

Postinfectious arthralgia

Low-grade polyarthralgia frequently follows some infections, e.g. glandular fever, rubella, *Mycoplasma pneumoniae*, viral hepatitis and meningococcal septicaemia and persist for months or years. The association of this with erythema chronicum migrans occurs in Lyme disease (p. 295) following tick-borne infection with the spirochaete *Borrelia burgdorferi*.

Osteoarthritis

This is a common degenerative disorder of synovial joints. There is damage to the hyaline cartilage, with sclerosis, cysts and osteophyte formation in underlying subchondral bone, and narrowing of the joint space. It is related to age, previous joint injury and deformity. Obesity increases the prevalence of osteoarthritis in the weight-bearing joints of the lower limb. There is a genetic component, especially in women.

Incidence

It is radiologically universal after the age of 55 years. The most common joints to be affected are the interphalangeal joints (50%), the thumb carpometacarpal joint (30%), the cervical spine (40%), lumbar spine (40%), knees (30%) and hips (20%).

Clinical features

There is joint pain, which is worse with move-ment and towards the end of the day. There is also stiffness, immobility, deformity and, occasionally, nerve root involvement. The joints may be red, warm and tender and even produce an effusion (beware of an infected effusion). Joint involvement is asymmetrical. Osteophyte formation, e.g. Heberden's nodes in the distal interphalangeal joints of the hands, can cause joint swelling and deformity sufficient to limit the range of movement. Involvement of the first metacarpophalangeal joint may interfere with manual dexterity and pinch grip. The stiffness tends to wear off in 10–15 min of exercise (cf. rheumatoid arthritis, 1–2 h).

Investigation

Joint X-rays show a loss of space, osteophytes and sclerosis of subchondral bone, sometimes with cyst formation. Synovial aspirates pro-duce < 100 WBC/mm^3 and these are chiefly monocytes.

Management

Use effective analgesia with or without anti-inflammatory agents including paracetamol and the non-steroidal anti-inflammatory drugs. Obese patients should lose weight if the arthritis affects weight-bearing joints. Graded exercise, particularly isometric exercise in which muscles are contracted against resistance, can improve symptoms in some patients.

A walking stick, and trainers or special orthopaedic shoes may be very effective in relieving symptoms. Orthopaedic surgery can offer arthrodesis, arthroplasty and joint replacement (hips, knees, fingers, shoulders and elbows).

Endocrine Disease

Diabetes mellitus (p. 153) and disorders of the thyroid gland are the only common forms of endocrine disease.

Thyroid

Some enlargement of the thyroid is common, especially in women, and large non-toxic goitres are not uncommon. Both hypothyroidism and hyperthyroidism are relatively common. Thyroid cancer is rare.

Non-toxic goitre

Aetiology
The enlargement of the gland (visible and palpable) is caused by an increased secretion of thyroid-stimulating hormone (TSH) secondary to diminished output of thyroid hormones. The causes are as follow.

• *Simple goitre.* Iodine deficiency, especially in areas of endemic goitre. Sporadic goitre is probably caused by relative iodine deficiency for that patient. Iodine requirement is increased at puberty in girls and during pregnancy. The gland tends to become nodular as age increases.

• *Goitrogens*, e.g. iodides in large doses, antithyroid drugs such as para-aminosalicylic acid (PAS) and lithium, are rare as causes (except when used therapeutically, e.g. carbimazole).

• *Inborn errors* of thyroid hormone synthesis (dyshormonogenesis). Six types of enzyme defect are known. All are rare and autosomal recessive. The most common is associated with nerve deafness (Pendred syndrome) and caused by impaired organic binding of iodine.

Clinical presentation
The patient or relatives usually notice a painless swelling of the thyroid. If untreated it may develop into a large nodular goitre and cause pressure on the trachea, oesophagus or veins, especially if there is retrosternal extension.

Differential diagnosis
• Autoimmune thyroiditis (Hashimoto disease).
• Toxic goitre.
• Cancer of the thyroid.
• Solitary nodule—benign or carcinoma (very rare).

Investigation
• Serum free triiodothyronine (T_3), free thyroxine (T_4) and TSH if hyperthyroidism is suspected, or free T_4 and TSH if hypothyroidism.
• Thyroid antibodies for Hashimoto disease.
• CT scan if pressure symptoms are present.
• Ultrasound will distinguish solid or cystic masses, whether single or multiple.
• Fine-needle aspiration with cytology may be diagnostic but some surgeons prefer excision.

Prophylaxis
Iodized salt, especially during pregnancy. Seafish in the diet.

Treatment
If the patient is euthyroid and malignancy excluded, treatment is not required unless the swelling is unsightly or causing pressure symptoms. If the TSH is raised, thyroxine may be given to suppress TSH hypersecretion. Surgery may be needed to remove nodules.

Thyrotoxicosis (hyperthyroidism)

Aetiology

The clinical picture results from an excess of thyroid hormones (T_4 and/or T_3). Graves' disease refers to the common form of hyperthyroidism in which eye signs and toxic symptoms accompany diffuse enlargement of the gland (female : male = 5 : 1) with antibodies and occasional pretibial myxoedema. Thyrotoxicosis is an autoimmune disease associated with thyroidstimulating immunoglobulins (TSI), against the TSH receptor site on the thyroid follicular cell membrane. There also appears to be a thyroid growth immunoglobulin (TGI), which may independently determine the size of any goitre. An ophthalmopathic immunoglobulin to eye muscle basement membrane may be causative and independent. There is an association with human leukocyte antigen (HLA) B8 and DR3. Rarely, a single toxic nodule may produce thyrotoxicosis. There is a strong genetic factor. Self-administered T_4 should not be forgotten as a cause of hyperthyroidism, particularly in doctors and nurses. A gross persistent excess of iodine in health foods and some cough medicines may precipitate hyperthyroidism.

Clinical presentation

The symptoms and signs, except the eye signs, can be deduced from knowledge of the pharmacological action of T_4 and T_3.

The most helpful symptoms are preference for cold weather, excessive sweating, increased appetite and weight loss, nervousness, tiredness and palpitations.

The most helpful signs are goitre, especially with a murmur, exophthalmos, lid retraction and lid lag, hot moist palms, tremor and excessive movements, tachycardia or atrial fibrillation.

Atypical presentations

• Atrial fibrillation, tachycardia or cardiac failure in middle age or older should always suggest thyrotoxicosis.
• Unexplained weight loss in apparently euthyroid patients.

Very rare. Toxic manic confusion. Severe proximal limb girdle myopathy. Diarrhoea.

Differential diagnosis

Thyrotoxicosis is often difficult to differentiate from an anxiety state, particularly when this is associated with a simple goitre. The palms tend to be moist but cold in anxiety state.

Investigation

Always carry out at least one, and preferably two, tests before starting treatment to confirm and document the diagnosis. Use serum free T_3, free T_4 (raised) and TSH (suppressed) in borderline cases. In exophthalmos, CT scan of the orbit demonstrates thickened external ocular muscle. The orbit contains excess mucopolysaccharide (and water).

Treatment

Antithyroid drugs

Carbimazole can be given in a titration regimen to block thyroid hormone synthesis sufficient to produce a euthyroid state. For this, give carbimazole 15 mg t.d.s. for 3 weeks, reducing to 5 mg t.d.s. or more according to the response and maintained for 12–18 months. Review at 6 months, 1 year and 18 months. When the drugs are stopped, relapse occurs in at least two-thirds within 1 or 2 years and either surgery or radioiodine is used (see below).

In the block–replacement regimen, enough carbimazole is given to block all thyroid hormone production with 40–60 mg in a single daily dose, plus replacement of normal thyroid requirements with L-thyroxine, 100–150 µg/day. Compliance is improved for some patients and relapse is possibly less common after treatment is stopped. Side-effects of carbimazole include skin rashes, loss of hair and neutropenia (sore throat is usually the first symptom) and patients must be warned to stop the drug and seek urgent medical advice. Propylthiouracil is a suitable alternative. In pregnancy, carbimazole in the usual dosage remains the treatment of choice. The baby can be breast-fed if the patient remains on the lowest effective dose of the drug.

Propranolol

Propranolol 20 mg t.d.s. may give rapid improvement in cardiac symptoms and a sense of well-being. It should not be used alone in thyrotoxic heart failure or as the sole therapy.

Radioactive iodine therapy

Radioactive iodine therapy is given after rendering the more toxic patient euthyroid with drugs, stopping them 4 days before administration, and reintroducing them 4 days afterwards while awaiting the 5-week delay before the effects of radiotherapy become apparent.

One strategy is to give an ablation, or near-ablation dose of radioiodine (about 550 MBq = 15 mCi) followed by standard replacement doses of thyroid hormone. Patients given more conventional doses of radioiodine experience an inexorable cumulative incidence of hypothyroidism of about 4% per year. Between 5 and 15% develop hypothyroidism in the first year.

Patients with a single toxic adenoma or a toxic multinodular goitre can have a large dose of radioiodine with relatively little chance of hypothyroidism, because the unaffected parts of the thyroid have been dormant following suppression of TSH by excessive thyroid hormone secretion, and do not take up the radioiodine.

Surgery

This requires adequate preoperative treatment with carbimazole and later potassium iodide. Subtotal thyroidectomy is advised for: (i) failure of medical treatment, and drug sensitivity in the young; and (ii) large multinodular goitres, especially with pressure symptoms as they may enlarge with medical therapy, and for cosmetic reasons. One year later about 80% are euthyroid, 15% hypothyroid and 5% have relapsed. Complications include hypothyroidism (eventually 10–15% in those with high antibody titres and long-term follow-up is required), recurrence of hyperthyroidism, recurrent laryngeal nerve palsy (rare), hypoparathyroidism (rare).

Treatment of complications
Eye
Lid retraction (sclera visible below the upper lid) usually responds to treatment of the thyrotoxicosis. Exophthalmos (sclera visible above lower lid) results from the swelling of retro-orbital tissues and may not improve and may progress. In malignant exophthalmos there is weakness of the external ocular muscles, often with diplopia, oedema of the conjunctivae and corneal damage from exposure. Treatment is difficult. The strabismus and lid retraction of dysthyroid ophthalmopathy may respond to local intramuscular injection of botulinum toxin (neurotoxin A) but the place of this in routine therapy is not yet determined. Local or systemic steroids may be required with tarsorrhaphy in severe cases. Orbital decompression may be required. The condition remits slowly over years with or without treatment.

Atrial fibrillation
Atrial fibrillation responds poorly to digoxin and larger doses are often needed until the patient is euthyroid. Cardioversion may then be used. Propranolol or other β-blocker may control severe tachycardia. Heart failure is unusual and responds to antithyroid drugs plus conventional treatment.

Thyrotoxic crisis
This is rare but dangerous and requires emergency treatment with i.v. hydrocortisone (100 mg qds) and i.v. propranolol (5 mg). Oral carbimazole (60–120 mg) is followed by potassium iodide (60 mg/day in divided doses). β-Blockade (propranolol 80 mg q.d.s.) is usually required. Oxygen should be given and particular attention paid to fluid balance because sweating is marked.

Hypothyroidism
This results from a low level of circulating thyroid hormone, either free T_4 or T_3. The term 'myxoedema' means that there is a deposition of a mucopolysaccharide beneath the skin, producing a non-pitting swelling of the subcutaneous tissues.

Aetiology
Autoimmune thyroiditis. This may present as Hashimoto disease when a goitre is present,

or as spontaneous or primary hypothyroidism if the gland atrophies without producing a goitre. Circulating thyroid antibodies are present.
• Destructive therapy for hyperthyroidism or carcinoma by operation or by radioiodine.
• Primary thyroid agenesis may produce cretinism in infants.
• Ingestion of goitrogens, usually an antithyroid drug such as carbimazole (or lithium, amiodarone) in too large doses or for too long.
• Secondary to hypopituitarism; this is rare.
• Inborn errors of thyroid metabolism.
• There may be a family history of thyroid disease or of autoimmune disease, e.g. 10% have pernicious anaemia.

Clinical presentation

The onset is insidious, difficult to distinguish from depression and the condition may be far advanced before it is recognized. All who have had destructive therapy to the thyroid should be followed up at 6-monthly intervals. Many of the symptoms also occur in euthyroid individuals, e.g. tiredness, loss of hair. Those which have the greatest diagnostic value are intolerance of cold, diminished energy, physical tiredness, slow cerebration, increase in weight, hoarseness of voice, diminished sweating, dry and rough skin, dry and unruly hair, deafness, constipation, muscular pains and paraesthesiae (carpal tunnel syndrome).

The physical signs include a typical facial appearance with periorbital puffiness and pallor, coarse and cold skin, slow movements, hoarse voice, slow pulse and a slowing of the recovery phase of the ankle jerk reflexes. Ischaemic heart disease is common. Central nervous system involvement may produce intellectual impairment and dementia (myxoedema madness) and coma (with hypothermia). Only 5% of patients presenting with hypothermia have hypothyroidism.

Investigation

• All suspected cases should be investigated: serum T_4 is reduced and this stimulates pituitary secretions of TSH (raised in primary hypothyroidism).

• The serum cholesterol is usually raised (p. 165) although not important in this diagnosis.
• Anaemia (normochromic or macrocytic).
• ECG shows slow rate and low voltage with flattened or inverted T waves.
• Rise in titre of thyroid antibodies.
NB Check for antithyroid drugs, e.g. lithium, amiodarone. Amiodarone is rich in iodine and also inhibits peripheral conversion of T_4 to T_3, making thyroid investigations difficult to interpret. Before starting treatment with amiodarone, basal T_3, T_4 and TSH levels should be checked to identify any underlying thyroid disease.

Treatment

T_4 is given in a dosage of 25–50 µg/day, starting with a low dose and raising it every month to achieve normal levels of TSH. The average maintenance dose is 125 µg/day. Free T_4 levels are above the normal range for the untreated patient. If ischaemic heart disease is present, the lowest dose should be used initially. Patients should be warned that treatment is for life. Osteoporosis is a long-term risk of overtreatment.

Autoimmune thyroiditis

This term usually refers to disorders of the thyroid gland in which circulating thyroid antibodies are present in the plasma; in addition, lymphoid and plasma cells are found in excess in the thyroid gland. The patients may be hypothyroid, euthyroid or hyperthyroid. Hashimoto disease refers to the condition in which autoimmune thyroiditis has produced a hard nodular goitre. Destruction of thyroid hormone-producing tissue causes a rise in TSH, which leads to thyroid enlargement. At this stage, the level of the circulating thyroid hormones, although reduced for that person, may be within the normal limits and there is no evidence of hypothyroidism. However, thyroid reserve is diminished, and later the free T_4 falls further and symptoms of hypothyroidism occur in about 2% per annum. By then the patient has a goitre that is often hard and sometimes nodular. In some patients the development of autoimmune hypothyroidism is associated with progressive fibrosis of the gland without the production of a goitre. These patients present with hypothyroidism without a goitre.

Clinical presentation
Hashimoto disease presents as a patient with a goitre who is either euthyroid or hypothyroid. The goitre must be distinguished from other types of non-toxic goitre and from carcinoma of the thyroid.

Investigation
Thyroid antibodies may be directed against thyroglobulin or the microsomal fraction of thyroid cells. The gland usually takes up a normal amount of iodine, i.e. the radioiodine uptake is within normal limits but there is faulty utilization of iodine, and the iodine is discharged from the gland by potassium perchlorate in about half the cases. The free T_4 is in the lower range of normal or in the hypothyroid free range.

Management
T_4 in full doses (p. 143) will suppress TSH, cause the gland to diminish in size and relieve any symptoms of hypothyroidism if present.

Acute thyroiditis
Although relatively uncommon, acute thyroiditis may often follow an upper respiratory tract infection or other microbial infection (e.g. measles, infectious mononucleosis, mumps, Coxsackie). There is fever and malaise, usually with some local swelling and tenderness of the gland and sometimes dysphagia. Initially there may be some hyperthyroidism. The serum T_4 may be normal or raised but the radioiodine uptake is suppressed. The differential diagnosis includes carcinoma (less tender but harder), haemorrhage into a cyst or Hashimoto thyroiditis. Pyogenic infection in the thyroid causes a more severe illness.

Management
Simple analgesia may suffice. Prednisolone 30 mg/day may be necessary and can usually be tailed off rapidly.

Thyroid cancer (p. 33)
All types are rare and some carry a relatively good prognosis. Ionizing radiation during childhood is a predisposing factor. The main types and their clinical features are as follow.

Papillary carcinoma is the most common type. It occurs in the relatively young and may present with neck lymph gland enlargement (p. 32). It is often TSH-dependent and regresses if thyroxine is given. The prognosis is relatively good.

Follicular carcinoma often produces functioning secondaries that are sensitive to radioiodine. It has a relatively good prognosis and is relatively common.

Anaplastic carcinoma usually presents with gland enlargement in the elderly and is highly malignant.

Medullary carcinoma is rare. It secretes calcitonin and may produce ectopic corticotrophin and other substances. It may be associated with a phaeochromocytoma in multiple endocrine neoplasia (MEN, p. 152). The prognosis is poor, although relatively better than anaplastic cancers. Relatives should be screened.

Thyroid nodules. A thyroid nodule that appears to be single is usually not single. Even if it is, the likelihood of malignancy is low. Ultrasound may distinguish solid from cystic lesions, but this does not distinguish between the presence and absence of thyroid carcinoma. Fine-needle biopsy and aspiration of fluid for cytology may miss a carcinoma and single cysts tend to refill. Surgical removal is preferred.

Pituitary

The hypothalamus controls the secretion of the anterior and posterior pituitary hormones. Hypothalamic nerve fibres liberate releasing factors that are carried in the portal blood stream to the pituitary gland and there cause release, synthesis or inhibition of pituitary hormones. At least nine factors have been suggested and three, corticotrophin-releasing hormone (CRH), thyrotrophin-releasing hormone (TRH) and gonadotrophin-releasing hormone (GnRH), have been isolated and their chemical structure determined. GnRH causes release of both luteinizing hormone (LH) and follicle-stimulating hormone (FSH). Prolactin (PRL) release is inhibited by dopamine.

The anterior lobe produces at least six types of hormone—growth hormone (GH), FSH, LH, TSH, adrenocorticotrophic hormone (ACTH) and PRL. The posterior lobe secretes two hormones, antidiuretic hormone (ADH) and oxytocin. The gland has a close anatomical and physiological relationship to the hypothalamus. The anatomical relationship to the optic chiasma is important and all patients with suspected pituitary tumours should have their visual fields plotted. X-ray of the pituitary fossa and computed tomography (CT) or magnetic resonance imaging (MRI) scan will accurately define the pituitary fossa.

The clinical features of pituitary disease differ according to the type of lesion and the region of the gland that is predominantly affected. All are rare and in examinations will have received some treatment. Failure of secretion is more common than increased secretion. Non-functional (chromophobe) adenoma is the most common cause of hypopituitarism. It also gives rise to increased intracranial pressure and to local pressure effects. Prolactinomas are the most common secreting tumours of the pituitary. They cause infertility and galactorrhoea in women, and impotence with gynaecomastia in men. The most common tumour in childhood is craniopharyngioma which often calcifies. Classically, eosinophilic tumours (rare) cause giantism in the child or acromegaly in the adult; basophil hyperplasia or adenoma produce Cushing syndrome. However, acromegaly may be associated with eosinophil, chromophobe or mixed-cell tumours.

Hypopituitarism

The pattern of deficiency depends on the nature of the lesion and its rate of progress. In general, deficiencies of GH, FSH and LH secretions occur early, TSH and ACTH next. Last of all, ADH secretion fails if the posterior lobe is involved by surgical intervention or suprasellar disease. Deficiency of each hormone is measured by suitable blood hormone assay and the integrity of the target organs assessed by applying the appropriate physiological stimulus, e.g. ACTH.

Aetiology

• Iatrogenic from hypophysectomy or irradiation—adequate replacement therapy prevents symptoms occurring.
• Non-functional (chromophobe) adenoma.
• Postpartum pituitary necrosis in the female (Sheehan syndrome). This is now extremely rare with improved standards of obstetric care.
• Other tumours (including secondary tumours), granulomas (sarcoid and tuberculosis) and head injury—all rare.

Clinical presentation

In children hypopituitarism produces pituitary infantilism (Peter Pan dwarfs—small but well-formed and in proportion). In adults the presentation depends upon the pattern of deficiency of the various hormones and associated pressure symptoms. The symptoms and signs can be worked out from knowledge of the functions of the target organs involved.

Hormone deficiency
Loss of sexual function occurs, both primary with amenorrhoea and loss of libido, and secondary with loss of body hair (male patients may find shaving unnecessary).

Adrenal insufficiency (p. 150) from failure of ACTH occurs but there is little change in electrolyte metabolism because aldosterone is still secreted.

Pallor and skin depigmentation occur.

Symptoms of hypothyroidism from lack of TSH appear but there is no myxoedema—the face is not coarsened.

Coma may occur from low cortisol levels, spontaneous hypoglycaemia or hypothermia.

Pressure effects
Compression of the optic chiasma produces bitemporal hemianopia and optic atrophy.

Pressure on the hypothalamus may cause somnolence and weight gain.

NB In the male, hypopituitarism is usually caused by a non-functional adenoma or large prolactinoma. In Sheehan syndrome, there is a history of postpartum haemorrhage, failure of lactation with atrophy of breast tissue and amenorrhoea in addition to the other effects described.

Investigation
Assessment of pituitary function involves:
• measurement of pituitary hormones (TSH, ACTH, FSH, LH, GH and PRL);
• measurement of target organ secretion (thyroid and adrenal, and sex hormones); and
• dynamic tests of hypothalamic pituitary function:
    (a) Synacthen (tetracosactrin) test (p. 151);
    (b) TRH stimulation test;
    (c) metyrapone test (p. 149);
    (d) LH-releasing hormone test;
    (e) the insulin hypoglycaemia test is potentially lethal in inexperienced hands.

Treatment
The pituitary is removed if there are pressure symptoms, particularly visual loss, unless a prolactinoma is present, when bromocriptine usually shrinks the tumour without surgery.

Replacement therapy by:
• cyclical oestrogen–progesterone therapy in women. Intramuscular depot testosterone esters every 2–4 weeks (e.g. Sustanon 250), or testosterone patches in men;
• hydrocortisone 20 mg in the morning and 10 mg at night. Fludrocortisone is not usually required;
• T_4 0.1–0.3 mg/day (100–300 μg/day);
• coma is treated as in Addisonian crisis (p. 150).

Acromegaly
Excess GH gives acromegaly in the adult (after the epiphyses have fused) and giantism in earlier life. The onset is between 20 and 40 years.

Giantism is almost always the result of the action of excessive secretion of GH before the epiphyses have united. Later in life pituitary failure tends to occur and giants are therefore not usually strong, aggressive or virile.

Aetiology
There is excessive secretion of GH from an adenoma of the pituitary, often of eosinophil cells. GH causes overgrowth of soft tissues, including the skin, tongue and viscera and of bones. It has an anti-insulin action.

Clinical presentation
The onset is insidious, often with early changes (look at old photographs). Headache occurs early because of stretching of the dura mater. Pressure effects with bitemporal hemianopia are rarer. Excessive secretion of GH causes the following.
• Face—increase in size of skull, supraorbital ridges, lower jaw (separation of teeth) and the sinuses.
• The tongue is enlarged.
• Vertebral enlargement, and kyphosis from osteoporosis.
• Hands and feet are spade-shaped and carpal tunnel syndrome may be present.
• Enlarged heart, liver and thyroid.
• Hypertension (15%).
• Diabetes mellitus (10%) and reduced glucose tolerance (30%).
• Arthropathy (50%).
    The following also occur:
• acne, hirsutes, excessive sweating;
• gynaecomastia and galactorrhoea (prolactin excess); and
• hypogonadism, oligomenorrhoea.

Investigation
• Assay of GH by radioimmunoassay; the levels are raised only in active disease and are not suppressed by glucose in a standard glucose tolerance test.
• Perimetry for bitemporal visual field defects (50%).
• X-ray of skull for enlargement of the sella, erosion of the clinoid processes, supraorbital ridges and lower jaw. The floor of the pituitary fossa may appear eroded or double in lateral-view tomograms.

- CT or MRI scan to show suprasellar extension.
- X-ray of hands for tufting of the terminal phalanges and increased joint spaces because of hypertrophy of the cartilage. The heel pad is usually thickened. These tests are interesting rather than diagnostic.
- Serum glucose may be raised.
- Fasting serum phosphate may be raised but is of no diagnostic value.
- Chest X-ray and ECG may show left ventricular hypertrophy from hypertension.

Prognosis and treatment

Life expectancy is halved as a result of cardiorespiratory complications. Successful management means destruction of the tissue producing excess GH. Surgery is indicated for progressive visual deterioration (regular perimetry is obligatory) and some would recommend it for all those with acromegaly who are fit for surgery. Transsphenoidal hypophysectomy is the treatment of choice. Craniotomy is sometimes used in those with suprasellar extension. Yttrium-90 implants or external irradiation are alternatives to surgical removal in active disease, but may cause further damage to the optic tracts, diabetes insipidus and aseptic bone necrosis, and have much lower cure rates. Cerebrospinal rhinorrhoea may result from yttrium implantation. Bromocriptine reduces GH and PRL levels and may be a useful adjunct to conventional therapy or used as sole therapy. Unlike destructive therapies, diabetes insipidus is not produced. Somatostatin analogues (octreotide) may be used, particularly for young patients, male or female, who wish to retain fertility.

Diabetes insipidus

A very rare disease caused by deficiency of ADH (vasopressin).

Aetiology

- Idiopathic, often familial and the most common form.
- Tumours: craniopharyngioma or secondary tumour.
- Surgery or radiation to pituitary gland.
- Head injury—usually mild and short-lived.

Rarely complete and permanent with transaction of the pituitary stalk with frontal vault fractures.
- Granulomas, e.g. sarcoid; or infections, e.g. basal meningitis.

Clinical presentation

Polyuria and polydipsia—5–20 l urine/24 h.

Investigation

The specific gravity of the urine is very low and fails to increase with water deprivation. Fluids are allowed overnight and stopped in the morning. It is dangerous to lose more than 2–3% of the body weight. In normal people plasma osmolality does not rise above 300 mosmol/kg and urine osmolality rises to 600 mosmol/kg during 8 h of water deprivation. In diabetes insipidus the former rises and the latter does not, or remains at about plasma level. Vasopressin corrects the abnormality in ADH-deficient diabetes insipidus but not in the nephrogenic type.

Differential diagnosis

Psychogenic polydipsia. Thirst dominates the picture. The patient resents the water deprivation test, and surreptitious drinking is common. Renal concentrating power may be moderately reduced because of the prolonged polyuria and consequent low medullary osmolality.

Nephrogenic diabetes insipidus. This refers to a vasopressin (ADH)-resistant polyuria. This is a rare sex-linked recessive inherited disorder with a primary renal tubular defect of water reabsorption. Secondary nephrogenic diabetes insipidus occurs with:
- diabetes mellitus (glycosuria);
- chronic renal failure;
- postobstructive uropathy;
- hypercalcaemia;
- hypokalaemia; and
- lithium toxicity.

Treatment

Desmopressin (DDAVP or arginine vasopressin) nasal spray 10–20 µg b.d. has replaced lysine vasopressin in the treatment of ADH deficiency.

Carbamazepine 200–400 mg/day may increase the renal response to ADH. Chlorpropamide (100–300 mg/day) acts similarly but is obsolescent because of the risk of hypoglycaemia.

Thiazide diuretics probably act by reducing glomerular filtration rate and are also used in nephrogenic diabetes insipidus.

Prolactinoma

These tumours cause galactorrhoea in both sexes and gonadal dysfunction—infertility in the female and impotence in the male. Measurement of PRL levels suggests the diagnosis usually before pressure symptoms occur. The tumours vary in size from pinhead (microadenoma) to very large (rare) and may necrose. Hyperprolactinaemia may be caused by a variety of physiological stimuli such as pregnancy and stress and by certain drugs such as oestrogens and tranquillizers. Dopamine receptor stimulants (e.g. bromocriptine and cabergoline) inhibit PRL secretion and are usually tried before surgery or radiotherapy. Visual fields need checking periodically because pituitary tumours may press on the optic chiasma to cause a bitemporal field loss. If the patient becomes pregnant, a small tumour may enlarge rapidly.

Adrenal

Adrenal glands

The medulla secretes adrenaline and noradrenaline (epinephrine and norepinephrine). The cortex produces steroid hormones, of which the most important are cortisol (hydrocortisone) and aldosterone. The secretion of most of the steroids is controlled by pituitary corticotrophin (ACTH) which itself is released by the hypothalamic hormone—corticotrophin-releasing hormone factor (CRF). The secretion of aldosterone is independent of the pituitary and controlled by the renin–aldosterone system. The adrenals also produce androgens and oestrogens. The effects of the three main groups of adrenocortical hormones differ. In summary, they are as follow.

Glucocorticoids (e.g. cortisol)

These raise the blood sugar and antagonize insulin. They have a permissive effect on the action of catecholamines on the heart and blood vessels and are essential for the body's response to shock. They suppress the reaction to injury, infection and inflammation. In excess they have a protein catabolic effect, atrophy skin and weaken capillaries. They reduce the circulating eosinophil and lymphocyte counts. They cause sodium retention and potassium depletion and alkalosis when given in large doses or over long periods.

Mineralocorticoids (e.g. aldosterone)

These cause sodium retention and potassium depletion, with hypertension, alkalosis and oedema. The synthetic steroids, fludrocortisone and deoxycorticosterone acetate, have similar actions.

Sex hormones

These produce effects depending on the dominance of male hormone, e.g. androsterone, or female hormone, e.g. oestrogens and progesterone. Hence, they may be virilizing or feminizing. Androgens antagonize some of the metabolic effects of the glucocorticoids.

Cushing syndrome
Aetiology

The syndrome is the result of excess corticosteroids and by far the most common cause is prolonged treatment with relatively large doses of oral corticosteroids. Most of the synthetic analogues of cortisone produce these side-effects but they are less liable to give rise to sodium retention. Apart from iatrogenic disease, this disorder is very rare.

Other causes are as follow.
• Basophil or chromophobe hyperplasia or adenoma of the pituitary gland, with excess production of corticotrophin (60%). This produces bilateral adrenal hyperplasia and is called pituitary-dependent Cushing syndrome but is properly called Cushing disease.
• Primary tumours of the adrenals, either adenoma (20%) or carcinoma (10%).
• Secondary to carcinoma elsewhere—usually

an oat cell carcinoma of the bronchus causing the ectopic ACTH syndrome. Other sites are the thymus, pancreas, thyroid or ovary. Pigmentation may occur in this condition.

Clinical presentation
The onset is insidious.
• Alteration in appearance with redistribution of body fat, 'mooning' of the face and truncal or 'buffalo' obesity (about 90%). The limbs are often spared but the obesity may be generalized. Growth is retarded in children.
• Protein breakdown leads to muscle weakness which may present as a proximal myopathy, wide purple striae (50%) on the abdomen, thighs and buttocks, and easy bruising (30%). The striae of obesity are pink.
• Osteoporosis with backache and vertebral collapse (50%).
• Disturbance of carbohydrate tolerance which may amount to diabetes (10%).
• Electrolyte disturbance with sodium retention, potassium loss and hypokalaemic alkalosis, especially in the ectopic ACTH syndrome, where ACTH levels are very high. Renal stones may occur (20%).
• Hypertension, probably related to sodium retention (60%).
• Masculinization caused by adrenal androgens —amenorrhoea, hirsutism, deep voice, greasy skin with acne in the female (80%).
• Mental disturbance—depression or mania and sometimes exaggeration of previous psychiatric abnormalities.
NB Almost all of these can be produced by large doses of corticosteroids.

Investigation
Screening tests for cortisol excess
Cortisol levels. Measuring random plasma cortisol levels is of little value. Loss of the normal circadian rhythm is commonly found. Twenty-four-hour urinary free cortisol reflects total cortisol production and is the most useful screening test.

Dexamethasone suppression test. Dexamethasone 2 mg at midnight normally suppresses plasma cortisol to < 200 nmol/l 8 h later.

If these tests suggest excess cortisol production, the following will confirm the diagnosis and establish the aetiology.
• ACTH levels are high in pituitary-dependent Cushing syndrome (Cushing disease) or ectopic production. ACTH levels are low in patients with adrenal adenomas.
• Dexamethasone 2 mg 6-hourly for 3 days suppresses urinary cortisol levels in Cushing syndrome, but not adrenal lesions, which are usually autonomous.
• Patients with Cushing disease demonstrate an exaggerated rise in ACTH and cortisol in response to CRH, whereas patients with ectopic ACTH secretion or adrenal adenomas fail to respond.
• CT or MRI scanning of the pituitary may demonstrate an adenoma, or abdominal CT scanning may reveal an adrenal lesion.

Management
Hypophysectomy is the treatment of choice for pituitary-dependent Cushing syndrome. When bilateral adrenalectomy is performed to treat Cushing syndrome caused by a pituitary basophil or chromophobe adenoma, Nelson syndrome may result with hyperpigmentation from excess β-lipotrophin activity (melanocyte-stimulating hormone (MSH) and ACTH) that is now not suppressed by high blood cortisol.

If the disease is primarily adrenal (yet to be called 'adrenal-dependent Cushing syndrome'), unilateral or bilateral adrenalectomy is performed and the latter is followed by replacement therapy with cortisol 20–40 mg/day and fludrocortisone 0.1 mg/day.

Removal of ectopic ACTH sources is rarely possible (bronchial carcinoma).

Metyrapone is a competitive inhibitor of 11 β-hydroxylation in the adrenal cortex, and can be used to help control symptoms of Cushing syndrome, or prepare patients for surgery. It inhibits cortisol production, leading to an increase in ACTH and can be used as a test of anterior pituitary function (p. 146).

Conn syndrome
(primary hyperaldosteronism)
This is a very rare condition caused by a

solitary benign adenoma or hyperplasia of the zona glomerulosa producing excess aldosterone.

Clinical presentation

Hypokalaemia results in muscle weakness, often in attacks. Polyuria and polydipsia are secondary to the hypokalaemia.

Sodium retention often leading to hypertension, but there is usually no oedema.

It may mimic hypertension from other causes, especially when potassium-losing diuretics are being given, or Cushing syndrome.

Investigation

The condition is marked by renal potassium wasting, i.e. serum potassium reduced often < 3 mmol and urinary potassium increased for serum blood level. It is usually associated with a metabolic alkalosis. The serum sodium is usually > 140 mmol.

Stop diuretics for 3 days and if potassium is still < 3.2 mmol check the urinary output of potassium: if it is < 20 mmol this is appropriate to the blood concentration and is probably normal; if it is > 30 mmol further investigation for primary hyperaldosteronism is required.

The serum renin is low and this differentiates it from secondary aldosteronism (which occurs in the nephrotic syndrome, cirrhosis of the liver with ascites and, rarely, in congestive cardiac failure and bronchial carcinoma).

The best screening test is a 24-h urinary aldosterone. If this is raised, take a plasma specimen at 7 a.m. from a rested and recumbent patient for renin and aldosterone.

Management

Surgical resection should be considered because some tumours are malignant. Spironolactone is an antagonist to aldosterone and may be given in primary or secondary aldosteronism.

Adrenogenital syndrome

This is a very rare condition of infancy or childhood caused by a congenital enzyme defect (usually of 21-hydroxylase) affecting cortisol synthesis. The resulting decrease in circulating cortisol stimulates overproduction of ACTH, which in turn stimulates the adrenals to produce an excess of androgenic steroids. Females show virilization early in life and are treated with cortisol. Males are less often diagnosed and may die in acute adrenal insufficiency but, if the infant survives, growth is excessive although precocious puberty results in a short final height. Treat with corticosteroids sufficient to suppress excess ACTH.

Adrenal insufficiency

(Addison's disease)

Acute

Adrenal crisis. There is apathy, coma and epigastric pain. The blood sugar is low. It occurs after trauma, severe hypotension and sepsis.

Less commonly, it may occur in patients previously (within 1–1 1/2 years) or currently being treated with corticosteroids when there is trauma, surgery or acute infection or withdrawal of steroids. It may follow surgical removal of the adrenals for Cushing syndrome or in the treatment of breast carcinoma unless there is adequate replacement therapy.

NB The Waterhouse–Friderichsen syndrome of severe acute meningococcal septicaemia, associated with purpura, is usually associated with raised levels of circulating corticosteroids despite the massive bilateral adrenal haemorrhage. Adrenal haemorrhage is frequently found at postmortem as a non-specific finding.

Chronic

There is insidious onset of weakness and fatigue with gastrointestinal symptoms of anorexia, weight loss, nausea, vomiting, intermittent abdominal pain and diarrhoea. Hypotension, often postural, and tachycardia occur late in the disease. Hyperpigmentation occurs in exposed areas, friction areas, hand creases and buccal mucosa.

Chronic adrenal insufficiency (Addison's disease) is rare (4/100 000 prevalence in UK) and causes include: autoimmune adrenal destruction; adrenal infiltration with secondary carcinoma, Hodgkin or leukaemic tissue;

destruction in tuberculosis, haemochromatosis, amyloidosis and histoplasmosis where prevalent. It may be associated with other organ-specific autoimmune disease, especially Hashimoto thyroiditis (Schmidt syndrome).

It may occur secondary to hypopituitarism (p. 145) during treatment of adrenal (or renal) tuberculosis and in the adrenogenital syndrome (p. 150).

Investigation
Plasma cortisol levels are usually low and show no diurnal variation.

No increase in output after tetracosactride (Synacthen). Serum electrolytes are usually normal but in impending crisis the sodium may be low, the potassium high and the blood urea raised.

There is a high plasma ACTH.

Screening of basal function
Both 24-h urinary free cortisol and 8 a.m. cortisol levels may be well in the normal range, even in strongly suspected cases.

A *single basal plasma ACTH assay* shows high levels in primary adrenal disease and undetectable values in pituitary disease.

Dynamic tests
Synacthen (tetracosactride) tests
• *Short Synacthen test.* Give 250 μg i.m. and take blood at 0, 30 and 60 min. In normal subjects, the initial level should be > 170 nmol/l (6 μg/dl), and rise by at least 190 nmol/l (7 μg/dl) to > 580 nmol/l (21 μg/dl). If the response is flat, proceed to a long Synacthen test.
• *Five-hour test* to 1 mg of depot tetracosactride. In normal patients, the serum cortisol more than doubles in the first hour.

Treatment
Maintenance therapy—hydrocortisone 20 mg a.m. and 10 mg p.m. and fludrocortisone 0.1 mg/day. The dosage is adjusted according to response as judged by lying and standing blood pressure, plasma urea and electrolytes and clinically.

In acute crisis—intravenous hydrocortisone 100 mg 6-hourly, intravenous saline and gluc-ose are required. Underlying infection must be treated.

Phaeochromocytoma
This is usually a benign tumour of the adrenal medulla. It can arise from other chromaffin tissues of the sympathetic nervous system, e.g. the para-aortic ganglia, and it may be associated with neurofibromatosis. Medullary thyroid carcinoma (calcitonin-producing) and parathyroid adenoma are associated with it (p. 152). Very rarely is it malignant.

It is a very rare cause of hypertension (< 1 in 200) but it is important to recognize, because it is treatable. It can be familial and bilateral.

Clinical presentation
The clinical features depend on the activity of the tumour and the relative amounts of adrenaline (epinephrine) with β- and some α-effects, and noradrenaline (norepinephrine) with α-effects. Usually, α-effects predominate. Some tumours secrete intermittently.

The β-effects include a rise in systolic blood pressure with an increase in heart rate, increase in the cardiac output and dilatation of muscle vessels. The α-effects include a rise in both systolic and diastolic blood pressure with reflex slowing of the heart rate and constriction of blood vessels.

A few patients have normal blood pressure between attacks of paroxysmal hypertension, but most are hypertensive all the time. In a typical attack there is pallor, palpitation, anxiety and sometimes angina, headache, sweating and nausea. The blood pressure may be very high and death may occur from myocardial infarction or a cerebrovascular accident. Hyperglycaemia may occur if adrenaline (epinephrine) is secreted.

NB Paroxysmal bradycardia (an α-effect) may occur.

Investigation
Estimation of catecholamines (adrenaline and noradrenaline (epinephrine and norepinephrine)) in the blood or urine or the urinary metabolite vanillylmandelic acid (VMA) or hydroxymethylmandelic acid (HMMA).

Abdominal CT or MRI scan will usually show the tumour. The patient must be fully α- and β-blocked before any interventional investigation or surgery.

Treatment

The tyrosine hydroxylase inhibitor metirosine blocks the synthesis of catecholamines and is used, together with an α-adrenoreceptor blocker, for preoperative management and for those unsuitable for surgery. Plasma volume must be monitored throughout the period and during surgery the central venous pressure should be monitored because changes in pulse and blood pressure are blocked.

In emergencies, α-effects may be antagonized by phentolamine and β-effects by propranolol.

Multiple endocrine neoplasia

(MEN syndromes)

There are two main autosomal dominant (chromosome 10) syndromes. Tumours originate from two or more endocrine (or neural) tissues and produce peptide hormones. They are very rare.

MEN type I refers to benign adenomas of parathyroid, pancreatic islets and anterior pituitary (PRL). The islet cell tumours produce effects which depend on their cellular origin: insulinoma (hypoglycaemia), gastrinoma (Zollinger–Ellison syndrome), glucagonoma (hyperglycaemia) and vasoactive intestinal polypeptide-secreting tumour (VIPoma, p. 233).

MEN type 2a refers to the association of calcitonin-producing medullary thyroid carcinoma (MTC), phaeochromocytoma, (commonly bilateral, and occasionally malignant) and, less commonly, parathyroid adenoma or hyperplasia. Over 90% have a defect in the proto-oncogene that encodes a tyrosine kinase receptor.

MEN type 2b refers to the very rare association of type 2a features with Marfanoid habitus, mucosal neuromas and multiple colonic diverticula with megacolon.

Families tend to run true. Patients with any one of the above tumours should be clinically, biochemically and genetically screened for others within the type and, if these are discovered, all other members of the family too. In type 2, perform a pentagastrin-stimulated calcitonin test plus serum calcium and assay of catecholamines. These are also used to assess complete removal of tumour and for early recognition of recurrence. Total thyroidectomy in infancy is performed prophylactically for those at risk of medullary thyroid carcinoma.

Shortness of stature

The common cause is short parents. Other causes are:
• Deficiency of GH—sometimes familial (see *Hypopituitarism*, p. 145), often associated with delayed or failure of sexual development. Bone age is retarded.
• Bone diseases, e.g. achondroplasia and rickets.
• Malnutrition, including the malabsorption syndrome.
• Renal (relatively common), liver or heart failure in early childhood.
• Large doses of steroids in childhood.
• Cretinism and childhood hypothyroidism.

Metabolic Disease

Diabetes mellitus

The prevalence of diabetes mellitus in adults worldwide was estimated to be 4.0% in 1995, and is expected to rise to 5.4% by 2025.

The American Diabetes Association/World Health Organization (WHO) recommend that the diagnosis of diabetes mellitus is based on positive findings from any two of the following on different days:

• symptoms of diabetes + casual plasma glucose > 11.1 mmol/l;
• fasting plasma glucose > 7.0 mmol/l;
• 2-h postprandial diabetes > 11.1 mmol/l (after 75 g oral glucose).

(Report of the Expert Committee on the Diagnosis and Classification of Diabetes Mellitus. *Diabetes Care* 1997; **20**: 1183–1197.)

Classification (Table 11.1)

The two major clinical syndromes called 'diabetes', type 1 and type 2, have little else in common apart from the raised blood glucose and the direct long-term consequences of this.

Type 1 diabetes mellitus (insulin-dependent diabetes mellitus; IDDM) is an autoimmune disorder in which the insulin-producing β cells of the pancreas are destroyed. Patients tend to be under 30 years old, experience an acute onset of the disease, are dependent upon insulin therapy, and prone to ketosis.

Type 2 diabetes mellitus is the more common form, accounting for 90% of patients with diabetes. Patients are typically obese, older adults with such mild symptoms that diagnosis may occur late in the disease, often from complications such as retinopathy or cardiovascular disease. Insensitivity of the tissues to insulin (insulin resistance) and inadequate pancreatic β-cell response to blood glucose are characteristic, leading to overproduction of glucose by the liver and under utilization by the tissues. Ketosis is unusual as patients have sufficient insulin to prevent lipolysis. Although initially controlled with diet and oral hypoglycaemics, many patients eventually need supplemental insulin, making them insulin-requiring type 2 diabetics. Those from the Indian Subcontinent and the Caribbean who move to the UK appear to be particularly at risk.

Gestational diabetes. Most women who develop diabetes during pregnancy have normal glucose homeostasis during the first half of the pregnancy and develop a relative insulin deficiency during the second half, leading to hyperglycaemia. The hyperglycaemia resolves in most women after delivery, but places them at increased risk of developing type 2 diabetes later in life.

Other specific types of diabetes

Secondary diabetes results from:

• hormonal antagonism of insulin: Cushing syndrome, acromegaly, phaeochromocytoma, hyperthyroidism and, more rarely, glucogonoma, somatostatinoma, aldosteronoma;
• pancreatic destruction: carcinoma of the pancreas, pancreatitis, pancreatectomy, cystic fibrosis, haemochromatosis;
• drugs: thiazide diuretics, α-interferon, tacrolimus, diazoxide; and
• infections: congenital rubella, cytomegalovirus.

TYPES OF DIABETES MELLITUS

Clinical classes	Distinguishing characteristics
Type 1 insulin-dependent diabetes mellitus (IDDM)	Patients are usually thin or have lost weight and usually have abrupt onset of signs and symptoms with insulinopenia before age 30. These patients often have strongly positive ketonuria and are dependent upon insulin to prevent ketoacidosis and to sustain life
Type 2 non-insulin-dependent diabetes mellitus (NIDDM; obese or non-obese)	Patients usually are older than 40 years at diagnosis, obese and have relatively few classic symptoms. They are not prone to ketoacidosis except during periods of stress. Although not dependent upon exogenous insulin for survival, they may require it for stress-induced hyperglycaemia, and hyperglycaemia that persists in spite of other therapy
Other specific types of diabetes	
	Diabetes mellitus caused by hormonal antagonism of insulin, pancreatic destruction, drugs, infections
GDM	Patients with GDM have onset or discovery of glucose intolerance during pregnancy

GDM, Gestational diabetes mellitus; IGT, impaired glucose tolerance.

Table 11.1 Types of diabetes mellitus and other categories of glucose intolerance.

Genetics

Type 1 diabetes mellitus

The identical twin of a patient with type 1 diabetes has a 30–50% chance of developing the disease, implying that both genetic and environmental factors are involved.

Two chromosome regions have been established as being associated with, and linked to, type 1 diabetes: the MHC class II region (designated IDDM1; 6p21) and the insulin gene region (IDDM2; 11p15). Genes at other loci are likely to be important, and IDDM was the first complex genetic disorder to be studied by genome-wide screening of affected sibling pairs. Several other loci have been identified by genome scanning, although different research groups have reported apparently conflicting results. However, it is likely that a consensus will emerge in the near future.

Type 2 diabetes mellitus

There is usually a family history, although inheritance is likely to involve interaction between multiple genes involved in both insulin secretion and insulin action. The identification of such genes has been aided by studies of an early-onset form of type 2 diabetes known as maturity onset diabetes of the young (MODY). MODY has an autosomal dominant inheritance, with different genetic defects being identified in different pedigrees. Mutations in the gene for insulin, the genes for insulin processing enzymes, and the gene for the insulin receptor have all been detected. For example, a defect in the insulin promoter factor-1 gene has been implicated as a cause of MODY4, and identified as a significant risk factor for type 2 diabetes.

Other genetic syndromes sometimes associated with diabetes include Down syndrome, Turner syndrome, Friedreich's ataxia, Huntington's chorea, Laurence–Moon–Biedl syndrome, myotonic dystrophy, porphyria and Prader–Willi syndrome.

Complications

Long-term complications occur in all forms of diabetes. Although the development of complications is unpredictable, good glycaemic control prevents or ameliorates diabetic microvascular complications in patients with type 1 and type 2 diabetes (see Trials Box 11.1).

TRIALS BOX 11.1

The **Finnish Diabetes Prevention Study Group** randomly assigned 522 middle-aged, overweight subjects (172 men and 350 women; mean age, 55 years; mean body mass index (BMI), 31) with impaired glucose tolerance to either an intervention group, which received individualized counselling aimed at reducing weight, total intake of fat, and intake of saturated fat and increasing intake of fibre and physical activity, or a control group. The cumulative incidence of diabetes after 4 years was 11% in the intervention group and 23% in the control group. During the trial, the risk of diabetes was reduced by 58% in the intervention group. *N Engl J Med* 2001; **344**: 1343–1350.

The **RENAAL (Reduction of Endpoints in NIDDM with Angiotensin II Antagonist Losartan) Study Investigators** assessed the role of the angiotensin-II-receptor antagonist losartan in patients with type 2 diabetes and nephropathy. A total of 1513 patients were randomized to losartan or placebo, both taken in addition to conventional antihypertensive treatment (calcium-channel antagonists, diuretics, α-blockers, β-blockers, and centrally acting agents) for a mean of 3.4 years. Losartan reduced the incidence of a doubling of the serum creatinine concentration and end-stage renal disease but had no effect on the rate of death. The benefit exceeded that attributable to changes in blood pressure. *N Engl J Med* 2001; **345**: 861–869.

The **Patients with Type 2 Diabetes and Microalbuminuria Study Group** evaluated the effect of the angiotensin-II-receptor antagonist irbesartan in 590 hypertensive patients with type 2 diabetes and microalbuminuria over a 2-year period. Irbesartan slowed progression to diabetic nephropathy, defined by persistent albuminuria in overnight specimens, independently of its blood-pressure-lowering effect. *N Engl J Med* 2001; **345**: 870–878.

Lewis *et al.* randomly assigned 1715 hypertensive patients with nephropathy caused by type 2 diabetes to treatment with the angiotensin-II-receptor blocker irbesartan, amlodipine, or placebo. Treatment with irbesartan over a mean of 2.6 years was associated with a relative risk of end-stage renal disease that was 23% lower than that in both other groups. This protection against the progression of nephropathy was independent of the reduction in blood pressure irbesartan caused. *N Engl J Med* 2001; **345**: 851–860.

The **United Kingdom Prospective Diabetes Study (UKPDS)** randomized 3867 newly diagnosed patients with type 2 diabetes into a conventional policy (aim at a fasting plasma glucose < 15 mmol/l) and an intensive glucose control policy (< 6 mmol/l). At 10 years, HbA1c values were 7.9 and 7.0%, respectively. The intensive policy reduced the risk of diabetes-related endpoints (microvascular, macrovascular and cataract extraction) by 12%; microvascular (chiefly retinal) by 25%. 1148 patients who also had hypertension were randomized into tight and less tight blood pressure control policies achieving mean levels of 154/87 and 144/82 respectively over 8.4 years. Captopril and atenolol were of similar effectiveness. The 'tight' policy reduced the risk of all diabetes-related endpoints by 24%, microvascular endpoints by 37%, strokes by 44%, and deterioration of vision by 47%. A log–linear relationship between the incidence of complications and increasing HbA1c or systolic blood pressure indicated that any reduction in glycaemic or blood pressure control would be advantageous. http://www.dtu.ox.ac.uk/ukpds.

The **Heart Outcomes Prevention Study** randomized 3577 patients with diabetes, who had a previous cardiovascular event or at least one other cardiovascular risk factor, but no clinical proteinuria, heart failure, or low ejection fraction to receive either ramipril or placebo, and vitamin E or placebo, according to a two-by-two factorial design. The study was stopped early because of a consistent benefit of ramipril. Ramipril lowered the risk of myocardial infarction by 22%, stroke by 33%, cardiovascular death by 37%, total mortality by 24%, revascularization by 17%, and overt nephropathy by 24%. The cardiovascular benefit was greater than that attributable to the decrease in blood pressure. *Lancet* 2000; **355**: 253–259.

STOP Hypertension-2 studied 6614 elderly patients aged 70–84 years, 719 of whom had diabetes mellitus at the start of the study (mean age 75.8 years). Patients were randomly assigned to one of three treatment strategies: conventional antihypertensive drugs (diuretics or β-blockers), calcium antagonists, or angiotensin-converting enzyme (ACE) inhibitors. Reduction in blood pressure and prevention of cardiovascular mortality was similar in the three treatment groups of diabetics. However, there were significantly fewer myocardial infarctions during ACE inhibitor treatment than during calcium antagonist treatment. *J Hypertens* 2000; **18**: 1671–1675.

The **Fosinopril vs. Amlodipine Cardiovascular Events Randomized Trial (FACET)** compared the effects of fosinopril and amlodipine on serum lipids and diabetes control in 380 patients with type 2 diabetes and hypertension over 3.5 years. Both treatments were effective in lowering blood pressure and there was no significant difference in total serum cholesterol, high-density lipoprotein (HDL) cholesterol, HbA1c, fasting serum glucose, or plasma insulin. The patients receiving fosinopril had a significantly lower risk of the combined outcome of acute myocardial infarction, stroke or hospitalized angina than those receiving amlodipine. *Diabetes Care* 1998; **21** (4): 597–603.

The **Appropriate Blood Pressure Control in Diabetes (ABCD) Trial** compared the effects of moderate control of blood pressure (target diastolic pressure, 80–89 mmHg) with those of intensive control of blood pressure (diastolic pressure, 75 mmHg) on the incidence and progression of complications of diabetes. The study also compared nisoldipine with enalapril as a first-line antihypertensive agent. The mean blood pressure achieved was 132/78 mmHg in the intensive group and 138/86 mmHg in the moderate control group. Blood pressure control of 138/86 or 132/78 mmHg with either nisoldipine or enalapril as the initial antihypertensive medication appeared to stabilize renal function in hypertensive type 2 diabetic patients without overt albuminuria over a 5-year period. The more intensive blood pressure control decreased all-cause mortality. *Diabetes Care* 2000; **23** (Suppl 2): B54–64.

The study found a significantly higher incidence of fatal and non-fatal myocardial infarction (a secondary endpoint) among those assigned to therapy with the calcium-channel blocker nisoldipine than among those assigned to receive enalapril. *N Engl J Med* 1998; **338**: 645–652.

The **Microalbuminuria Collaborative Study Group, United Kingdom** compared the effects of intensive therapy with continuous subcutaneous infusion or multiple daily injections of insulin with conventional therapy in 70 insulin-dependent diabetics with microalbuminuria. Intensive therapy had no impact on the progression of albuminuria. Blood pressure, rather than glycaemic control, seemed to be the main determinant of progression of microalbuminuria. *Br Med J* 1995; **311**: 973–977.

The **European Microalbuminuria Captopril Study Group** compared the effect of captopril and placebo in 92 non-hypertensive patients with insulin-dependent diabetes and microalbuminuria. Captopril impeded progression to proteinuria and prevented any increase in albumin excretion rate. *J Am Med Assoc* 1994; **271**: 275–279.

The **Diabetes Control and Complications Trial Research Group** compared intensive and standard treatment in 1441 patients with type 1 diabetes (mean age 27) over a 6.5-year period. In all, 726 patients had no retinopathy (primary prevention), whereas 715 had mild retinopathy (secondary prevention). Intensive treatment involved insulin given by a pump, or by three or more injections daily, with dosages adjusted according to blood glucose measured at least four times daily. Standard treatment involved insulin given once or twice daily, with once-daily monitoring of blood or urinary glucose. Intensive treatment reduced the risk of developing retinopathy by 76% in the primary prevention group, and reduced the risk of worsening retinopathy by 54% in the secondary prevention group. In both groups the risk of developing albuminuria was reduced by 54%, and the risk of neuropathy by 60%. *N Engl J Med* 1993; **329**: 977–986.

Mathiesen *et al*. studied the effect of captopril in 44 normotensive insulin-dependent diabetics with microalbuminuria. Captopril postponed the development of clinical proteinuria when compared with no treatment. *Br Med J* 1991; **303**: 81–87.

The UK Prospective Diabetes Study (UKPDS, p. 155) showed that after 10 years of type 2 diabetes patients have a twofold greater mortality than the general population, and one-third of patients have a macro- or microvascular (eyes or kidneys) complication that requires clinical attention.

Vascular complications
Large-vessel disease. Vascular complications account for 75% of deaths. The incidence of coronary artery occlusion at postmortem is five times higher in diabetics than non-diabetics, regardless of age or sex. There is a 2–3 times increased risk of coronary heart disease and myocardial infarction. Peripheral artery occlusion in the legs is 40 times more common in diabetics, leading to claudication, rest pain, ulcer formation and gangrene.

Small-vessel disease (diabetic microangiopathy) produces renal failure, invariably associated with retinopathy, and gangrene of the skin and feet with wedge-shaped infarcts—arterial pulses in the feet are usually present and the skin is warm.

Eye

Diabetic eye disease is the most common cause of visual loss in adults of working age in the UK. Fifty per cent of patients have *background retinopathy* after 10 years of diabetes. In the early stages, when treatment is most effective, there are no warning visual symptoms. Routine expert screening of the retina is part of good diabetic care. Controllable risk factors include hypertension and smoking. It is characterized by:

- microaneurysms—focal dilatations of capillary walls, not visible with the ophthalmoscope;
- dot or blot intraretinal haemorrhages;
- soft (cotton-wool) exudates caused by microinfarction of superficial nerve fibres;
- hard exudates caused by leakage of plasma into the retina; and
- retinal oedema.

In *proliferative* retinopathy new vessels proliferate in response to ischaemia, mainly near the disc margins. These fragile vessels are prone to haemorrhage into the retina and vitreous. Vitreous haemorrhage gives sudden blindness, followed by fibrosis and contraction leading to retinal detachment and glaucoma. Laser photocoagulation destroys new vessels and reduces oxygen requirements throughout the retina, thereby retarding new vessel proliferation.

Kidney

Thirty per cent of patients with type 1 diabetes develop end-stage renal failure.

Hyperfiltration and increased creatinine clearance occur early after the onset of diabetes.

After several years, microvascular changes (basement membrane thickening, hyaline degeneration of afferent and efferent arterioles) are associated with increased glomerular permeability and proteinuria. Kimmelstiel–Wilson nodules (nodular glomerulosclerosis) are pathognomonic of diabetic nephropathy.

Microalbuminuria heralds the onset of diabetic renal disease, and indicates progressive generalized vascular disease. Normal 24-h urinary albumin excretion rate (AER) is < 15 mg (concentration < 20 mg/l). Microalbuminuria is defined as an AER of 30–300 mg (concentration < 20–200 mg/l). Once persistent proteinuria occurs (> 300 mg in 24 h), end-stage renal failure usually develops within 5 years.

The progression of microalbuminuria is closely associated with changes in blood pressure, and control of blood pressure may be more important than glycaemic control in preventing renal disease. Angiotensin-converting enzyme inhibitors prevent progression of microalbuminuria to proteinuria in non-hypertensive patients with IDDM. They are generally favoured, alone or in combination with other agents, in the treatment of hypertension in diabetics (see Trials).

Pyelonephritis is more common in diabetics. Renal papillary necrosis can occur as a result of ischaemia of the papillae, which may slough and cause obstruction.

Neuromuscular complications

Up to 50% of patients with long-standing diabetes have neuromuscular complications.

- Peripheral neuropathy is the most common, initially causing loss of ankle jerks and absent vibration sense in the lower limbs. Later there is loss of touch and pain sensation. Patients often complain of numbness, and a burning sensation that is worse at night. Chronic painless ulcers develop in areas of repeated trauma (e.g. pressure points with ill-fitting footwear). Painless neuropathic arthropathy (Charcot joints) most commonly affects the tarsometatarsal joints.
- Painful peripheral neuropathy may respond to oral gabapentin or tricyclic (antidepressant) or topical capsaicin cream.
- Mononeuritis is thought to result from ischaemia following occlusion of vasa nervorum. The 3rd cranial nerve, ulnar nerve or lateral popliteal nerves are the most commonly affected. More than one nerve can be involved. It is often transient, and spontaneous recovery of function usually occurs over a period of months.
- Diabetic amyotrophy usually occurs in middle-aged diabetics who develop painful, asymmetrical weakness and wasting of the quadriceps muscles. Improving diabetic control is often associated with recovery.

AUTONOMIC FUNCTION TESTS

Parasympathetic
Heart rate response to deep breathing
Heart rate response to standing
Heart rate response to the Valsalva
    manoeuvre

Sympathetic
Blood pressure response to standing
Blood pressure response to muscle exercise
    such as sustained hand grip

Table 11.2 Tests of autonomic function.

• Autonomic neuropathy (Table 11.2) produces: erectile dysfunction (impotence) in 25% of male patients; diarrhoea, often nocturnal; gastroparesis; postural hypotension; gustatory sweating; and neuropathic bladder.

Skin
• Insulin sensitivity may occur in the first month of insulin therapy with production of tender lumps after each injection. Spontaneous recovery occurs, and no change of therapy is indicated.
• Lipodystrophy is painless atrophy or hypertrophy at injection sites. It is uncommon since the introduction of recombinant human insulins.
• Necrobiosis lipoidica (diabeticorum) is virtually pathognomonic of diabetes, occurs in 1%, and may precede it. It is characterized by atrophy of subcutaneous collagen, usually over the shins. The lesions start as small, brownish, shiny patches and may develop to become violet rings with yellow masses at the periphery and scarring, atrophy and sometimes ulceration at the centre. The most important management is to protect the lesions from trauma. Cosmetic camouflage can reduce emotional trauma. There is no curative therapy.
• Photosensitivity may occur with chlorpropamide.

Diabetic foot disease
A hospital foot care team includes chiropodists (podiatrists), vascular surgeons, physicians, radiologists and nurses. The major risk factors

of hyperglycaemia, smoking and hypertension, are identified and controlled where necessary. Neuropathy and peripheral vascular disease and callus are assessed and vascular reconstruction considered. Ulceration, gangrene and amputation rates can be much reduced by patient education in foot care.

Intercurrent infection
Intercurrent infection is common in diabetics, particularly of the urinary tract and skin. Tuberculosis and candidiasis (vulvitis and balanitis) are more common in diabetes.

Clinical supervision of people with diabetes mellitus
Supervision is best coordinated by diabetes care teams in primary care and at the hospital. In addition to the patient, they consist of doctors (GP, diabetologist, ophthalmologist, and other specialists according to complications), nurses (diabetes specialist and practice nurse), dietitian, chiropodist and pharmacist.

At least once a year, in a diabetic clinic at hospital or in primary care, there should be a discussion with the patient about the following.
• Diet and eating.
• The patient's understanding of diabetes, its impact on life at home or at work, general well-being, the drugs or insulin, its control with home blood glucose monitoring results, any other problems including sexual (contraception, preconception, erectile dysfunction), alcohol, work, sport, driving, insurance and hypoglycaemic attacks. The risk factors of smoking, hypertension, obesity, hyperglycaemia and dyslipidaemia must be assessed and controlled.
• Glucose control from the patient's routine blood glucose testing records obtained with a glucose–oxidase-impregnated stick read on a meter or by eye, and symptoms of low or high blood glucose. Ideally, the blood sugar should be normal (4–6 mmol/l) at all times and the patient symptomless. Realistically, the patient should aim to keep the blood glucose under 10 mmol/l at all times while avoiding hypoglycaemic symptoms.

Hyperglycaemia produces polyuria with nocturia and thirst. There may be intermittent blurring of vision, weight loss, genital pruritus from genital candidiasis or hospital admissions with ketoacidosis.

Hypoglycaemia ('hypo') produces 'warning' symptoms, although in late type 2 diabetes mellitus, 25% of patients may lose these and therefore have 'hypoglycaemic unawareness'. Hypoglycaemic awareness involves 'autonomic' symptoms, thought to be caused by a physiological response to the hypoglycaemia by adrenaline (epinephrine), noradrenaline (norepinephrine) and the sympathetic nervous system such as tremor, sweating, anxiety, palpitation and shivering. If plasma glucose levels drop below 3–4 mmol/l, 'neuroglycopenic' symptoms develop (caused by a deficiency of brain glucose), with tiredness, dizziness, drowsiness, difficulty in speaking, inability to concentrate and confusion, sometimes aggressive. Determine at what time of day in relation to food (not enough), exercise and insulin (too much) they occur. Early morning headaches may be the only indication of nocturnal hypoglycaemia. Weight gain can occur.

Examination should include:
• weight, which, with height, will provide the body mass index (BMI: weight in kilograms per square of height in metres);
• blood pressure, lying and standing;
• legs and feet for sensory neuropathy, including ankle reflexes, and for arterial disease, including the four major arterial foot pulses and evidence of reduced capillary circulation. Note the temperature of the feet and check them for infection and care of nails—regular expert chiropody may prevent serious complications such as ulcers;
• injection sites; and
• eyes—visual acuity (Snellen chart) and examine the retinae through dilatated pupils (tropicamide).

Investigations:
• Blood for:
   (a) glycosylated haemoglobin (HbA1c), which gives an index of average blood glucose control over the previous 2–3 months: aim for 7% or less
   (b) glucose with the timing of the last meal
   (c) creatinine (and/or urea)

   (d) lipid screen, aiming for a total cholesterol of < 5.2 mmol/l and a fasting triglyceride < 2.0 mmol/l.
• Urine for albumin and microalbumin (p. 157).

Type 1 diabetes

Type 1 diabetics require insulin to control blood glucose. Good control decreases the incidence of coma, intercurrent infection, retinopathy and probably neuropathy and nephropathy (see Trials). Hypoglycaemia is the most common complication of insulin therapy.

The new patient is advised about diet, the effects of exercise, insulin therapy, injection technique, urine testing for ketones and home blood glucose monitoring and recording. Insulin regimens need to be individualized according to the patient's lifestyle, motivation and comprehension. A knowledge of insulin preparations and their duration of action (Table 11.3) is essential. Premixed insulins are convenient for patients with poor sight or problems with dexterity.

The normal pancreas secretes about half its insulin at a continuous basal level, and the other half as boluses in response to food. Most diabetic patients are managed with twice-daily medium-acting preparations to provide continuous basal insulin levels, and two or three injections of short-acting insulin (often using a pen device) before main meals. Dietary caloric intake (unless excessive) is best chosen by the patient with professional dietetic advice, and insulin therapy adjusted for the chosen diet.

Control is best monitored by home blood glucose estimations, with periodic HbA1c at the clinic.

NB After pancreatectomy patients usually need 0.6 U/kg/day.

Type 2 diabetes

Type 2 diabetes can be prevented by changes in the lifestyles of high-risk subjects (see Trials Box 11.1). Reduction of dietary calorie intake to roughly 1200–1500 kcal with weight loss may be sufficient to reduce the blood sugar to normal. If not, use an oral hypoglycaemic agent in the form of a sulphonylurea or metformin, alone or in combination.

INSULINS

Name	Onset (h)	Peak (h)	Duration (h)
Neutral soluble Actrapid Velosulin Humulin S Insuman rapid	0.5–1	2–6	6–8
Isophane Insulatard Humulin I	2	4–12	12–24
Insulin zinc suspension (Lente) Monotard Humulin Lente	2	2–8	16–24
Insulin zinc suspension crystalline (Ultra-Lente) Ultratard Humulin Zn	4–8	12–20	24–28
Biphasic Mixtard 10, 20, 30, 40 50 (%sol to isophane) Humulin M2 (20% sol/80% isophane, M3 (30% sol) M5 (50% sol)	$^1/_2$–1	2–8	

Isophane insulin is a suspension of insulin with protamine.

Table 11.3 Commonly used insulins.

Sulphonylureas augment any residual pancreatic insulin secretion. Chlorpropamide has a long duration of action and is thus more likely to cause hypoglycaemia. It can also cause facial flushing after alcohol. Glibenclamide is usually given as a single dose before breakfast, whereas the short-acting tolbutamide is given in divided doses. Tolbutamide may be used in renal impairment, as may gliclazide, which is principally metabolized in the liver.

Thirty per cent of patients have a poor response to sulphonylureas, and the failure rate in the remaining 70% is 5% per year.

Metformin inhibits hepatic glucose production, mainly by inhibiting gluconeogenesis. It is particularly useful in the obese because it promotes weight loss. It has beneficial effects on plasma lipid level with reductions in total and low-density lipoprotein (LDL) cholesterol and in triglycerides. It is generally well tolerated and improves glucose control as either monotherapy or in combination with a sul-phonylurea. Weight gain and hypoglycaemia can limit its use in combination with insulin. Gastrointestinal side-effects are initially common, but usually subside. It should be avoided in patients with renal impairment (serum creatinine > 120 μmol/l) because of the risk of lactic acidosis. Vitamin B_{12} deficiency can occasionally occur as a result of decreased absorption.

The α-*glucosidase inhibitor, acarbose*, has only a small effect on plasma glucose by delaying the digestion and absorption of starch and sucrose.

Repaglinide stimulates insulin release. It is very short acting and is taken before food.

Thiazolidinediones (commonly termed *glita-zones*) activate nuclear peroxisome proliferator activated receptor-γ (PPAR-γ), which is expressed predominantly in adipose tissue. Thiazolidinediones increase transcription of genes involved in adipocyte differentiation and lipid and glucose metabolism. They reduce insulin resistance and tend to improve lipid profiles with decreased triglycerides and increased high-density lipoprotein (HDL) cholesterol. *Troglitazone* was withdrawn because of reports of hepatotoxicity. *Rosiglitazone* and *pioglitazone* can be used in combination with metformin in obese patients with insufficient glycaemic control and in combination with sulphonylureas if metformin is either not tolerated or contraindicated (e.g. renal impairment). In the USA both drugs are licensed for use as montherapy. Insulin requirements can be reduced by thiazolidinediones, but an increased incidence of cardiac failure was reported in trials in which rosiglitazone was used in combination with insulin.

The use of insulin is complicated by the invariable insulin resistance that is associated with type 2 diabetes. In addition, insulin stimulates appetite and can lead to weight gain in already obese patients. However, many patients with type 2 diabetes eventually require insulin therapy to control blood glucose.

Insulin should be given to patients at times of stress (e.g. infection, surgery, myocardial infarction).

Diabetic emergencies

There are two common types of diabetic coma:
• hypoglycaemia, the more common; and
• hyperglycaemic ketoacidosis.
There is rarely any difficulty in differentiating between these two situations. If in doubt, blood sugar can easily be estimated at the bedside with 'stix'.

Hypoglycaemia

Patients are usually known diabetics on insulin or, less commonly, sulphonylurea therapy, and very rarely have insulinoma or Addison's disease. In diabetics hypoglycaemia is caused by excess therapy, excess exercise, decreased food intake or an alcoholic binge. The rate of onset of symptoms is rapid. Most patients are aware of impending coma and may prevent it by taking sugar. Hypoglycaemic symptoms may be reduced by autonomic neuropathy. One-third of those who have had diabetes for more than 15 years may experience little or no warning. Patients present either in precoma with agitated, often aggressive confusion, or

in coma when marked sweating is usually present.

The differential diagnosis of hypoglycaemia involves the following considerations:
• excess insulin, which may be exogenous, endogenous (usually from insulinoma) or sulphonylurea therapy (frequently chlorpropamide or glibenclamide, because of their long duration of action);
• after excess alcohol;
• postgastrectomy;
• hypopituitarism and hypoadrenalism; and
• 'hungry neoplasm', e.g. hepatic carcinoma.

Oral glucose or, if necessary, intravenous glucose (20–40 ml of 50%) will reverse symptoms within minutes. Glucagon 1 mg intramuscularly acts as rapidly and can be given by relatives.
NB Hypoglycaemia must be treated immediately because it may produce irreversible brain damage. Fluid replacement and corticosteroids are required in addition to glucose if Addison's disease is present.

The hypoglycaemia of chlorpropamide therapy may require continued glucose administration for several days (the drugs effects last up to 60 h).

Rarely, warning symptoms of hypoglycaemia may be absent in those on β-blockers or human insulin.

Hyperglycaemic ketoacidotic coma

This appears to be occurring less frequently, perhaps because of better education of patients.

Onset is gradual over hours or days. There is often evidence of infection (25–35%), particularly of the renal, respiratory or gastrointestinal tracts. Septicaemia and meningitis are uncommon but important causes. The patient may not have been eating properly, and has often stopped taking insulin.

Symptoms include thirst and dry mouth, polyuria, air hunger, nausea and vomiting, weakness, myalgia, headache and abdominal pain. Drowsiness may progress to confusion and coma.

Signs are those of confusion and dehydration, with hyperventilation (Kussmaul respiration) and the characteristic smell of ketones. There is fever, hypotension and tachycardia.

Management:
• replace fluids;
• correct electrolytes;
• give insulin; and
• look for and treat any underlying cause.

Fluid replacement

Venous blood should be taken for glucose, urea and electrolytes, and haemoglobin and intravenous fluid therapy started immediately. No fixed regimen can be given, and therapy depends upon an assessment of the degree of dehydration. (The average deficit is 6–8 l, to be replaced in the first 24 h in addition to the daily requirement.)

Ketoacidotic patients are water, sodium and potassium-depleted and acidotic. For moderate to severe cases, in young people, 1 l of normal (0.9%) saline may be given in the first half-hour and repeated in the following hour and continued at a rate of 0.5–2 l/h for the first 2 h.

Electrolytes

Nearly all patients have low total body potassium with a deficit of 200–400 mmol on admission. Treatment will tend to exacerbate the dangers of this situation (acidosis will have caused a shift of intracellular potassium into the blood, and treatment causes it to move back into the cells again).

If the serum potassium is > 5.5 mmol/l, then no potassium chloride is added to the initial intravenous fluids, but serum potassium is measured at least every 2 h.

If the serum potassium is normal, then 20–40 mmol of potassium chloride is given hourly.

If the serum potassium is < 3.5 mmol/l, then 40–80 mmol of potassium chloride is given hourly.

Aim to keep plasma potassium between 4 and 5 mmol/l.

The use of bicarbonate to correct acidosis is controversial. Rapid correction of the acidosis leads to a rise in arterial $P\text{CO}_2$ and a paradoxical fall in cerebrospinal fluid pH, exacerbating central nervous system depression. In addi-

tion, a shift of the haemoglobin oxygen dissociation curve to the left increases tissue hypoxia.

Insulin

Soluble insulin must be given immediately. A low-dose regimen, given as an intravenous infusion or as hourly intramuscular injections, is preferred. The subcutaneous route is avoided as reduced skin blood flow in shocked patients leads to unpredictable absorption. A suggested regimen is a loading dose of 8 U followed by an infusion of 6 U/h until the blood sugar falls below 15 mmol/l (monitor glucose hourly), when the amount of insulin infused is reduced. The patient is not returned to the normal insulin regimen until awake and able to eat and drink.

Underlying cause

Intercurrent infection must always be considered and treated. It is advisable to perform urine microscopy and culture, blood culture and chest X-ray.

Special measures

• *Aspiration.* There is usually gastric dilatation, and death can occur from aspiration pneumonia. If the conscious level is depressed, a nasogastric tube should be inserted and the gastric contents aspirated.

• *Catheterization.* Urinary catheterization should be avoided in mild cases where confusion is minimal, but is required in those who are in a coma. Urine is sent to the laboratory for culture.

Hyperosmolar non-ketotic coma

This occurs in the elderly, obese diabetic, often previously undiagnosed. There is often a precipitating factor such as myocardial infarction, stroke or infection. The onset is slow with polyuria over 2–3 weeks and progressive dehydration. Blood glucose levels are very high (often above 45.0 mmol/l) and plasma osmolality is increased (often above 400 mosmol/l). Plasma bicarbonate is usually normal with no ketonuria. If plasma bicarbonate is low, think of lactic acidosis.

These patients need large quantities of fluid (up to 10 litres) given as normal saline.

Monitoring of central venous pressure or pulmonary wedge pressure is usually required. Insulin is required over the acute episode, often in small doses (10–20 U may suffice). The mortality is high (50%) and cerebral oedema from overhydration is a real risk. Prophylactic heparin may reduce the increased risk of thrombosis, arterial and venous. Unlike in patients with ketoacidosis, subsequent insulin therapy is not mandatory—survivors may do well on diet and oral hypoglycaemics.

Lactic acidosis
This usually occurs in the elderly diabetic, precipitated by alcohol or metformin. It may occur in shocked patients or those with uraemia. Patients are very acidotic and hyperventilating. Blood lactic acid levels are raised. Blood glucose may be normal and there is little or no ketonuria.

There is an increased anion gap in which the cation total (predominantly Na^+ plus K^+) exceeds the anion total (predominantly Cl^- plus HCO_3^-) by up to 25 mmol/l, the difference being lactate.

These patients require insulin, glucose, bicarbonate, and fluid replacement. A rough guide to the infusion of sodium bicarbonate in adults is 50 mmol bicarbonate for every 0.1 units of pH below. The mortality is very high (over 50%).

NB Cerebrovascular accidents and aspirin overdosage may both produce the combination of coma plus glycosuria.
NB Diabetics also have strokes, take overdoses and become concussed.

Diabetes and pregnancy
A specialist team of diabetologist, obstetrician and midwives usually reviews patients regularly. There should be a neonatal intensive treatment unit (ITU) on site for delivery.

Pre-existing diabetes in the mother
Diabetic control should be optimized before conception. Daily oral folic supplements (5 mg) should be taken before conception and for at least the first 12 weeks of pregnancy to reduce the risk of neural tube defects. Good glycaemic control should be maintained throughout pregnancy. Regular fetal ultrasound assesses gestation and growth. The more rigid regimens insist on plasma glucose levels below 5.5 mmol/l for most of the day, with a postprandial level below 7–8 mmol/l. Urine testing is not useful because of the fall in renal glucose threshold. Insulin requirements tend to fall in the first trimester, stabilize in the second trimester, and rise again in the last trimester, only to fall abruptly on delivery. The patient may be admitted for accurate diabetic control and delivery at term (see *Diabetes and surgery*, below). The risks to the fetus are considerable, with a high perinatal mortality that is related to the degree of diabetic control. If fasting and postprandial blood glucose levels are within normal limits, fetal loss is probably no greater than in the normal population. Babies tend to be large (macrosomia) if glycaemic control is poor. In non-insulin dependent diabetes mellitus (NIDDM), insulin is used if the above control levels are not achieved by diet alone.

Gestational diabetes mellitus
Gestational diabetes mellitus (GDM) is diabetes with onset or first recognition in pregnancy. In the UK, it occurs in about 4% of pregnancies. Diagnosis is usually established by an oral glucose tolerance test, using a 75 g glucose load, when fasting plasma glucose is > 5.5 mmol/l or rises to > 9 mmol/l at 2 h. Treatment usually involves insulin as well as diet (if plasma glucose > 6 mmol/l). Glucose tolerance returns to normal after delivery although 60% develop diabetes within 16 years, with the associated long-term risks.

Diabetes and illness
Even with vomiting, hepatic glycogenolysis can provide enough glucose during most illnesses. Normal doses of insulin are continued and blood glucose estimated 2–4-hourly. Soluble insulin is taken 5 units 2-hourly if the blood

glucose is in the range 12–20 mmol/l and not climbing. Ketonuria must be monitored every time urine is passed. Diabetics who have been properly educated in diabetes will know a number of suitable 10 g carbohydrate exchanges, such as a 5-ml spoonful of glucose or sucrose, 50 ml Lucozade or 200 ml whole milk.

Diabetes and surgery

The main danger is that the patient becomes hypoglycaemic while anaesthetized. However, with increases in cortisol, glucagon, growth hormone and catecholamines, plus a decrease in insulin, surgery tends to produce hyperglycaemia even in the non-diabetic subject. With elective surgery, the patient should be first on the operating list. No food or insulin is given on the morning of the operation. Routine bladder catheterization is not indicated. Good postoperative monitoring is mandatory.

Diabetes and driving

In the UK, the licensing authority and insurance company must be informed when diabetes that requires treatment with insulin or tablets is diagnosed. Diabetic patients treated with insulin will be given a group 1 entitlement licence for up to 3 years depending upon the quality of control, the regularity of medical surveillance and the state of complications. Patients with diabetes managed with tablets and/or diet and without complications may be issued with a 'till 70' licence. Patients treated with insulin are given a licence when the patient is not subject to frequent or sudden attacks of hypoglycaemia. This implies that the patient must carry glucose tablets (or equivalent) and recognize and avoid situations in which there is increased risk of hypoglycaemia. The complications of reduction of visual acuity, sensory neuropathy and peripheral vascular disease must be assessed. Patients receiving insulin will not normally obtain a vocational driving licence (for heavy goods vehicles and public service vehicles), but patients treated with tablets and/or diet normally will.

From the guide to UK medical standards of fitness to drive:

1 *Insulin-treated.* The applicant must recognize warning symptoms of hypoglycaemia and meet visual standards.
2 *Diet and tablet-treated.* There is no restriction unless there is a relevant disability (e.g. visual disturbance).
3 *Diet alone.* The applicant need not notify DVLA unless there is a relevant disability.

Hyperlipidaemia

The major plasma lipids, cholesterol and triglyceride, are absorbed from dietary fat, and also synthesized by the liver. Both are insoluble in water, and are thus transported in the plasma as water-soluble lipoproteins particles, in which a lipid droplet of insoluble cholesterol ester and triglyceride is surrounded by a coat of more polar substances such as phospholipid, free cholesterol and specific proteins known as apoproteins. In addition to this stabilizing of the lipoprotein complex, apoproteins (apos A–F) act as enzyme cofactors and interact with cell-surface receptors. The density of lipoproteins decreases as the triglyceride content increases.

Low-density lipoprotein (LDL) is the major carrier of cholesterol in plasma. It transports cholesterol to peripheral cells for membrane synthesis and hormone production, and to the liver for bile acid production.

High-density lipoproteins (HDLs) return cholesterol from peripheral tissues to the liver for excretion.

Dietary lipids

In the intestinal mucosa, triglycerides are coated with cholesterol, lipoprotein and phospholipid to form *chylomicrons* which are secreted into mesenteric lymphatics. Chylomicrons in the circulation are gradually depleted of triglyceride by lipoprotein lipase, an enzyme found on vascular endothelium in both muscle and fat. Triglyceride-depleted chylomicron remnants are taken up by the liver. Chylomicrons are normally absent after a 10-h fast. Apolipoprotein CII (apo-CII) in chylomicrons activates lipoprotein lipase, whereas apolipoprotein E mediates hepatic uptake of chylomicron remnants.

Hepatic synthesis of lipids

Cholesterol is synthesized in the liver from acetyl-coenzyme A. The enzyme 3-hydroxy-3-methylglutaryl coenzyme A (HMG CoA) reductase catalyses an early step in cholesterol synthesis. Triglycerides are formed by binding three fatty acids to glycerol.

Triglyceride-rich very-low-density lipoproteins (VLDLs) are synthesized in the liver and depleted of triglyceride in the circulation to form intermediate-density lipoproteins (IDLs). IDLs have a short half-life (< 30 min) in the circulation. They are either taken up by the liver, or further depleted of triglyceride to form LDLs which have a half-life of several days. LDLs can deliver cholesterol to the tissues, in part by interacting with the LDL receptor on the surface of cells. Lipoprotein a resembles LDL, but contains apoprotein a, which is structurally similar to plasminogen. In addition to being a source of cholesterol, lipoprotein a may also interfere with fibrinolysis.

HDL is synthesized in gut and liver, and has a relatively high apoprotein content. HDL accepts cholesterol from other lipoproteins and cells.

Hence, LDL is the chief form of cholesterol in the blood, and VLDL the chief form of fasting serum triglyceride.

Classification

The most common problem is elevated cholesterol. Although this is usually polygenic, or secondary to other diseases, less common familial causes of hyperlipidaemia should be considered so that screening of family members can be performed.

The Fredrickson WHO classification (Table 11.4) is still sometimes referred to.

Polygenic hypercholesterolaemia

This is the most common cause of raised cholesterol. Triglycerides may be normal (WHO type IIa) or raised (type IIb). Coronary heart disease risk is increased, and can be reduced by lowering cholesterol levels (see Trials Box 11.2).

Familial hypercholesterolaemia

In familial hypercholesterolaemia a deficiency of the receptor for LDL results in hypercholesterolaemia (severe in the homozygous form, less marked in heterozygotes) leading to atherosclerosis. Corneal arcus, xanthelasma and tendon xanthomas are characteristic. Patients die prematurely, usually from myocardial infarction. Prevalence is estimated at 1 in 500.

Familial defective apolipoprotein B-100

This is caused by a single amino-acid substitution in apolipoprotein B, resulting in defective binding of LDL to its receptor. It is clinically indistinguishable from familial hypercholesterolaemia.

Familial hypertriglyceridaemia

This may be caused by increased hepatic VLDL production or a failure of triglycerides to be cleared from chylomicrons by lipoprotein lipase. Marked hypertriglyceridaemia (> 10 mmol/l) is associated with eruptive xanthomas, lipaemia retinalis and acute pancreatitis.

Familial combined hyperlipidaemia

This condition is inherited as an autosomal dominant trait. Cholesterol and triglycerides are both increased. Corneal arcus and xanthelasmas (but not tendon xanthomas) are frequently present, and the risk of atherosclerosis is increased.

Dysbetalipoproteinaemia

This is a rare disorder in which mutations in the apolipoprotein E gene lead to elevations in triglycerides and total cholesterol.

Secondary hyperlipidaemia

This may occur in hypothyroidism, nephrotic syndrome, oral oestrogen or thiazide diuretic therapy, alcohol abuse and liver disease. These conditions should be excluded when investigating lipid abnormalities.

Associations between lipids and vascular disease

There is a strong association between plasma total cholesterol or LDL cholesterol and

HYPERLIPIDAEMIAS

Type of hyperlipidaemia	Prevalence	Fredrickson/ WHO lipoprotein phenotype	Typical lipid levels (mmol/l)	Lipoproteins	Chronic heart disease risk	Pancreatitis risk	Clinical signs
Polygenic hypercholesterolaemia	—	IIa	Cholesterol: 6.5–9.0 Triglyceride: normal	LDL↑ HDL→↓	+	—	Xanthelasma, corneal arcus
Familial combined hyperlipidaemia	1 : 200	IIb (IIa or IV)	Cholesterol: 6.5–10.0 Triglyceride: 2.5–12.0	VLDL↑→ LDL↑→ HDL→↓	+ +	—	Corneal arcus, xanthelasma
Familial hypercholesterolaemia (heterozygous)	1 : 500	IIa (or IIb)	Cholesterol: 7.5–16.0 Triglyceride: < 5.0	LDL↑ VLDL→↑ HDL→↑	+ + +	—	Tendon xanthomas, corneal arcus, xanthelasma
Remnant particle disease	1 : 10 000	III	Cholesterol: 9.0–14.0 Triglyceride: 9.0–14.0	IDL↑ HDL→↑	+ + +	+	Palmar tuberous and occasional tendon xanthomas
Chylomicronaemia syndrome	—	I	Cholesterol: < 6.5 Triglyceride: 10.0–30.0	Chylomicrons ↑	—	+ + +	Eruptive xanthomas, lipaemia retinalis, hepatosplenomegaly
Familial hypertriglyceridaemia	—	IV (or V)	Cholesterol: 6.5–12.0 Triglyceride: 10.0–30.0	VLDL↑ Chylomicrons→↑	?	+ +	Eruptive xanthomas, lipaemia retinalis, hepatosplenomegaly

Table 11.4 Classification of hyperlipidaemias. (Modified from *Mims* (Supplement) 1989, with the permission of Haymarket Medical Publications, London.)

TRIALS BOX 11.2

Fibrates

The **Helsinki Heart Study** compared the effect of gemfibrozil on cardiac endpoints in 4081 asymptomatic middle-aged men with non-HDL cholesterol > 5.2 mmol/l. The incidence of coronary heart disease was 34% lower in patients treated with gemfibrozil than those receiving placebo. *N Engl J Med* 1987; **317**: 1237–1245.

Resins

The **Lipid Research Clinics Coronary Primary Prevention Trial (LRC-CPPT)** compared the incidence of coronary heart disease in 3806 middle-aged hypercholesterolaemic (cholesterol > 265 mg/dl) men treated with colestyramine and diet, with that in similar men treated with placebo and diet. The incidence of coronary heart disease was 19% lower in those receiving colestyramine. *J Am Med Assoc* 1984; **251**: 351–364.

Statins

The **Scandinavian Simvastatin Survival Study (4S)** studied 4444 patients (mostly men) aged 35–70 years with serum cholesterol above 5.5 mmol/l, despite 2 months' dietary advice, and angina or previous myocardial infarction.

Patients were randomized to receive simvastatin (20–40 mg/day) or placebo. Simvastatin reduced total cholesterol by 25% and total mortality by 30%. Major coronary events (non-fatal myocardial infarction, resuscitated cardiac arrest, death) were reduced by 44%. Risks of developing unstable angina or needing coronary artery revascularization, or suffering a stroke or transient ischaemic attack were reduced by about 30%. *Lancet* 1994; **344**: 1383–1389.

The **Pravastatin Limitation of Atherosclerosis in the Carotid Arteries (PLAC-I)** trial studied 408 patients with coronary artery disease and a serum low-density lipoprotein (LDL) cholesterol of 130–190 mg/dl. Fatal and non-fatal myocardial infarctions were reduced in patients receiving pravastatin 40 mg/day compared with placebo. *J Am Coll Cardiol* 1994; **131A**: 1–484.

The **Pravastatin, Lipids and Atherosclerosis in the Carotid Arteries (PLAC-II)** trial studied 151 patients with coronary artery disease and a serum LDL cholesterol of 130–190 mg/dl. Coronary events and all deaths, when combined, were lower in patients receiving pravastatin 20–40 mg compared with placebo. *Am J Cardiol* 1995; **75**: 455–459.

The **Regression Growth Evaluation Statin Study (REGRESS)** studied the effect of pravastatin 40 mg/day or placebo in 885 symptomatic men with significant coronary atherosclerosis and serum cholesterol 4–8 mmol/l. There were fewer cardiovascular events, and less progression of atherosclerosis, in patients receiving pravastatin. *Circulation* 1995; **91**: 2528–2540.

The **West of Scotland Coronary Prevention (WOSCOP) Group** compared the effect of treatment with pravastatin and placebo for an average of 4.9 years in 6595 men aged 45–65 with a mean plasma cholesterol level of 7.0 mmol/l and no history of myocardial infarction. Pravastatin lowered plasma cholesterol and reduced the incidence of myocardial infarction and death from cardiovascular causes without adversely affecting the risk of death from non-cardiovascular causes. *N Engl J Med* 1995; **333**: 1301–1307.

The **Cholesterol and Recurrent Events (CARE) Investigators** studied the effect of pravastatin or placebo in 3583 men and 576 women with myocardial infarction who had plasma total cholesterol levels below 240 mg/dl. Pravastatin reduced the need for coronary bypass surgery and coronary angioplasty over a 5-year period. *N Engl J Med* 1996; **335**: 1001–1009.

The **Long-Term Intervention with Pravastatin in Ischaemic Disease (LIPID) Study Group** compared pravastatin with placebo over a mean 6.1 years in 9014 patients who were 31–75 years of age. The patients had a history of myocardial infarction or hospitalization for unstable angina and initial plasma total cholesterol levels of 155–271 mg/dl. Pravastatin therapy reduced mortality from coronary heart disease and overall mortality, as well as the incidence of all prespecified cardiovascular events in patients with a history of myocardial infarction or unstable angina who had a broad range of initial cholesterol levels. *N Engl J Med* 1998; **339**: 1349–1357.

Air Force/Texas Coronary Atherosclerosis Prevention Study compared lovastatin with placebo for prevention of the first acute major coronary event in 5608 men and 997 women without clinically evident atherosclerotic cardiovascular disease with average total cholesterol and LDL-C levels, and below-average HDL-C levels over a mean of 5.2 years. Lovastatin reduced the incidence of first acute major coronary events, myocardial infarction, unstable angina, coronary revascularization procedures, coronary events and cardiovascular events. Lovastatin (20–40 mg/day) reduced LDL-C by 25% to 2.96 mmol/l (115 mg/dl) and increased HDL-C by 6% to 1.02 mmol/l (39 mg/dl). *J Am Med Assoc* 1998; **279**: 1615–1622.

Heart Protection Study (see p. 265).

Diet
A systematic review of controlled trials stating intention to reduce or modify fat or cholesterol intake in healthy adult participants over at least 6 months revealed a small but potentially important reduction in cardiovascular risk with reduction or modification of dietary fat intake, seen particularly in trials of longer duration. *Br Med J* 2001; **322**: 757–763.

coronary heart disease, whereas there is an inverse relationship between HDL cholesterol and risk of coronary heart disease. As 60–70% of plasma cholesterol is present in LDL, total cholesterol is often used as a surrogate measure of LDL cholesterol. Raised levels of lipoprotein a also predict the risk of coronary heart disease.

Raised plasma triglyceride levels are associated with coronary heart disease. However, increased triglyceride levels are commonly found with hypercholesterolaemia, and it is less clear whether triglyceride levels are independent predictors of coronary heart disease risk. Xanthelasma and corneal arcus usually indicate hypercholesterolaemia, although they can occur with normal cholesterol levels. Tendon and palmar xanthomas only occur in hypercholesterolaemia, whereas eruptive xanthomas and lipaemia retinalis are found in hypertriglyceridaemia.

Management of hyperlipidaemia

There is good evidence that lowering raised cholesterol in patients at risk of coronary artery disease improves morbidity and mortality. Some primary prevention studies have also shown a benefit in lowering cholesterol in asymptomatic individuals (see Trials Box 11.2). The indication for treatment to lower cholesterol in patients who do not have existing disease which puts them at high risk of atherosclerotic disease is often based on calculation of the overall risk of coronary heart disease. This can be calculated according to cholesterol level, age, sex and blood pressure using risk tables. Tables produced jointly by the British Cardiac Society, British Hypertension Society, British Hyperlipidaemia Society and British Diabetic Association are available at http://www.hyp.ac.uk/bhs/risktables.html.

Diet typically lowers cholesterol by only 5–10%; less than 15% of cholesterol is dietary in origin. The longer chain saturated fatty acids raise, and mono- and polyunsaturated fatty acids lower, LDL cholesterol. Alcohol tends to increase plasma HDL cholesterol, reduce platelet aggregation and promote the effects of fibrinolytic factors.

Fibrates reduce serum triglyceride levels, principally through increased lipoprotein lipase activity. They tend to reduce LDL cholesterol and raise HDL cholesterol. Clofibrate increases biliary cholesterol secretion, predisposing to gallstones. Gemfibrozil has been shown to be effective in reducing both cholesterol and coronary heart disease (Helsinki Heart Study; see Trials). Bezafibrate, ciprofibrate and fenofibrate reduce both lipid and fibrinogen levels. All fibrates can cause myositis.

Resins reduce LDL levels by sequestering bile acids in the small intestine. Colestyramine and colestipol are both effective in reducing cholesterol, but their use is limited by gastrointestinal side-effects.

Statins are competitive inhibitors of HMG CoA reductase. They are potent in lowering LDL cholesterol, but less effective than fibrates in reducing triglycerides or increasing HDL cholesterol. Myositis is a rare but severe side-effect of statins.

Nicotinic acid derivatives reduce synthesis of both cholesterol and triglyceride. Their use is limited by side-effects, particularly vasodilatation leading to flushing.

Porphyrias

There are six main inborn errors of metabolism in which there is increased intermittent excretion of porphyrins in the urine and/or faeces.

Physiology

Porphyrins are intermediates in the biosynthesis of haem. The precursors are glycine and succinyl-CoA, which are converted to δ-aminolaevulinic acid (δ-ALA) by δ-ALA synthetase. Two molecules of δ-ALA condense to form the single pyrrole ring, porphobilinogen. Four porphobilinogen molecules are then cyclized by porphobilinogen deaminase to form the four-pyrrole ring structure which is characteristic of porphyrins. Porphyrins are divided into uro-, copro- and protoporphyrins according to the structure of side chains around the ring. Porphyrin biosynthesis occurs predominantly in the liver and bone marrow.

Classification

Porphyrias are classified as hepatic or erythropoietic according to the principal site of the enzyme defect and excess precursor production. They can also be classified as acute or non-acute. Porphyrins are colourless, but become coloured on oxidation. Porphyrins in urine darken on standing. Porphobilinogen is detected by Ehrlich's aldehyde reagent, which produces a pink colour with both urobilinogen and porphobilinogen. When chloroform is added, urobilinogen, but not porphobilinogen, moves into it. Porphyrins fluoresce in ultraviolet light.

Acute porphyrias (all inherited as autosomal dominant traits)

These disorders of haem synthesis have a prevalence of 1 in 10 000 in the population.

The biosynthesis of haem (from glycine and succinyl CoA) involves eight stages and enzymes, and is controlled by negative feedback of the haem concentration. Hereditary reduction of an intermediary enzyme makes patients susceptible to an increased demand for haem, which reduces the negative feedback so that excess toxic precursors (e.g. porphobilinogen and 5-aminolaevulinic acid (5-ALA)) are produced. Attacks are usually precipitated by drugs (such as alcohol, oral contraceptives and hormone replacement therapy (HRT), benzodiazepines, anabolic steroids, tricyclic and monoamine oxidase inhibitor (MAOI) antidepressants, most thiazide diuretics, sulphonylureas, non-selective antihistamines, many anticonvulsants, some antibiotics especially cephalosporins, and gold salts). Less commonly, acute attacks are precipitated by fasting or infection.

The symptoms are characterized by gastrointestinal, neuropsychiatric and cardiovascular features. The neuropsychiatric features may result in permanent sequelae.

Clinical features

Clinical features are very variable in severity.
• Abdominal pain, vomiting and constipation. This mimics obstruction so that patients are at risk of unnecessary and potentially dangerous surgery.
• Tachycardia and hypertension, or severe postural hypotension.
• Peripheral neuropathy with weakness or paralysis, including respiratory paralysis.
• Confusion with agitation or depression, hallucination and psychosis. Seizures may occur, even in between attacks, and may be difficult to treat because many anticonvulsants are contraindicated.
• Occasionally, inappropriate antidiuretic hormone syndrome with severe hyponatraemia, sweating, pallor and fever.

Attacks are rare before puberty, and in females may be related to the menstrual cycle. Ask about the family history. Check the urine (and stool) for porphyrins, 5-aminolaevulinic acid (5-ALA), and porphobilinogen.

Acute intermittent porphyria
(the Swedish type)

This is caused by a defect in porphobilinogen deaminase. Onset is usually between 15 and 35 years, and abdominal pain and vomiting are the most common presenting features. The skin is 'never' affected. There may be a family history. The urine turns red-brown on standing, and the diagnosis is confirmed by detecting excess porphobilinogen in the urine.

Variegate porphyria
(the South African type)

This is caused by a defect in protoporphyrinogen oxidase. Clinical features are similar to those of acute intermittent porphyria, together with cutaneous features. The skin, photosensitized by porphyrins, is fragile, particularly on the backs of the hands.

Hereditary coproporphyria

This is caused by a defect in coproporphyrinogen oxidase. Features are similar to variegate porphyria. It is extremely rare.

Management of acute porphyric crisis

During acute attacks a high carbohydrate intake (glucose polymer drinks or intravenous infusion of glucose) provides nourishment and rehydration, and suppresses ALA synthase activity. Haem arginate (Normosang) infusion, 3–4 mg/kg/day for 4 days, as haem replacement, restores negative feedback and shortens acute attacks. Pain is controlled with paracetamol or pethidine; agitation, nausea and vomiting with chlorpromazine; constipation with co-danthramer or neostigmine; tachycardia and hypertension with propranolol, seizures with diazepam or valproate; and respiratory paralysis with assisted ventilation. Check with the patient about future avoidance of precipitant drugs and alcohol. The patient should carry a complete list of relevant drugs, and wear a medical bracelet. Relatives should be screened and advised.

Non-acute porphyrias
Porphyria cutanea tarda
This is caused by a defect in hepatic uroporphyrinogen decarboxylase. It may be acquired or, less commonly, inherited. It is usually secondary to liver disease (particularly alcoholic), although in such cases there may be a genetic predisposition. Patients are not usually sensitive to drugs, although they may present after an alcoholic binge. The features are predominantly cutaneous with porphyrin-induced photosensitivity leading to bullae on exposed areas and hyperpigmentation. Urinary uroporphyrin excretion is increased, but urinary porphobilinogen is normal.

Congenital porphyria
This is caused by a defect in uroporphyrinogen cosynthase. It is inherited as an autosomal recessive trait and characterized by extreme skin manifestations plus red staining of the teeth and bones which presents before the age of 5 years. It is extremely rare.

Erythropoietic porphyria
This is relatively common and inherited as an autosomal dominant trait. It is caused by a defect in ferrochetalase activity. It presents in childhood with cutaneous photosensitivity of varying severity. It is distinguished by the presence of free protoporphyrin in the red cells which fluoresce in ultraviolet light.

Carcinoid syndrome

Carcinoid tumours originate from argentaffin cells, usually in the small bowel. *Carcinoid syndrome* results from a malignant carcinoid tumour, usually of the ileum, which has metastasized to the liver. Carcinoid of the appendix rarely metastasizes. Most bronchial adenomas are carcinoid but only a few produce the syndrome.

Physiology
Carcinoid tumours secrete serotonin (5-hydroxytryptamine) and kinin peptides. These are normally metabolized in the liver, so the syndrome only occurs if they are released from the liver by hepatic metastases. 5-Hydroxytrypamine is metabolized to 5-hydroxyindoleacetic acid (5-HIAA), which is excreted in the urine.

Clinical features
Symptoms of the primary tumour may be present, e.g. episodic diarrhoea or recurrent haemoptysis. The carcinoid syndrome is characterized by episodes of facial flushing, fever, dyspnoea from bronchospasm, nausea, vomiting, colic and diarrhoea. Later, valvular stenosis of the pulmonary and tricuspid valves may develop. There may be evidence of malignancy with cachexia and irregular hepatomegaly from metastases.

Investigation
The 24-h urinary excretion of 5-HIAA is measured on a low-serotonin diet (excluding bananas, tomatoes, walnuts, etc.). Normal range: 2–10 mg in 24 h.

Management
Cyproheptadine 4 mg t.d.s., α-blockade, octreotide (somatostatin analogue) or methysergide 1–2 mg q.d.s. (serotonin antagonist) and tumour chemotherapy may be given, but usually with disappointing results. Surgery is used to remove localized carcinoid, and can be of benefit in reducing bulk of liver tumour.

Hepatic arterial embolization is helpful in some. Treat diarrhoea symptomatically.

Metabolic bone disease

Physiology

Bone normally consists of 60% mineral and 40% organic matter (matrix). The former is mostly calcium and the latter mostly collagen. In all, 99% of total body calcium is contained within the skeleton. Cortical (compact) bone comprises 80% of the skeleton and forms the shafts of long bones and the surface of flat bones. Cortical bone is arranged concentrically around channels, known as the Haversian system, containing blood vessels, lymphatics and nerves. Trabecular bone is found at the end of long bones and inside flat bones.

Osteoblasts—derived from bone marrow stromal cells. Synthesize and mineralize bone matrix. About 20% of osteoblasts become calcified into lacunae and differentiate terminally into osteocytes.

Osteoclasts—derived from haematopoietic cells. Large, multinucleated cells which resorb bone. Osteoclasts express receptors for calcitonin, but not for vitamin D or parathyroid hormone. However, osteoclast activity is modulated by these agents, probably through signals generated by osteoblasts.

Bone remodelling occurs continuously at the endosteal surface (interface between bone and marrow), and to a lesser extent at the periosteal surface. In the normal young adult the amount of bone resorbed and formed in the skeleton is similar.

Parathyroid hormone (PTH) secretion is predominantly controlled by the concentration of ionized calcium in extracellular fluid. Intact PTH is rapidly cleared from the circulation by the liver and kidney (half-life < 4 min), but inactive C-terminal fragments persist longer, and account for about 90% of circulating PTH.

Increased PTH levels are associated with bone resorption, which releases calcium.

Osteoclastic cell number and activity are increased. However, intermittent administra-

tion of low doses of PTH increases formation of trabecular bone.

PTH decreases renal tubular phosphate reabsorption, and increases renal tubular calcium reabsorption. It indirectly increases intestinal calcium absorption through increased formation of 1,25-dihydroxyvitamin D.

PTH-related protein (PTHrP) is secreted by tumours that are associated with hormonal hypercalcaemia, including squamous, breast and renal carcinoma. It is only homologous to PTH in its amino terminus. PTHrP binds to the same receptor as PTH and shares its biological activities. Circulating levels of PTHrP are normally very low.

Vitamin D is principally synthesized from 7-dehydrocholesterol in the skin on exposure to ultraviolet light (Fig. 11.1). Dietary intake is only important when ultraviolet irradiation does not occur. Because of this, vitamin D is often regarded as a steroid hormone rather than a vitamin. The major circulating form is 25-hydroxyvitamin D3, which is converted to either 1,25-dihydroxyvitamin D3 or 24,25-dihydroxyvitamin D3 in the kidney. 1,25-Dihydroxyvitamin D3 is the most potent vitamin D metabolite. 1,25-Dihydroxyvitamin D3 decreases 1-hydroxylase activity and increases 24-hydroxylase activity, whereas PTH increases 1-hydroxylase activity and decreases 24-hydroxylase activity.

Vitamin D is thought to diffuse across the plasma membrane of target cells and interact with an intracellular receptor. The ligand–receptor complex regulates gene expression by binding to regulatory DNA sequences in the promoter region of genes, thereby acting directly as a transcription factor.

Calcitonin is secreted by C cells of the thyroid. Its principal action is to inhibit osteoclastic bone resorption. It has been used in the treatment of Paget disease, osteoporosis and hypercalcaemia of malignancy.

Osteoporosis

Osteoporosis refers to a loss of bone mass rather than an alteration in its constituents. It is characterized by increased risk of fragility fracture. The most common fracture sites are

METABOLISM OF VITAMIN D

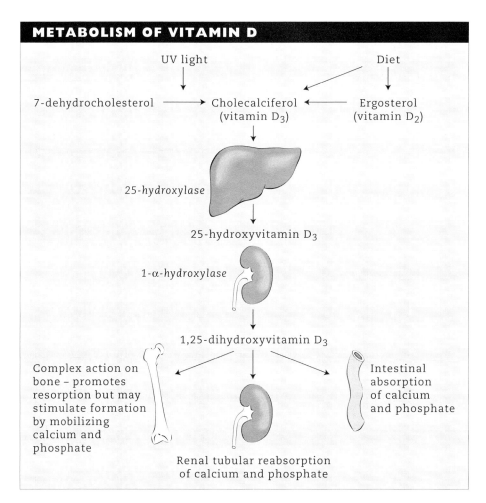

Fig. 11.1 Metabolism and actions of vitamin D.

the spine, femoral neck and radius. The WHO defines osteoporosis as bone density 2.5 standard deviations below the mean for young white adult women.

Aetiology

Pathogenesis is multifactorial. The risk is increased by ageing, female sex, race (white and Asian) and small body build. Oestrogen deficiency is a major factor in postmenopausal women, and women with premenopausal oestrogen deficiency (premature menopause, oophorectomy, anorexia, chronic illness, excessive physical exercise) are at risk. Family history of osteoporosis is a weak risk factor. Immobilization, often caused by arthritis,

appears to contribute. Some drugs, including steroids, thyroid hormones and alcohol, adversely affect bone mass. The role of calcium intake, calcium absorption and vitamin D is less clear.

Classification

Generalized

Normal ageing, especially in women:

1 *Postmenopausal (type 1)*, with trabecular bone loss giving vertebral lesions of end-plate collapse, wedging and crush fracture, up to about 70 years.

2 *Senile (type 2)*, with additional cortical bone loss giving fractures characteristic of the neck of femur, usually in women over 75 years. This

fracture is partly caused by the normal increase in body sway with age and resultant instability with falls.

Idiopathic—any age, but excessive in degree when compared within the age group. It is usually more dramatic therefore in the young.

Secondary
Endocrine
- Cushing syndrome (including steroid therapy).
- Thyrotoxicosis (including thyroid therapy).
- Pregnancy.
- Hypogonadism.
- Hyperparathyroidism.

Drugs
- Corticosteroids, thyroxine, heparin, alcohol, anticonvulsants.

Malignancy
- Myeloma.

Gastrointestinal
- Malabsorption.
- Chronic liver disease.

Localized
- Immobilization and paralysis.
- Rheumatoid arthritis.

Clinical features
Clinical features are related to fracture. Vertebral fractures (wedge or crush) are most common in the mid dorsal spine and the dorsolumbar junction (T12 and L1). They may be asymptomatic, or cause sudden severe back pain. Spinal cord compression is not a feature, and suggests other causes such as metastases or Paget disease. Multiple fractures cause loss of height and spinal deformity. Hip fractures invariably follow a fall and are often associated with prolonged hospital admission. Mortality at 6 months is around 15%. Colles' fracture usually follows a fall on to the outstretched hand.

Investigation
Biochemistry
Serum calcium, phosphate and alkaline phosphatase and urinary calcium are normal.

(Alkaline phosphatase may be elevated following a fracture.)

Radiology
Lateral X-rays of lumbar and dorsal spine. There may be wedging or concave deformities (codfishing) of the vertebral bodies. Discs may rupture into the vertebral bodies (Schmorl's nodes). Loss of bone density may be evident but radiological evaluation of bone mass is unreliable. Unequivocal osteopenia on X-ray signifies advanced bone loss.

Bone densitometry
Quantitative computed tomography (CT), single- and dual-photon absorptiometry to dual-energy X-ray absorptiometry (DXA) assesses bone density by measuring the absorption of γ- or X-rays at clinically relevant sites such as the radius, hip or spine. Where available, DXA is the preferred method, providing a rapid method of assessment which is associated with low-radiation exposure.

Histology
This is not indicated routinely, but shows a diminished number of normally calcified trabeculae.

Prevention and treatment
A number of agents have been shown to have beneficial effects on bone density or fracture rates in postmenopausal women. Efforts should be directed towards prevention in those with identifiable risk factors. These include late menarche, early menopause, oophorectomy before age 50, slimness, long-term corticosteroid therapy, alcoholism and smoking.

Hormone replacement therapy
Oestrogen therapy slows bone loss and reduces the occurrence of fractures when started at menopause. The increased risk of endometrial carcinoma is countered by cyclical progestogen for 10–12 days each month in women who have not undergone hysterectomy. Prolonged use (> 10 years), which is probably necessary to prevent bone loss, appears to increase risk of breast cancer. Oestrogen therapy also protects against ischaemic heart

disease and stroke, although this effect may be blunted by cyclical progestogen. There is a small (2–3%) increased risk of venous thromboembolism, which disappears after hormone replacement therapy is stopped. Absolute contraindications to hormone replacement therapy are breast cancer, endometrial cancer, malignant melanoma and pregnancy.

Bisphosphonates

Bisphosphonates, which are synthetic analogues of inorganic pyrophosphate, have been shown to increase vertebral bone density and may reduce vertebral fracture rate (see Trials Box 11.3). They have a high affinity for hydroxyapatite and inhibit bone resorption. However, with prolonged use they can inhibit bone mineralization. Cyclical administration is therefore recommended for etidronate. Alendronate has less effect on mineralization and can be given continuously.

Calcium

A daily calcium intake of 1–1.5 g is recommended (0.5 l of milk contains about 0.75 g). Those who are unable to achieve this through diet should receive calcium supplements.

Vitamin D

Studies suggest that small doses of vitamin D can reduce bone loss and prevent fractures in women with postmenopausal osteoporosis.

TRIALS BOX 11.3

Oestrogens

Many prospective and retrospective studies have shown beneficial effects of oestrogens, alone or in combination with other agents, on postmenopausal osteoporosis. Examples include the following.

Nordin et al. studied the effects of various treatments prospectively in 95 postmenopausal women with vertebral fracture. Calcium, hormonal treatment (ethinylestradiol or, where contraindicated, norethisterone) and vitamin D with hormonal treatment appeared to be useful in reducing cortical bone loss. Vitamin D alone was of no value. Br Med J 1980; **280**: 451–455.

Genant et al. prospectively studied 37 premenopausal women for 24 months following hysterectomy and oophorectomy for benign conditions. Spinal quantitative CT demonstrated bone mineral loss after oophorectomy which was prevented by conjugated oestrogens (Premarin up to 0.6 mg/day). Ann Intern Med 1982; **97**: 699–705.

Ettinger et al. measured spinal bone mass prospectively in 73 women immediately after the menopause. Bone loss was reduced by treatment with conjugated oestrogens (Premarin 0.3 mg/day) with calcium supplements, but not calcium supplements alone. Ann Intern Med 1987; **106**: 40–45.

Felson et al. performed a cross-sectional study of bone density in 670 postmenopausal women. Bone density was higher in women who had taken oestrogen therapy, but this effect was only apparent in women who had received treatment for 7 or more years. N Engl J Med 1993; **329**: 1141–1146.

The **Multiple Outcomes of Raloxifene Evaluation (MORE) Investigators** studied the effect of raloxifene, a selective oestrogen receptor modulator, on risk of vertebral and non-vertebral fractures in a multicentre, randomized, blinded, placebo-controlled trial of 7705 women aged 31–80 years who had been postmenopausal for at least 2 years and who met World Health Organization criteria for having osteoporosis. Raloxifene increased bone mineral density in the spine and femoral neck and reduced risk of vertebral fracture. J Am Med Assoc 1999; **282**: 637–645.

Bisphosphonates

Storm et al. compared the effect of intermittent cyclical etidronate (400 mg/day for 2 weeks followed by 13 weeks with no drugs repeated 10 times over 150 weeks) and placebo on bone mass and fracture rate in 66 women with postmenopausal osteoporosis. All patients received calcium and vitamin D supplements. Etidronate significantly increased vertebral bone mineral content, and after the first year reduced the risk of vertebral fracture. *N Engl J Med* 1990; **332**: 1265–1271.

Watts *et al.* compared cyclical etidronate (400 mg/day for 14 days within a 91-day cycle, which was repeated eight times) with placebo in 429 postmenopausal women with osteoporosis. All patients received calcium supplements, and some received supplemental phosphate. Etidronate increased spinal bone mass and reduced the incidence of new vertebral bone fractures. There were no additional benefits from phosphate. *N Engl J Med* 1990; **323**: 73–79.

The **Alendronate Phase III Osteoporosis Treatment Study Group** studied the effect of oral alendronate, an aminobisphosphonate that inhibits bone resorption without impairing mineralization, in 994 women with postmenopausal osteoporosis. Daily alendronate with calcium supplementation increased bone mass and reduced vertebral fractures over a 3-year period. *N Engl J Med* 1995; **333**: 1437–1443.

The **Vertebral Efficacy With Risedronate Therapy (VERT) Study Group** studied the effect of risedronate, a potent bisphosphonate, in a randomized, double-blind, placebo-controlled trial of 2458 ambulatory postmenopausal women younger than 85 years with at least one vertebral fracture at baseline. All subjects received calcium, and vitamin D was provided if baseline levels of 25-hydroxyvitamin D were low. Treatment with 5 mg/day of risedronate, compared with placebo, decreased the cumulative incidence of new vertebral fractures by 41% over 3 years. Bone mineral density increased significantly compared with placebo and bone formed during risedronate treatment was histologically normal. *J Am Med Assoc* 1999; **282**: 1344–1352.

The **Fracture Intervention Trial Research Group** examined the effect of alendronate treatment for 3–4 years on risk of new fracture among 3658 women with osteoporosis enrolled in the Fracture Intervention Trial. Reductions in risk of clinical fracture were statistically significant by 12 months into the trial, and reductions in fracture risk during treatment with alendronate were consistent in women with existing vertebral fractures and those without such fractures but with bone mineral density in the osteoporotic range. *J Clin Endocrinol Metab* 2000; **85** (11): 4118–4124.

The **Hip Intervention Program Study Group** studied the effect of risedronate in 5445 women 70–79 years old who had osteoporosis and 3886 women at least 80 years old who had at least one non-skeletal risk factor for hip fracture or low bone mineral density at the femoral neck. The women were randomly assigned to receive treatment with oral risedronate or placebo for 3 years. Risedronate significantly reduced the risk of hip fracture among elderly women with confirmed osteoporosis but not among elderly women selected primarily on the basis of risk factors other than low bone mineral density. *N Engl J Med* 2001; **344**: 333–340.

Calcitonin
In the **PROOF (Prevent recurrence of osteoporotic fracture) Study** 1255 postmenopausal women with established osteoporosis were randomly assigned to receive salmon calcitonin nasal spray or placebo daily. All participants received elemental calcium and vitamin D; 783 women completed 3 years of treatment, and 511 completed 5 years. Salmon calcitonin nasal spray at a dosage of 200 IU/day significantly reduced the risk of new vertebral fractures in postmenopausal women with osteoporosis. *Am J Med* 2000; **109**: 267–276.

Calcium and vitamin D
Dawson-Hughes *et al.* studied the effect of calcium supplementation (500 mg/day) on bone loss in 301 postmenopausal women. Calcium supplementation was only of benefit in reducing bone loss in older women (> 6 years postmenopausal) with a daily dietary calcium intake of < 400 mg. *N Engl J Med* 1990; **323**: 878–883.

Chapuy *et al.* studied the effect of vitamin D_3 (20 µg/day) and calcium (1.2 g/day) on the frequency of hip fractures and other non-vertebral fractures in 3270 healthy elderly women (mean age 84 years). Vitamin D_3 and calcium supplementation reduced the risk of hip fracture by 43% and other non-vertebral fractures by 32%. *N Engl J Med* 1992; **327**: 1637–1642.

Tilyard *et al.* compared the effect of 1,25-dihydroxyvitamin D_3 (0.25 µg twice daily) or supplemental calcium (1 g/day) for 3 years in 622 postmenopausal women who had one or more vertebral compression fractures. Calcitriol reduced the number of new vertebral fractures. *N Engl J Med* 1992; **326**: 357–362.

Calcitonin

Calcitonin prevents bone resorption. Although it may prevent postmenopausal bone loss, it is often used to treat bone pain following fracture. Its use is limited by side-effects (nausea, flushing, tingling, unpleasant taste), the need for parenteral administration and cost.

Fluoride

Sodium fluoride stimulates osteoblast proliferation. It increases bone mass, but bone formation may be abnormal and the effect on fracture rate is unclear.

Osteomalacia

In osteomalacia (soft bones) there is inadequate mineralization of bone. In childhood, osteomalacia presents as rickets.

The most common cause is vitamin D deficiency. It may also result from:
• vitamin D resistance or abnormal vitamin D metabolism;
• phosphate depletion; or
• chronic metabolic acidosis.

Clinical features

Adult osteomalacia patients may present with:
• bone pain and tenderness;
• pathological fracture;
• weakness, most marked in the quadriceps and glutei, which results in a waddling gait and difficulty rising from a chair; and
• the signs of underlying disease, e.g. malabsorption—the osteomalacia being diagnosed in the course of investigation.

Rickets patients present differently, because the reduced mineralization affects growing bones, causing:
• deformities in the legs (bow-legs, knock-knees);
• deformities in the chest (prominent costochondral junctions—ricketic rosary);
• deformities in the skull (craniotabes, open fontanelles and delayed eruption of the teeth); and
• hypotonia, weakness, tetany.
NB Rickets in the UK occurs chiefly in Asian immigrants caused by a combination of poor sunlight and a diet poor in vitamin D.

Aetiology

• Reduced intake of vitamin D—either dietary calciferol or cutaneous cholecalciferol (from 7-dehydrocholesterol), but usually both (dark skin, northern climate, poor diet).
• Malabsorption, especially gluten-sensitive enteropathy and postgastrectomy states.
• Abnormal vitamin D metabolism. Failure of 1-hydroxylation by the kidney is common in chronic renal failure. In type I vitamin D-dependent rickets there is a recessively inherited defect in the 1-hydroxylase enzyme. Hepatic enzyme induction with long-term anticonvulsant therapy can increase vitamin D metabolism and inactivation.
• End-organ resistance to vitamin D. Vitamin D-dependent rickets type II is an autosomal recessive disorder of the vitamin D receptor. 1,25-Vitamin D levels are markedly elevated.
• Phosphate depletion. X-linked hypophosphataemic rickets (familial vitamin D-resistant rickets) is a dominant disorder in which there is a renal phosphate leak and abnormal 1,25-vitamin D production. In Fanconi syndrome the phosphate leak is accompanied by aminoaciduria and glycosuria.
• Chronic metabolic acidosis. Usually as a result of chronic renal failure or renal tubular defects.

Investigation

Biochemistry

Reduced serum phosphate with increased alkaline phosphatase. Plasma calcium is usually low normal (maintained by secondary hyperparathyroidism).

X-ray

Rickets. In addition to bone deformities there are widened and irregular metaphyses ('cupping, splaying and fraying').

Pseudofractures (Looser's zones) are translucent bands ($\approx$ 2 mm) perpendicular to the surface of the bone, extending from the surface inwards, best seen in the pubic rami, the necks of the humeri and femurs and in the outer borders of the scapulae which are points of stress.

Generalized osteopenia with cortical thinning may be associated with multiple fractures, particularly in the ribs.

Bone scan
There is a generalized diffuse increase in uptake. Occasionally, Looser's zones show multiple areas of increased uptake. In osteoporosis bone scanning is normal, whereas in Paget's disease there is strong focal uptake.

Histology
The number of bone seams is normal. There is excess volume of osteoid tissue. Calcification fronts (identified by tetracycline labelling) are absent. There is usually some evidence of hyperparathyroidism.

Investigation of underlying disease (malabsorption, uraemia) may be required.

Treatment
Vitamin D (calciferol). The dosage and formulation depend on the aetiology. Serum calcium must always be monitored.
NB Calciferol 10 µg = 400 units.
• Deficiency states: 1000 units/day. Maintenance requirements in the normal individual, including children, are around 500 units/day.
• Malabsorption states: water-soluble hydroxylated metabolites can be absorbed by the small intestine, e.g. 1α-hydroxycholecalciferol (alfacalcidol) or 1,25-dihydroxyvitamin D (calcitriol).
• Vitamin D-resistant states: in familial vitamin-resistant (hypophosphataemic) rickets treatment is with oral phosphate supplements with calcitriol. Type II vitamin D-dependent rickets (end-organ resistance) responds poorly to treatment, although huge doses of calcitriol (20–60 µg/day) with calcium supplements are sometimes effective.
• In uraemia there is failure of 1α-hydroxylation. Treatment is with alfacalcidol or calcitriol.

Calcium supplements are not usually required unless there is severe osteomalacia or poor dietary intake. In these circumstances calcium uptake into bone may precipitate hypocalcaemia.
NB About 1 g calcium is contained in 850 ml (1 1/2 pints) of milk or 1 tablet of Sandocal 1000.

Paget's disease (osteitis deformans)
James Paget, 1814–1899, Great Yarmouth.

Increased bone remodelling, in which both resorption and production of bone are accelerated, leads to deformity and fragility. It is a disease chiefly of the elderly, affecting 10% of 95-year-olds (4% of 50-year-olds). In only about 5–10% is the disease clinically important.

Aetiology
Familial clustering and the finding of viral inclusions in osteoclastic nuclei suggest the disease may be triggered by slow viral infection of osteoclasts in genetically predisposed individuals.

Histology
Initially, bone resorption is associated with increased numbers of large osteoclasts which contain up to 100 nuclei. Numerous osteoblasts are then recruited to the site of bone resorption, and produce abnormal new bone. This consists of woven bone in which collagen fibres are laid down in an irregular fashion, and patches of mature lamellar bone which lack the normal Haversian systems. The overall appearance gives a characteristic mosaic pattern.

Biochemistry
Increased bone resorption leads to increased urinary hydroxyproline. Increased osteoblastic activity is reflected in increased levels of plasma alkaline phosphatase. Involvement of 10% of the skeleton is associated with a doubling in alkaline phosphatase.

Serum calcium levels are usually normal. In immobilized patients the stimulus to new bone formation may be lost, and hypercalcaemia may result from uncoupled resorption if there is extensive Paget's disease.

Radiology
Expansion and disorganization of bone with both lytic and sclerotic lesions are characteristic. There is cortical thickening and coarsening of trabeculae. The pelvis and lumbar spine are most frequently affected, followed by sacrum, thoracic spine, skull, lower limbs and upper limbs. Bowing deformity occurs in weight-

bearing long bones, and osteoarthritis is common in adjacent joints.

Bone scintigrams show increased uptake at affected sites.

Clinical features

Many patients are asymptomatic, the diagnosis being made by an incidental finding on X-ray. Pain is the most common symptom, sometimes with a rise in temperature over the site of the lesion. Pain may result from arthritis in adjacent joints. Bone deformity is most obvious when there is enlargement of the skull or bowing of the legs.

Complications

• Fractures: up to 15% of patients suffer pathological fractures in abnormal bone. Fissure fractures are small fractures on the convex surface of long bones. They may be asymptomatic, but can cause pain or progress to clinical fractures. Compression of affected vertebrae is common.
• Deafness is common in patients with skull involvement. It may result from involvement of the ossicles or compression of the cochlea or internal auditory canal. Occlusion of other foramina of the skull leading to compression of other cranial nerves occurs less often. Platybasia or flattening of the base of the skull may, rarely, lead to brainstem compression or obstructive hydrocephalus.
• Spinal involvement may cause cord compression, particularly in the cervical and thoracic regions where the canal is narrower, and paraparesis may result.
• Less than 1% of patients develop osteogenic sarcoma in Pagetic bone. The pelvis and femur are the most common sites. It may be heralded by increasing pain. Lesions are typically osteolytic and X-rays may reveal a soft-tissue mass. Diagnosis is confirmed by open or needle biopsy.
• High-output cardiac failure is a rare complication of extensive disease.

Treatment

Pain may be controlled with analgesics and non-steroidal anti-inflammatory drugs. Physiotherapy maintains mobility.

A number of specific treatments are now available. These agents are effective in relieving symptoms. They may also be of benefit in preventing complications in asymptomatic patients.

Calcitonin

Salmon calcitonin (salcatonin) given subcutaneously is the most widely used. It inhibits osteoclastic activity and is of use in relieving pain. It may also be of benefit in relieving complications such as deafness. Calcitonin is safe, but side-effects, including nausea, flushing, unpleasant taste and pain at the injection site, are common.

Bisphosphanates

Bisphosphanates reduce bone turnover in Paget's disease, probably by binding to hydroxyapatite crystals on the surface of newly deposited bone. Administration of high doses for long periods inhibits new bone formation as well as bone resorption. Periods without treatment are therefore important in prolonged usage.

Etidronate is usually given as a single oral dose of 5 mg/kg/day for 6 months, followed by 6 months without treatment. Pamidronate can be given as a single intravenous infusion of up to 60 mg; this can induce remission for many months.

Plicamycin

Plicamycin (mithramycin) is now rarely used in the treatment of Paget's disease because of hepatic, renal and bone marrow toxicity.

Serum alkaline phosphatase and 24-h urinary hydroxyproline measurement can be used to monitor response to treatment. Urinary hydroxyproline levels reflect bone resorption and give a more rapid indication of response and an earlier warning of relapse.

Uraemic bone disease

(renal osteodystrophy)
In renal failure, there is reduced 1,25-dihydroxyvitamin D_3 (1,25-$(OH)_2D_3$) with increased PTH. In addition there is reduced renal phosphate excretion. The mechanisms of renal osteodystrophy are as follow.

Phosphate retention
This has two secondary effects:
• reciprocal depression of serum calcium level (mediated at the bone surface); and
• rise in the calcium × phosphorus product (despite the serum calcium depression), which may lead to ectopic calcification.

Lack of vitamin D
The diseased kidneys fail to hydroxylate 25-hydroxycholecalciferol to $1,25-(OH)_2D_3$. This failure is expressed at two important sites:
• the gut, where there is reduced calcium absorption; and
• the bone, to produce osteomalacia and hypocalcaemia.

Hypocalcaemia produced by these mechanisms is a stimulus to the parathyroid glands which are thus in a state of continuous hypersecretion, tending to return the serum calcium levels towards normal. This (secondary) hyperparathyroidism (p. 180) may be demonstrated on bone X-rays (p. 181), and the serum level of parathyroid hormone is elevated.

The hypocalcaemia only rarely leads to tetany because acidosis reduces the protein binding of calcium, and thus increases the level of ionized calcium.

The clinical consequences of renal failure on calcium metabolism are thus:
• osteoporosis produced by hyperparathyroidism;
• osteomalacia caused by lack of vitamin D; and
• ectopic calcification.

Management
There are five chief therapeutic manoeuvres.
1 *Restriction of dietary phosphate.* Aluminium or calcium-containing antacids (aluminium hydroxide or calcium carbonate or calcium acetate) are used as phosphate-binding agents to prevent intestinal absorption. Aluminium-containing agents are now rarely used because of concerns about aluminium toxicity. Calcium-containing agents are contraindicated if hypercalcaemia is present. Sevelamer is a phosphate binding agent that does not contain calcium or aluminium.
2 *Dialysis* against a suitable ionized calcium concentration (about 1.5 mmol/l) and no phosphate should return the calcium and phosphate levels towards normal.
3 *Vitamin D* increases calcium levels, and reduces hyperparathyroidism. It may be used to treat muscular weakness, bone pain and biochemical or radiological osteomalacia. Unwanted effects are increased absorption of phosphate from the gut, and hypercalcaemia. 1α-Hydroxylated forms (alfacalcidol or calcitriol) are used.
4 *Parathyroidectomy* should reduce calcium and phosphate levels and permit vitamin D therapy without the risk of hypercalcaemia.
5 *Renal transplantation*, if successful, returns renal function to normal and corrects deficient $1,25-(OH)_2D_3$ production. Persistent hyperparathyroidism can lead to marked hypercalcaemia. In the long-term, the side-effects of immunosuppressive drugs may influence the skeleton adversely.

Hypercalcaemia

The normal range of serum calcium is 2.2–2.6 mmol/l. Calcium is bound to albumin and 'correction' should be performed when albumin levels are abnormal. For every 1 g/l that the albumin is lower than 40 g/l, add 0.025 to the serum calcium (or subtract if serum calcium is raised above 40 g/l).

Acidosis increases ionized calcium by decreasing binding of calcium ions to albumin, whereas alkalosis has the reverse effect.

Aetiology
Common:
• Malignancy
  (a) bone metastases, commonly breast, lung, prostate, ovary, kidney
  (b) multiple myeloma, leukaemia, Hodgkin's.
• Primary hyperparathyroidism (p. 180).
Much less common:
• Familial benign hypocalciuric hypercalcaemia, characterized by slight, life-long, asymptomatic hypercalcaemia.
• Chronic renal failure, if complicated by tertiary hyperparathyroidism (p. 180).

- Drug-induced—excess vitamin D.
- Granulomatous disease—increased sensitivity to vitamin D (the hypercalcaemia may be precipitated by exposure to sunlight). Sarcoidosis, rarely others, such as tuberculosis, leprosy, histoplasmosis.
- Endocrine very rarely: thyrotoxicosis, phaeochromocytoma, Addison's disease.
- As a complication of total parenteral nutrition.

Clinical features

The clinical features depend on the rapidity of onset and the severity of the rise in serum calcium concentration. Slow-onset, mild hypercalcaemia is usually asymptomatic (see *Hyperparathyroidism*, below). Severe hypercalcaemia, usually caused by malignant disease, with an onset over only a few weeks or months, may produce the following features.
- *Neurological*—tiredness, depression, confusion, muscle weakness, fatigue and hypotonicity.
- *Gastrointestinal*—anorexia, nausea and vomiting, constipation, thirst.
- *Renal*—polyuria (impaired distal tubular function), stones, nephrocalcinosis.
- *Cardiovascular*—bradycardia, and atrioventricular block (cardiac repolarization is increased, leading to shortening of the QT interval).
- *Psychiatric disorders* (3%) include depression and confusion.

Investigation

Malignancy and hyperparathyroidism account for 90%. Malignancy can often be detected clinically or radiologically. PTH, performed by radiometric immunoassay (IRMA), is absent in all non-parathyroid causes. Normal or elevated levels of parathyroid hormone in the presence of hypercalcaemia are inappropriate, and imply hyperparathyroidism: the serum phosphate is at or below normal levels. Sarcoid should be considered. Protein electrophoresis should be performed to exclude myeloma.

Treatment

Emergency
Rehydrate with intravenous 0.9% saline and give furosemide (frusemide). Loop diuretics inhibit sodium and calcium reabsorption from the thick ascending limb of the loop of Henle. Dialysis (haemo- or peritoneal) against a low calcium dialysate is reserved for severe hypercalcaemia or those with renal impairment.

Intravenous bisphosphonates (pamidronate or clodronate) inhibit osteoclast-mediated bone resorption and can be used with rehydration to treat hypercalcaemia of malignancy. Corticosteroids can be used in haematological malignancies (myeloma, lymphoma) and sarcoid. They are ineffective in parathyroid disease.

Endocrine bone disease

Hyperparathyroidism

Parathyroid hormone increases serum calcium by:
- increasing calcium absorption from the gut;
- increasing mobilization of calcium from bone by osteoclast-mediated resorption; and
- reducing renal calcium clearance.

It also increases renal phosphate clearance and this may also indirectly increase mobilization of calcium from bone.

Primary hyperparathyroidism results from a single adenoma (85%) or hyperplasia of the parathyroid glands. It is more common in females than males (3 : 1) and has a peak incidence at about 50 years old. Very rarely, a functioning carcinoma may occur. Ectopic PTH may be produced by carcinoma elsewhere, particularly of the lung and kidney. It may be part of a multiple endocrine neoplasia (MEN) syndrome (p. 152).

Secondary hyperparathyroidism is a physiological response to hypocalcaemia produced by another disease, e.g. chronic renal failure and hypovitaminosis D (dietary deficiency or malabsorption). The calcium may be normal or low.

Tertiary hyperparathyroidism refers to the situation where chronic secondary hyperparathyroidism has resulted in an autonomous adenoma. This, as in primary hyperparathyroidism, is characterized by hypercalcaemia, although the hyperphosphataemia of renal failure may persist.

Clinical presentation

Hyperparathyroidism usually produces a slight hypercalcaemia that develops slowly over many months or even years. It is usually asymptomatic.

• The hypercalcaemia is usually found during routine investigation (0.1% of the general population; up to 8% of hospital admissions).
• The chronic hypercalciuria can produce renal calculi, nephrocalcinosis and, later, renal failure.
• Skeletal changes (see *Radiology*, below).
• Severe hypercalcaemia, which is unusual, may produce anorexia, nausea, vomiting, thirst, polyuria, constipation, muscle fatigue and hypotonicity. Rarely, calcium deposition may occur in the conjunctiva usually at the medial limbus of the eye (3%). Dyspepsia and peptic ulceration may occur (5%).
• Psychiatric disorders (3%) include depression and confusion.

Hence the frequently quoted mnemonic: 'Bones, stones, groans (peptic ulcer) and moans (psychiatric disease).'

Differential diagnosis

This is from other causes of hypercalcaemia (p. 179) and hypercalciuria.

Investigation

Biochemistry

In primary hyperparathyroidism the serum calcium is raised and the phosphate reduced. A raised serum alkaline phosphatase indicates increased bone activity. There is a high renal clearance of phosphate and a mild renal tubular acidosis (with a high serum chloride level). The serum calcium level is not reduced by corticosteroids. The serum PTH is raised. In the secondary hyperparathyroidism of renal failure, the serum phosphate is high and the serum calcium tends to be low.

Radiology

More specific changes include loss of the lamina dura of the teeth (25%) and small subperiosteal

bone resorption cysts most marked in the middle phalanges of the hands (and feet). Osteitis fibrosa cystica with bone cysts is relatively rare. Bone density is measurably reduced in the lumbar spine, femora and radii. CT scan and isotopic subtraction scan of the neck and mediastinum (up to 20% are ectopic) seldom helps to localize the abnormal gland.

Treatment

The diseased parathyroid glands should be resected by an experienced surgeon if the serum calcium is persistently over 3.0 mmol/l (after correction for serum albumin level). Surgery is also recommended for patients with lower levels if they are under 50 years old or have any of the clinical presenting features given. It is important to visualize and probably biopsy all four parathyroid glands to determine whether they are normal or hyperplastic. A single enlarged gland is removed or, if all are enlarged, three and a half, the remaining half either being left *in situ* or implanted in the forearm. Some advocate the removal of all hyperplastic glands and subsequent treatment with alfacalcidol. A postoperative 'hungry bones syndrome' can develop with tetany and hypomagnesaemia.

Prognosis

Patients with uncomplicated disease and serum calcium levels consistently < 3 mmol/l do not show deterioration in any of the clinical features over several years.

Hypoparathyroidism

Aetiology

Secondary to thyroid surgery.

Primary idiopathic. This appears to be an organ-specific autoimmune disease and is associated with an increased incidence of Addison's (hypoadrenal) disease, pernicious anaemia and malabsorption. Parathyroid agenesis occurs in DiGeorge syndrome with thymic hypopolasia as a result of maldevelopment of the third and fourth pharyngeal pouches. There is T-cell deficiency and children die from infection in infancy.

Pseudohypoparathyroidism (very rare) is caused by a failure of end-organ response in bone and kidney to endogenous PTH which is thus present in excess amounts. Unlike patients with true idiopathic hypoparathyroidism, there is no increase in urinary cyclic adenine monophosphate when PTH is injected.

Clinical presentation

This depends upon its speed of onset and its degree. Acute hypocalcaemia gives paraesthesia around the mouth and in the extremities followed by cramps, tetany, stridor, convulsions, and death if untreated.

Trousseau's (twitching of the angle of the mouth on tapping over the 7th nerve) and Chvostek's (carpopedal spasm) signs may be present.

Ectodermal changes: teeth, nails, skin and hair. There is an excessive incidence of cutaneous moniliasis in primary hypoparathyroidism.

Ocular changes: cataract and, occasionally, papilloedema.

Calcification in the basal ganglia and, less commonly, other soft tissues.

NB The hereditary syndrome of pseudohypoparathyroidism is caused by tissue resistance to PTH and usually presents in childhood. The patients have a moon face, are short, mentally retarded, have calcification of the basal ganglia and often have short fourth or fifth metacarpals. The biochemistry is similar to idiopathic hypoparathyroidism. Pseudopseudo-hypoparathyroidism refers to patients who have the somatic manifestations of pseudohypoparathyroidism but normal biochemistry.

Tetany may also occur rarely in rickets, the malabsorption syndrome, alkalosis, especially hyperventilation (p. 252) and, very rarely, in osteomalacia and uraemia.

Investigation

There is a low serum calcium and a high serum phosphate level with normal alkaline phosphatase. There is no common diagnostic radiological skeletal abnormality. X-ray of the skull may show calcification of the basal ganglia. If the patient is thought to have idiopathic hypoparathyroidism investigate for the associated pathologies.

The differential diagnosis of hypocalcaemia is that of the causes of PTH deficiency and of hypovitaminosis D—reduced intake or absorption, and resistance (p. 176).

Treatment

Emergency
Treat tetany with 10–20 ml 10% calcium gluconate intravenously.
NB Rebreathing from a bag is effective if there is hyperventilation.

Intravenous magnesium chloride may also be required if there is also hypomagnesaemia.

Long-term therapy involves the use of vitamin D analogues, alfacalcidol or calcitriol supplements to raise the serum calcium towards normal levels.

Gout and hyperuricaemia

A disease characterized by episodes of acute arthritis, at first affecting only one joint and associated with hyperuricaemia. Hyperuricaemia is 10 times more common without clinical gout than with it.

Primary gout
An error of purine metabolism that occurs in men and postmenopausal women (10 : 1) with a prevalence in the UK of 3/1000. The hyperuricaemia is familial and there is a family history of gout in 30%. Hyperuricaemia can also result from increased consumption of purine-containing foods and excess alcohol, especially in predisposed individuals who are often also obese.

Secondary gout
This occurs at all ages in both sexes.

Ten per cent of all gout is associated with myeloproliferative disease which causes increased purine turnover and release, and hence a rise in serum uric acid (e.g. myeloid leukaemia, myelofibrosis, polycythaemia rubra vera, multiple myeloma and in Hodgkin's disease). This occurs particularly after treatment with antimetabolite drugs when the serum uric acid and urea rise as a result of tissue destruction.

Drug-induced hyperuricaemia may follow treatment with diuretics, particularly thiazides, and salicylates in small doses.

Chronic renal failure may be associated with hyperuricaemia and, rarely, clinical gout, secondary to reduced renal uric acid excretion.

Clinical features

In the first attack, the big toe is affected in 75% of cases, the ankle or tarsus in 35%, and knee in 20%. In 40% it involves more than one joint. The onset is usually sudden and the joint is red, hot, shiny and exquisitely tender. The patient is febrile, irritable and anorexic. Attacks, at first monarticular in most patients, tend to be recurrent and to become polyarticular. They may be precipitated by trauma (including surgery), exercise, dietary excess, alcohol and starvation. Chronic gouty arthritis remains asymmetrical and tophi appear, especially on the cartilages of the ears and close to joints in 20% of untreated patients.

Complications

Renal disease. Uric acid stones occur in 10% of patients in the UK and may produce renal colic. Chronic renal failure may follow long-standing hyperuricaemia (chronic urate nephropathy).

Hypertension, obesity and coronary artery disease are more common in patients with hyperuricaemia. Secondary pyogenic infection of gouty joints is uncommon.

Investigation

The serum uric acid is raised.
NB Five per cent of men have levels of 0.42 mmol/l or more, but only 0.6% have clinical gout.

Leukocytosis is common and the erythrocyte sedimentation rate (ESR) is raised.

Radiology: asymmetrical soft-tissue swelling may be the only abnormality in acute gout. Chronic disease produces irregular punched-out bony erosions near but not usually involving the articular margins. Tophi may be seen if calcified. Osteoarthritic changes are common

in gouty joints. Uric acid renal stones are radiolucent.

Aspirates of joint fluid contain negatively birefringent needle crystals of monosodium urate when viewed by polarized light.

Differential diagnosis

Acute gout must be distinguished from other causes of acute arthritis, particularly septic staphylococcal arthritis and rheumatic fever. Pseudogout may occur in chronic renal failure.

Chronic gout, particularly if widespread, may resemble rheumatoid or osteoarthritis.

Hyperuricaemia may be secondary to diuretic therapy.

Treatment

Acute episodes

Indometacin 100 mg followed by 25 mg t.d.s. or naproxen 750 mg followed by 250 mg t.d.s. Hydrocortisone 100 mg intramuscularly repeated as required, may be given in resistant cases and may relieve pain almost instantaneously.

Colchicine (0.5–1 mg 2-hourly until pain is relieved, vomiting and diarrhoea begin or a total of 8 mg) may be given if non-steroidal anti-inflammatory drugs are contraindicated. Allopurinol may be started a fortnight after the acute attack has subsided but must be covered by continuation of non-steroidal anti-inflammatory drug therapy or colchicine 0.5 mg b.d. until at least 1 month after hyperuricaemia is corrected, because acute gout may otherwise be precipitated.

Chronic recurrent gout and hyperuricaemia

Probenecid 0.5 g two or three times a day and sulfinpyrazone 100 mg t.d.s. act by increasing renal clearance of uric acid and urates.

Allopurinol 300 mg/day is of particular value in the treatment of chronic tophaceous gout or chronic hyperuricaemia and when renal disease is present. It blocks the metabolic pathway at xanthine and hypoxanthine (by inhibiting xanthine oxidase), both of which are more soluble than uric acid and less liable to form stones. The dosage is adjusted between 100 and 900 mg/day to keep the serum uric acid normal. It should be given well before starting cytotoxic chemotherapy, otherwise the release of uric acid in the tumour lysis syndrome can precipitate acute renal failure.

These drugs may precipitate an acute attack and cover with colchicine or anti-inflammatory agent (steroidal or non-steroidal) is advised when allopurinol is started.

Indications for long-term therapy are the presence of clinical gout, urate nephropathy, tophaceous gout, myeloproliferative disorders under therapy, or non-symptomatic but persistent plasma uric acid levels over 0.8 mmol/l.

Overeating and overdrinking (of alcohol) should be corrected (not only for gout), the obese should lose weight, and drug therapy, particularly thiazides and aspirin-containing drugs, assessed and modified where necessary.

Pseudogout (articular chondrocalcinosis or calcium pyrophosphate gout)

This is rare and sometimes familial. It is less uncommon in females (male : female = 2 : 1) than gout. The patients are usually elderly. It is associated with diabetes mellitus (40%), hyperparathyroidism (p. 180) and haemochromatosis (p. 215). It may occur in chronic renal failure. Chondrocalcinosis is frequently found by chance on X-ray of the knees and may be symptom-free. It may present as osteoarthritis. However, there may be episodic pain and effusions into large joints and it may thus mimic gout, although the big toe is seldom affected and the symptoms are usually less acute, less severe and more prolonged. The effusions contain calcium pyrophosphate crystals which are rod- or brick-shaped and positively birefringent (whereas crystals in gout are negatively birefringent). The disease is associated with radiological calcification of the joint capsule and cartilage. The cartilages of the knee are characteristically outlined by calcium but calcification may occur in any cartilaginous joint. The patient may develop osteoarthritis secondary to the destruction of joint cartilage. Intra-articular steroids have been used. Indomethacin may be needed in acute episodes.

Diagnosis is established by calcification on X-ray of the joint, a normal serum uric acid and the characteristic crystals in the aspiration of joint fluid.

Osteogenesis imperfecta

A hereditary connective tissue abnormality with involvement of collagen-containing tissues such as the skeleton (fragile), sclerae (blue), skin (thin), teeth (thin dentine), tendons (hypermobile joints), heart (valve disorders) and ear (deafness).

Osteogenesis imperfecta tarda is a more common, mild, autosomal dominant disease and fractures are rare.

Osteogenesis imperfecta congenita is a rare, severe, autosomal recessive disease with the above features plus scoliosis, bowed legs and multiple fractures.

Nutrition

Obesity

Excess body fat can be measured only indirectly and weight in relation to height and age is used as a measure. BMI is increasingly used. The normal range is 20–25 kg/m^2. The distribution of fat is important. Central obesity (with a waist : hip ratio of > 1.0) is particularly associated with insulin resistance and diabetes mellitus.

Aetiology

It is impossible to differentiate between genetic, environmental and socioeconomic factors. Most fat people have at least one fat parent. There are likely to be controlling endocrine factors yet to be determined—fat people have high plasma insulin and cortisol with low levels of growth hormone.

Ultimately, obesity is perpetuated by ingestion of calories in excess of needs and reduced by lowering the calorie intake and maintaining this reduced level.

Differential diagnosis

Weight gain is a feature of myxoedema and Cushing syndrome and a rapid weight gain occurs with fluid retention in heart failure, renal failure and the hypoalbuminaemia of chronic liver disease.

Prognosis

Mortality is increased in obesity. Actuarial figures suggest that weight reduction to normal reduces the increased mortality to normal.

Common complications include hypertension, myocardial infarction, diabetes mellitus, risk from surgery, osteoarthritis, herniae, gallstones, hiatus hernia and varicose veins. In women there is also an increased incidence of hirsutism and breast and endometrial carcinoma. Perhaps the saddest complications are psychological.

Treatment

The principle is simple: eat less. Therapy is aimed at encouraging and supporting patients during the period when they readjust to a reduced calorie intake. Many patients lose 5–10% weight after starting a diet, and this is mainly water. Losing more weight is often very difficult but the initial weight loss is always encouraging. Exercise is of limited benefit in using calories because, for instance, walking at normal speed for 1 h uses the energy equivalent of about three chocolate biscuits. However, it does improve general fitness and morale. In trials, orlistat can lead, over 1 year, to losses of weight 2–5 kg more than is achieved with placebo.

The embarrassment and sometimes depression felt by the patient and the irritation of many clinicians based on poor results and poor patient compliance make successful treatment very difficult. Self-care groups (e.g. Weight Watchers) are usually more successful in the short term. If depression is a feature this will invariably prevent successful attempts at weight reduction unless the cause disappears or it responds to therapy. There is probably no role for anorectic drugs, and certainly none for thyroxine.

Malnutrition

Malnutrition is a major problem of the developing world. *Marasmus* refers to severe protein-energy malnutrition. Children are grossly underweight with muscle wasting and no fat. There is no oedema. In kwashiorkor there is protein deficiency with adequate calorie intake. There is oedema from hypoproteinaemia, and lipids accumulate in the liver, causing hepatomegaly.

In industrialized countries, malnutrition occurs during any acute illness, but particularly of the gastrointestinal tract, e.g. carcinoma of the stomach, ulcerative colitis, Crohn disease, malabsorption. Protein loss is marked following burns from cutaneous loss, and also postoperatively from reduced intake and increased catabolism.

Enteral or intravenous feeding may be indicated.

Vitamin deficiencies

Vitamins (vital amines) are organic substances with specific biochemical functions. They are found in food, and are only required in small amounts.

Fat-soluble vitamins

Vitamin A (retinol) is found in liver, fish and dairy products. It is also produced in the intestine by cleavage of β-carotene found in carrots and other vegetables. Vitamin A is required for night vision (11-*cis*-retinaldehyde combines with rhodopsin in retinal rods). It is also important for epithelial keratinization.

Deficiency is rarely seen in industrialized countries. It causes night blindness and xerophthalmia (metaplasia of the cornea), a common cause of blindness in the developing world. Overdosage reduces keratinization of skin and sebum production. It causes rough, dry skin and hair, and liver enlargement. The recommended daily intake for adults is 750 µg.

Vitamin D (see p. 177).

Vitamin E (α-Tocopherol and related compounds) is found in vegetable oils. It is antioxidant, and present in all cell membranes. Severe deficiency causes haemolytic anaemia, and muscle and neurological disorders. The recommended daily intake for adults is 10 mg.

Vitamin K is found in green vegetables. It is a cofactor for the synthesis of clotting factors

(II, VII, IX and X), and deficiency causes prolonged prothrombin time and bleeding. The recommended daily intake for adults is 100 μg.

Water-soluble vitamins

Vitamin B$_1$ (thiamine) is found in many foods, including wheat, cereals and meat. Deficiency rapidly occurs if intake is low as body stores are small. It is a cofactor of many metabolic pathways. The recommended daily intake for adults is 1 mg.

Deficiency causes:

• *Wernicke–Korsakoff* syndrome occurs in chronic alcoholics. There is ataxia, nystagmus and ophthalmoplegia, and confusion. The inability to retain new memories is accompanied by confabulation (Korsakoff's psychosis). Ischaemia and capillary haemorrhages occur in the mammillary bodies and around the aqueduct in the midbrain. Red cell transketolase levels are reduced. The disorder usually responds to parenteral thiamine (50–100 mg), although the memory defect often persists.
• *Beriberi* is now rare outside Asia. In addition to Wernicke's encephalopathy there is cardiomyopathy and peripheral neuropathy.

Vitamin B$_2$ (riboflavin) is found in most foods. Rich sources are dairy products, liver and cereals. It is a cofactor for cellular oxidation. Deficiency causes angular stomatitis, atrophic glossitis and seborrhoeic dermatitis. It usually occurs with other B vitamin deficiencies. The recommended daily intake for adults is 1 mg.

Nicotinamide forms part of the coenzymes nicotinamide adenine dinucleotide (NAD) and nicotinamide dinucleotide phosphate (NADP). It is found in many foods, including liver, meat, fish and cereals. It can also be synthesized from the amino acid tryptophan. Deficiency causes pellagra with dermatitis, diarrhoea and dementia. The adult daily requirement of nicotinamide is 20 mg, although this can partly be supplied by tryptophan (60 mg tryptophan is converted to 1 mg nicotinamide). *Nicotinic acid* can also be given, although its use is limited by vasodilatation.

Vitamin B$_6$ (pyridoxine) is found in many foods, including liver, meat, fish and cereals.

Dietary deficiency is rare, but a number of drugs, including isonizid, penicillamine and hydralazine, antagonize its effects. Isoniazid peripheral neuropathy is prevented by pyridoxine. It may also be of benefit in hyperoxaluria and sideroblastic anaemia. The normal adult daily requirement is 3 mg/day.

Vitamin B$_{12}$ and *folic acid* (see p. 301).

Vitamin C (ascorbic acid) is an antioxidant. The main sources are fresh fruits and vegetables. One of its many roles is the reduction of proline to hydroxyproline, which is necessary for collagen formation. Impaired collagen production is the principal defect in scurvy, which is characterized by:

• swollen, spongy gums;
• spontaneous bleeding—bruising, bleeding gums, perifollicular haemorrhages, subperiosteal haemorrhages;
• anaemia; and
• hair follicle keratosis with 'corkscrew hairs'.

The normal adult daily requirement is 30–60 mg/day.

Enteral feeding

Indications

Patients who cannot eat sufficient food, but have a functioning gut.

• Unconsciousness.
• Dysphagia—neurological, oesophageal obstruction, head and neck surgery.
• Loss of nutrients from fistulas or stomas.
• Any major illness, e.g. postoperatively, following radiotherapy or chemotherapy, burns.

Administration

A fine-bore nasogastric tube is usually well-tolerated. If there is oesophageal obstruction, or prolonged feeding is necessary, a tube can be inserted directly into the stomach across the abdominal wall.

Requirements

An average patient needs:

• 2000–3000 kcal, of which 30–40% should be provided by fat; and
• 10–15 g nitrogen (60–90 g protein).

A number of commercial preparations are available. Most contain milk or soya proteins.

Protein hydrolysates or free amino acids are only necessary if the ability to break down protein is limited by pancreatic or bowel disease. The mixture should contain vitamins and trace elements.

Complications
- Vomiting.
- Aspiration.
- Diarrhoea.
- Electrolyte and metabolic disturbances.

Parenteral nutrition
Parenteral nutrition is indicated when feeding via the gut is not possible because of:
- a reduction in functioning gut mass, either because of parenchymal disease or loss of small intestine—the short-bowel syndrome;
- ileus—usually postoperatively; or
- loss of intestinal contents via fistulas.

It may supplement oral or enteral feeding, or be the only source of nutrition—total parenteral nutrition.

Requirements
Protein is provided as essential and non-essential L-amino acids. Energy is given as 150–250 kcal/g nitrogen. Glucose is the usual source of carbohydrate. Insulin may be necessary, particularly if more than 180 g of glucose is given daily. Some 30–40% of required energy is provided as fat. Fat emulsions provide essential fatty acids, and have a high energy : volume ratio.

The mixture of amino acids, glucose and fat together with trace elements and vitamins is prepared under sterile conditions by pharmacy, usually in a 3-l bag.

Administration
The tendency for peripheral veins to thrombose makes administration through a central venous catheter necessary. The catheter is inserted under full aseptic conditions. Tunnelling reduces the risk of infection. Patients requiring long-term parenteral nutrition can be taught to administer infusions overnight at home.

Complications
- Catheter-related—infection, blockage, venous thrombosis.
- Air embolism.
- Metabolic problems—hyperglycaemia, electrolyte imbalance, trace element or vitamin deficiencies.
- Fluid overload if renal insufficiency or cardiac problems.

Anorexia nervosa
This is a relatively common disorder of young women (incidence 1 in 250 schoolgirls aged 16 or under in the UK) who fast, vomit and/or purge to maintain a markedly low weight. Bulimia nervosa is habitual vomiting or purging, with eating binges between.

Anorexia nervosa is associated with extreme thinness, anovular amenorrhoea and fine hairs on the arms and legs (lanugo). Such patients have a markedly altered body image, and a craving to be very thin after considering themselves overweight. The cause is not known.

There is evidence of hypothalamopituitary dysfunction with low levels of lutenizing hormone (LH), follicle-stimulating hormone (FSH) and oestradiol. LH and FSH levels respond to gonadotrophin-releasing hormone injections, indicating an intact anterior pituitary. The levels of circulating hormones return to normal with recovery.

Treatment requires expert psychiatric advice and often periods of hospitalization with the aim of readjusting abnormal psychopathology, and increasing weight. Improvement of varying degrees, and often complete, occurs in most patients, although treatment may be necessary for many years. The mortality is 5–15%, often from suicide.

Renal Disease

Disease of the renal tract presents in only a few ways. Urinary tract infection is the most common, especially in females. In males it is prostatic hypertrophy and its consequences. Proteinuria, haematuria and disorders of excretory function often cause no symptoms if mild, being picked up during routine screening (e.g. insurance medical).

Urinary tract infection

There are two main clinical syndromes.

1 *Cystitis*, which is characterized by suprapubic tenderness, dysuria and frequency. NB These symptoms can occur without infection (the urethral syndrome). Other causes include non-specific urethritis, gonococcus, interstitial cystitis, drug-induced cystitis (e.g. cyclophosphamide), bladder stones or tumours, vaginitis (infections or senile).

2 *Acute pyelonephritis* presents with dysuria, frequency, loin tenderness and fever, often with rigors and vomiting. Fever may be the only feature in children, in whom recurrent infection may be associated with vesicoureteric reflux that tends to diminish with age.

Bacteriuria is confirmed by finding a urinary excretion of more than 100 000 organisms/ml urine (counts < 10 000/ml are usually caused by contamination). Infection may be symptom-free. *Escherichia coli* is the most frequent organism (70–80% of cases). Other organisms (*Proteus*, *Staphylococcus*, *Streptococcus*, *Klebsiella* and *Pseudomonas*) are usually associated with structural abnormality or catheterization, and reinfection. Tuberculosis classically causes a sterile pyuria.

Pyuria can almost always be detected by careful microscopic examination of fresh unspun urine. Microscopic haematuria is common.

Management

Uncomplicated cases are treated with oral antibiotics such as trimethoprim or ampicillin (3-day course for cystitis, at least 7 days for pyelonephritis) after obtaining urine for culture and antibiotic sensitivity. Resistant organisms can be treated with co-amoxiclav (Augmentin) or ciprofloxacin. Patients with acute pyelonephritis who are vomiting, pregnant or have evidence of septicaemia (blood cultures are positive in 20%) require intravenous antibiotics.

There may be an obvious predisposing cause, e.g. pregnancy, urinary obstruction or catheterization. Diabetes mellitus must be excluded. Acute pyelonephritis or more than two episodes of cystitis in a woman, or any infection in a man, suggest a structural abnormality. Ultrasound of the renal tract is performed to look for perinephric abscess, renal scarring, stone, tumours or obstruction. Intravenous urography (IVU) and possibly cystoscopy may be necessary (frequent infections, persistent haematuria, dysuria or loin pain) to exclude small stones/tumours or bladder diverticula.

Women prone to recurrent infections should be given advice about complete emptying of the bladder (double micturition), and voiding soon after intercourse. Low-dose antibiotic prophylaxis (e.g. trimethoprim 100 mg/day or nitrofurantoin 100 mg/day) reduces the incidence of infection, and can be used safely for long periods.

Children always require investigation as infection in the presence of ureteric reflux leads to permanent kidney damage.

KIDNEY SIZE

Causes of small kidneys	
Unilateral	Hypoplasia, chronic pyelonephritis, obstructive atrophy, tuberculosis, renal artery stenosis
Bilateral	All of the above plus chronic glomerulonephritis, hypertension, diabetes, analgesic nephropathy
Causes of enlarged kidney	
Unilateral	Compensatory hypertrophy, bifid collecting system, renal mass, hydronephrosis, renal vein thrombosis
Bilateral	Polycystic kidneys, amyloid, acute glomerulonephritis

Table 12.1 Causes of small and large kidneys.

Imaging the kidneys

A *plain abdominal film* usually shows the renal outlines, and identifies any calcification in the renal tract.

Renal ultrasound is useful in determining renal size and contour, and defining the size, location and consistency (solid or cystic) of any renal mass, and looking for pelvicalyceal dilatation of obstruction.

IVU has the advantage of demonstrating the whole urinary tract, but its usefulness has been replaced in many cases by ultrasound, computed tomographic (CT) scanning and radionuclide scanning. Ultrasound and CT are particularly useful for anatomical studies, and radionuclide scanning for providing functional information. IVU should not be performed if there is a history of sensitivity to contrast media. Dehydration prior to the examination should be avoided in renal failure, diabetes or myeloma.

The patient fasts for 6 h. A supine plain abdominal film is taken and inspected to identify the renal areas and look for opacities. Contrast medium is injected as an intravenous bolus and images of the renal areas obtained. A compression band is applied to the lower abdomen to compress the ureters and distend the pelvicalyceal system. The compression is then released and further films taken.

Timed serial X-rays should be available. First, inspect the plain film for renal tract calcification. Contrast is normally visible in the parenchyma as a nephrogram after 1 min (delayed in renal artery stenosis), and in the pelvicalyceal system by 5 min. Measure the size

(Table 12.1; normal adult kidneys are 11–15 cm, or three vertebrae in length), and look for the normally smooth outline. An irregular outline because of renal scarring is a feature of *chronic pyelonephritis*, *tuberculosis* and *analgesic nephropathy*. The calyces are usually cupped, but become dilatated and clubbed in *urinary tract obstruction* and *papillary necrosis*. Look for filling defects caused by *carcinoma*. After 10–20 min the compression bands are removed and contrast should fill the ureters and bladder. Look for dilatation resulting from *obstruction*, or filling defects because of *calculi* or *carcinoma*. Look at the postmicturition film to assess emptying of the bladder and urinary tracts.

Isotope scanning (most commonly ^{99m}Tc-diethylenetriaminepentacetic acid (DTPA) or ^{99m}Tc-dimercaptosuccinate (DMSA) can be used to assess renal blood flow, renal function and transit time of filtrate across the parenchyma into the collecting system. It is useful in the diagnosis of renal artery stenosis and obstruction. In addition, the renal parenchyma can be visualized for evidence of scarring.

Stones

Eighty per cent of urinary tract stones contain calcium, usually as calcium oxalate. Less common constituents are uric acid (10%) or cystine. Staghorn calculi contain struvite, made up of calcium, ammonium and phosphate. Classical features are severe loin pain, with microscopic or macroscopic haematuria.

Clinical features

The most common presentation is with severe loin pain radiating to the groin (renal colic), with microscopic or macroscopic haematuria. About 1 in 1000 men and 1 in 3000 women present with their first kidney stone in a single year. Fifteen per cent of patients develop recurrent stones within a year of first presentation, 30% by 5 years.

Recurrent stones should be investigated for a metabolic cause:

• hypercalciuria—50% of stone-formers have increased urinary calcium excretion;
• elevated serum calcium—usually caused by hyperparathyroidism in stone-formers;
• hyperuricaemia; and
• cystinuria.

Management

The diagnosis is confirmed by imaging. Abdominal X-ray may detect calcium-containing stones. Ultrasound usually identifies stones, and will detect dilatation of the renal pelvis or ureter, indicating obstruction. IVU or CT scanning provide the most sensitive methods of detecting stones. Most small stones (< 5 mm) will pass spontaneously. Stones between 5 and 9 mm may also pass, but those > 9 mm are rarely passed. In such cases stones are cleared by extracorporeal shock wave lithotripsy, endoscopic removal, either percutaneously or through cystoscopy with retrograde urethroscopy, or open surgical procedure.

Measures to prevent stone formation

• Increased fluid intake—at least 2 l/day.
• Diet—increased risk of stone formation is associated with low rather than high calcium diet, and with diets high in sodium and protein.
• Thiazide diuretics reduce urinary calcium in hypercalciuria.
• Allopurinol reduces urinary uric acid excretion.
• Penicillamine and captopril form a complex with cystine, which renders it more soluble, and can be used to prevent or dissolve stones.
• Alkalinization of urine increases solubility of uric acid and cystine and may be of value in preventing uric acid or cystine stone formation by increasing solubility of these compounds.

Chronic interstitial nephritis

The term *chronic pyelonephritis*, which implies infection, has been replaced by *chronic interstitial nephritis*, which is characterized by a chronic tubulointerstitial inflammatory infiltrate. Interstitial involvement is usually secondary to papillary or tubular damage by infection, ischaemia, radiation, toxins or metabolic disease. The most common cause is reflux nephropathy (see below). Other causes include obstructive uropathy, drugs (cyclosporin, lithium, chronic analgesic ingestion), renovascular disease, sickle-cell disease, long-standing hypokalaemia, hypercalcaemia or hyperuricaema, tuberculosis, sarcoid, heavy metal poisoning (lead, cadmium), radiation nephritis, Sjögren syndrome and hereditary nephritides (e.g. Alport syndrome).

Clinical features

There is usually altered tubular function (glycosuria, aminoaciduria, renal tubular acidosis and tubular proteinuria) with a variable degree of renal failure. Ultrasound and radionuclide scans may show obstruction, and the kidneys are often small and scarred.

Management

Treat any underlying cause. Antibiotics (prophylactic if necessary) for infection. Patients are commonly unable to concentrate their urine, and need a high fluid intake.

Reflux nephropathy

Reflux of urine through a congenitally abnormal vesicoureteric junction occurs in about 1% of infants. Reflux of sterile urine into the kidney may cause renal damage through hydrostatic injury, but there is clear evidence that reflux of infected urine leads to renal scarring. Reflux is present in 50% of infants who develop urinary infection during their first year, and one-third of children who have infection before the age of 12 years. Reflux can also present with enuresis, hypertension and proteinuria. There is a familial incidence.

Management
Children with urinary infections (and possibly those with affected siblings or parents) should be screened with an ultrasound of the renal tract followed by a micturating cystourethrogram. In some centres radionuclide cystography is used. Ureteric reimplantation and conservative treatment with antibiotics to prevent infection are equally effective in preventing scarring. Without surgery reflux generally resolves as the child grows older.

Proteinuria

Small amounts of low-molecular-weight proteins are normally filtered by the glomerulus, and reabsorbed or catabolized by proximal tubular cells. The kidneys normally excrete 50–80 mg protein daily, of which 30–50 mg is Tamm–Horsfall protein, a mucoprotein secreted by tubular cells. Proteinuria > 150 mg/day is abnormal. Proteinuria detected by dipstick should be quantified on a 24-h collection. Dipsticks primarily detect albumin, and are relatively insensitive at detecting immunoglobulins or Bence Jones protein (immunoglobulin light chains). Microalbuminuria (urinary albumin excretion of 30–300 mg/day) is an early sign of diabetic nephropathy (p. 157).

Causes of proteinuria
• Glomerular disease: glomerulonephritis, glomerulosclerosis (diabetic and hypertensive), glomerular amyloid deposition.
• Tubular disease (because of impaired reabsorption of filtered proteins): chronic interstitial nephritis, polyuric phase of acute tubular necrosis, Fanconi syndrome, tubular toxins (aminoglycosides, lead, cadmium).
• Non-renal disease: fever, heavy exercise, heart failure. Orthostatic proteinuria, a benign condition in 2% of adolescents who have proteinuria when upright but not when recumbent.
• Urinary tract disease: infection, tumours, calculi.

• Increased production of filterable proteins: immunoglobulin light chains (Bence Jones protein) in myeloma, myoglobinuria, haemoglobinuria.
    Renal vein thrombosis is both a cause and consequence of proteinuria.

Clinical presentation
Often asymptomatic (routine screening). Nephrotic syndrome if severe. There may be evidence of underlying cause (e.g. urinary infection, diabetes, hypertension).

Assessment
The history should include enquiries about recent infections (urinary or as a cause of glomerulonephritis), renal disease (including any family history), drugs and occupation. Examination may be normal but there may be oedema, hypertension, heart failure or evidence of renal failure.

Investigation
Serum creatinine, urea and electrolytes and 24-h urine collection for protein content and creatinine clearance.
    Serum proteins for albumin and protein electrophoresis (serum and urine) for monoclonal gammopathy. Blood glucose for diabetes.
    Serum complement (may be low in glomerulonephritis, p. 199), antinuclear antibodies (systemic lupus erythematosis, SLE), antineutrophil cytoplasmic antibodies (systemic vasculitis), cryoglobulin levels.
    Plain abdominal X-ray and ultrasound of renal tract for stones, structural abnormalities and renal size.
    In the majority of cases these investigations fail to define the underlying cause, and renal biopsy may be necessary, particularly if proteinuria exceeds 2 g/day or there is impaired excretory function. This usually establishes the diagnosis, and may identify a treatable cause (particularly some forms of glomerulonephritis).
    In the absence of oedema, treatment should be directed towards any underlying cause or associated conditions (e.g. hypertension).

Nephrotic syndrome

The triad of:
- proteinuria;
- hypoalbuminaemia; and
- oedema.

Aetiology

Any cause of severe proteinuria. Usually it is a consequence of glomerular disease—commonly glomerulonephritis (p. 199), diabetic glomerulosclerosis, renal amyloid. More than 75% of childhood and 25% of adult nephrotic syndrome is a result of minimal-change disease (p. 201). Tubular proteinuria is usually less than 2 g/day and does not cause nephrotic syndrome.

It is associated with thrombosis (loss of anticoagulant proteins such as antithrombin III, protein S, protein C), infection (loss of immunoglobulins) and hyperlipidaemia.

Management

Identify and treat any underlying cause.

Diabetic glomerulosclerosis—angiotensin-converting enzyme inhibitors reduce proteinuria by lowering glomerular capillary pressure, and slow progression of diabetic nephropathy.

General management is aimed at the following.
- Reducing oedema with salt restriction and diuretics. Salt-free albumin (to restore intravascular volume) with diuretics is sometimes used in resistant cases.
- Angiotensin-converting enzyme inhibitors reduce proteinuria, probably by lowering glomerular capillary pressure. Non-steroidal anti-inflammatory drugs also reduce proteinuria, but these agents reduce renal blood flow and glomerular filtration rate and cause salt retention.
- Treatment of hypertension: angiotensin-converting enzyme inhibitors and diuretics in the first instance, but additional agents may be required.
- The optimum dietary protein intake is controversial. Most physicians recommend a normal protein intake. Any protein restriction should allow for urinary protein loss.

- Anticoagulate if immobile or thrombotic episode. Look for and treat intercurrent infection.
- Hyperlipidaemia may be severe. Very-low-density lipoprotein cholesterol, low-density lipoprotein cholesterol and total plasma cholesterol are elevated, as are triglyceride levels. Although this pattern is associated with increased cardiovascular risk, the value of treatment with diet or lipid-lowering agents (3-hydroxy-3-methyl glutaryl coenzyme A (HMG CoA) reductase inhibitors are usually effective, p. 168) has not been fully assessed.

Haematuria

Isolated haematuria on dipstick testing of urine can occur in normal individuals.

Microscopic haematuria is confirmed by finding more than three red cells per high-power-field of spun urine. Macroscopic haematuria is always abnormal.

Aetiology

Common
- Renal tract infection.
- Renal tract stones (calcium oxalate 80%, triple phosphate 10%, urate 10%, cystine < 1%).
- Tumours of the bladder, kidneys and prostate.
- Glomerulonephritis.
- Schistosomiasis is common worldwide.

Uncommon
- Hypertension.
- Renal trauma.
- Papillary necrosis.
- Renal infarction.
- Drugs—cyclophosphamide (haemorrhagic cystitis), anticoagulants.
- Medullary sponge kidney (usually benign developmental abnormality with medullary cysts which may be complicated by infection or calculi).

Familial causes
- Polycystic kidneys (p. 195).
- Alport syndrome (p. 196).

- Thin basement membrane disease (a generally benign condition in which haematuria is usually the only clinical feature).
- Medullary cystic disease (tubulointerstitial nephritis with medullary cysts that usually progresses to renal failure).

The causes vary with age. Glomerular causes predominate in children and young adults, whereas tumours and calculi are common in the elderly.

Investigation

The likely source may be suspected from the history and examination.

Microscopy of a fresh urine sample is performed in all patients to confirm the presence of red cells. The presence of red-cell casts or dysmorphic (abnormally shaped) red cells indicates glomerular bleeding (red cells are deformed by mechanical and osmotic stress as they pass through the tubules). Heavy proteinuria suggest a glomerular lesion, while white-cell casts indicate renal inflammation. Bacteria may be seen and culture should be performed. Urine should also be sent for cytology.

Plasma urea and *creatinine* to assess renal function.

Plain abdominal film and *ultrasound of the renal tract* to assess renal size and look for structural lesions (calculi, tumours, cysts).

If glomerular bleeding is suspected (young age, hypertension, proteinuria, renal impairment, absence of structural lesion), consider *renal biopsy*.

If a lesion of the renal tract is suspected (older age, no evidence of intrinsic renal disease) proceed to *cystoscopy* with *IVU* if the upper renal tract has not been clearly identified by ultrasound.

NB Normal urine (centrifuged deposit) contains:
- Red cells 1×10^6 cells/24 h (3 per high-power-field).
- White cells 2×10^6 cells/24 h (6 per high-power-field).
- Hyaline casts are composed of uromucoid (Tamm–Horsfall protein which is excreted by normal tubular cells).
- Cellular casts result from adherence of either red cells (implying glomerular bleeding) or white cells (implying tubular inflammation) to the surface of hyaline casts.
- Epithelial cells may be found in normal urine as a result of contamination by cells from the vulva or prepuce.

Acute renal failure

Characterized by a rapid rise in serum creatinine, usually with a decrease in urine output. The causes can be divided into prerenal, renal and postrenal.

PRERENAL
Aetiology
- Sepsis—the most common cause, usually complicating surgery or pneumonia.
- Hypovolaemia from any cause (e.g. haemorrhage, burns, severe diarrhoea or vomiting).
- Cardiogenic shock.
- Drug-induced hypotension (e.g. following drug overdose).

NB Angiotensin-converting enzyme inhibitors may reduce glomerular perfusion sufficiently to cause renal failure if given in the presence of bilateral renal artery stenosis (p. 275). In accelerated (malignant) hypertension acute, severe hypertension is associated with marked renal abnormalities. The most striking of these is gross intimal hyperplasia, leading to occlusion of the lumen in small arteries and arterioles. Renal failure is a rapid consequence of this condition if the blood pressure is not controlled.

Renal failure commonly complicates advanced liver disease. Plasma urea and creatinine may be normal because of reduced hepatic urea synthesis, low dietary protein intake and loss of muscle mass. There is often a precipitating cause (e.g. hypovolaemia following diuretic therapy, paracentesis or gastrointestinal bleeding, sepsis). Unexplained renal failure complicating liver disease is the *hepatorenal syndrome*. The prognosis is poor. Reinfusion of ascites into the internal jugular vein via a peritoneovenous shunt can expand plasma volume and improve renal function, but does not improve survival.

Pathophysiology

Despite high blood flow (20% of cardiac output) the kidneys are particularly susceptible to ischaemia. Factors contributing to ischaemic or toxin-induced renal cell injury include cellular adenosine triphosphate depletion (as a result of hypoxia and mitochondrial injury), and free radical generation.

The medulla receives less than 10% of renal blood flow, and is at greatest risk of injury. The common response to severe injury (regardless of cause) is *acute tubular necrosis* (ATN). The necrosis of tubular epithelial cells is most prominent in the proximal tubules and thick ascending limb of the loop of Henle. The tubular lumen may be obstructed by cell debris and casts. Regeneration of tubular cells leading to recovery can take weeks. Severe prolonged ischaemia can cause acute cortical necrosis from which there is little chance of recovery.

The distinction between prerenal failure (in which concentrating powers are retained) and ATN (in which concentrating powers are lost) can be made on urinalysis. In prerenal failure urine osmolality is high (> 500 mosmol/kg), urine sodium is low (< 20 mmol/l) and urine : plasma urea ratio is $> 10 : 1$. In ATN urine is isotonic with plasma (< 400 mosmol/kg), urine sodium is > 40 mmol/l and urine : plasma urea ratio is $< 10 : 1$.

RENAL

Causes

- Glomerulonephritis (p. 199).
- Nephrotoxic drugs (e.g. aminoglycosides, cyclosporin A, amphotericin B).
- Poisoning (e.g. heavy metals).
- Myoglobinuria—following rabdomyolysis myoglobin may cause tubular toxicity or form tubular casts. Creatine kinase is markedly elevated.
- Acute tubular (or cortical) necrosis complicating prerenal disease.
- Acute interstitial nephritis (usually drug-induced hypersensitivity reaction which responds to withdrawal of the drug and a short course of corticosteroids. Eosinophils may be present within the predominantly mononuclear cell interstitial infiltrate).

- Intrarenal obstruction (e.g. urate or oxalate crystals, calcium precipitation, tubular casts in myeloma).

NB Hypercalcaemia causes renal failure through renal vasoconstriction, direct tubular cell toxicity and distal tubular calcium phosphate precipitation.

Haemolytic–uraemic syndrome (HUS) is characterized by thrombocytopenia (platelet consumption), microangiopathic haemolytic anaemia (red cell fragments on film) and acute renal failure. Commonly follows a diarrhoeal illness in infants infected with a verotoxin-producing strain of *Escherichia coli*. In adults it may follow an upper respiratory tract infection or be associated with cyclosporin A, the oral contraceptive pill or cytotoxic agents. Familial forms occur. Renal biopsy shows occlusion of glomerular capillaries with fibrin and thrombi, without evidence of complement or immunoglobulin deposition. Recovery usually occurs over a few weeks in children, but the prognosis for adults is poor. Responses to plasma exchange with fresh frozen plasma have been reported. *Thrombotic thrombocytopenic purpura* (TTP, p. 310) is closely related to HUS, but is most common in women and central nervous system involvement and fever are typical additional features.

POSTRENAL

Acute urinary tract obstruction from:
- prostatic hypertrophy;
- renal and ureteric stones;
- tumour of renal pelvis, ureters or bladder;
- blood clot;
- sloughed papillae;
- external compression from retroperitoneal fibrosis or tumours; and
- surgical mishap (e.g. ureteric involvement in hysterectomy).

NB Lesions above the bladder must involve both urinary tracts.

Investigation

Where there is no obvious cause following careful history and examination, and preliminary biochemical and haematological assessment.

• Check that there is no obstruction. Rectal examination is obligatory to exclude prostatic disease in men, or a pelvic mass. The bladder is enlarged in urethral obstruction. Ultrasound to look for urinary tract dilatation is the simplest method of excluding obstruction. This will also give information about renal size (small kidneys indicate chronic renal disease; scarring usually indicates chronic interstitial nephritis or ischaemia).

• If renal size is normal and there are no clues on investigations, including urinalysis (exclude infection; heavy proteinuria, granular or red cell casts indicate intrinsic renal disease), calcium, uric acid, protein electrophoresis (myeloma), antineutrophil cytoplasm antibodies (vasculitis), antiglomerular basement membrane antibodies (Goodpasture disease), antinuclear antibodies (SLE), platelet, eosinophil count and coagulation (disseminated intravascular coagulation (DIC), TTP, HUS, drug-induced hypersensitivity).

• Proceed to renal biopsy providing there are no contraindications.

Management

Should be undertaken in a specialized unit where facilities for renal replacement therapy are available.

Identify and correct underlying causes—often multiple (e.g. hypotension, sepsis, DIC and aminoglycoside toxicity).

Rapid correction of prerenal causes (intravenous fluids or blood for hypovolaemia, antibiotics for sepsis, inotropes, avoidance of nephrotoxic drugs) may prevent ATN and restore renal function. Loop diuretics (e.g. furosemide (frusemide)) are often given, and may prevent tubular cell ischaemia through inhibition of active sodium chloride reabsorption, thereby reducing oxygen requirements.

Relieve urinary tract obstruction from below (urethral catheterization with or without ureteric stents) or above (nephrostomy). Prostatic obstruction in elderly men is the most common cause.

Initiate treatment for any intrinsic renal disease (e.g. immunosuppression for certain forms of glomerulonephritis, p. 199).

Continuing assessment of fluid status through input–output records, physical examination, daily weight, lying and standing blood pressure. Fluids should be restricted if there is oliguria or anuria, but patients are usually catabolic and nutrition should not be neglected. A protein intake of 0.6–0.8 g/kg/day with 30 kcal/kg/day should be maintained. In severely ill patients parenteral nutrition may be necessary.

Careful monitoring of electrolytes, urea, creatinine and acid–base status.

If renal failure persists, renal replacement therapy with haemodialysis, peritoneal dialysis or haemofiltration will be required. Absolute indications include hyperkalaemia (potassium above 6–7 mmol/l), markedly elevated plasma creatinine (> 1000 μmol/l, but absolute level must take clinical state into account), severe acidosis (bicarbonate below 10–15 mmol/l) and fluid overload with pulmonary oedema.

Chronic renal failure

Common causes
• *Chronic glomerulonephritis* (p. 199).
• *Diabetic nephropathy* (p. 157).
• *Chronic interstitial nephritis* (p. 190).
• *Hypertension*: estimates of the prevalence of chronic renal failure caused by essential hypertension vary widely from 0.002 to 20% of all cases of renal failure, reflecting the fact that the diagnosis of renal disease caused by hypertension depends on the exclusion of other causes. Many cases may have undiagnosed renal disease. Renal failure because of hypertension is much more common in black people than white people, and within the black population there appears to be familial clustering of renal disease caused by hypertension, suggesting a genetic susceptibility to hypertensive renal damage.
• *Renovascular disease* (p. 275).
• *Hereditary renal disease.*

• *Polycystic kidney disease*
An autosomal dominant condition in which renal failure results from progressive cystic degeneration of the kidneys. Patients present with hypertension, abdominal pain, haematuria

or chronic renal failure. The diagnosis is confirmed by ultrasound, and family members should be screened. Progression to renal failure with hypertension is usual, although the age at which renal replacement therapy becomes necessary varies. Approximately 85% of cases are caused by a defect in *PKD1* which maps to 16p13.3. The *PKD2* gene, responsible for most non-16p-linked polycystic kidney disease, has been localized to 4q13–q23.

The disease should be considered a multisystem disease in which cysts occur in other organs (liver, pancreas, testes). There is an increased incidence of cardiac valve disease, cerebral aneurysms, hernias and diverticular disease. The underlying cellular defect is at present unknown. Analysis of the DNA sequence available so far has not revealed homologies to other known proteins. Characterization of the protein should help clarify the molecular pathology.

• *Alport syndrome*
X-linked hereditary nephritis—associated with sensorineural deafness and eye lesions. Characterized by thinning and splitting of glomerular basement membrane (GBM). There is an abnormality of type IV collagen (α5 chain; gene locus Xq22).
• Long-standing urinary tract obstruction.
NB About 20% of patients with chronic renal failure present with bilaterally small kidneys and no diagnosis is reached. Under these circumstances renal biopsy is hazardous and unlikely to show reversible changes.

Clinical features
Screening for renal disease and the availability of dialysis mean that the classical manifestations of *uraemia* (literally *urine in the blood*) are now seen infrequently. Chronic renal failure is, by definition, slow to progress and usually presents with lethargy, general malaise, anorexia and nausea. Generalized pruritus is common. Impotence, menstrual irregularities and loss of fertility are common complaints in younger patients. In severe uraemia there is a characteristic fishy fetor, hiccups, vomiting, severe

pruritus with skin excoriations, skin pigmentation, peripheral neuropathy and central nervous system derangements leading to lethargy, stupor and coma with fitting. Pericarditis may be associated with effusion and tamponade.

Investigations
Biochemical
Plasma urea and creatinine provide a guide to the severity of renal failure.

Urea. Although there is little evidence that urea ($H_2N\text{-}CO\text{-}NH_2$; molecular mass 60 Da) is toxic, it is the most abundant nitrogenous compound to accumulate in renal failure. It is the end-product of protein metabolism and is synthesized primarily in the liver. It is freely filtered by the glomerulus, but approximately 50% is reabsorbed so urea clearance is less than glomerular filtration rate (GFR). Urea production increases with cellular catabolism (infection, trauma, steroid therapy) or following protein load (dietary or following gastrointestinal haemorrhage). It is reduced in liver failure.

Creatinine is derived from metabolism of creatine in muscle. The rate of production correlates with muscle mass, and depends little on protein intake. Fifty per cent loss of renal function is needed before the serum creatinine rises above the normal range; it is therefore not a sensitive indicator of mild to moderate renal injury.

Creatinine clearance provides a more accurate assessment (if performed correctly). The patient performs a 24-h collection of urine (the first urine passed on waking is discarded, and all urine passed up until and including emptying the bladder the following morning is collected). A single measurement of plasma creatinine is made during this time. Creatinine clearance is measured as:

(urine creatinine concentration ÷ plasma creatinine) × urine volume per minute.

In addition to being filtered by the glomerulus, small quantities of creatinine are excreted by the tubules. The creatinine clearance therefore slightly overestimates the GFR. ^{51}Cr *ethylene diaminetetra-acetic acid (EDTA) clearance* more accurately reflects the GFR. It is calculated from the rate of disappearance of a bolus injection of ^{51}Cr EDTA from the blood. The normal GFR is 110–130 ml/min per 1.73 m^2.

Hyperkalaemia (p. 204) is common.

A number of abnormalities of *calcium* and *phosphate* homeostasis occur.

Phosphate retention leads to:
• reciprocal depression of serum calcium level; and
• rise in the calcium x phosphate product which may lead to ectopic calcification.

The diseased kidneys fail to hydroxylate *25-hydroxycholecalciferol* (25-HCC) to the more active form 1–25-dihydroxycholecalciferol (1–25-DHCC). This results in:
• reduced calcium absorption from gut; and
• osteomalacia.

Hypocalcaemia stimulates the parathyroid glands which are thus in a state of chronic hypersecretion, tending to return the serum calcium level to normal.

Thus, dihydroxycholecalciferol is reduced (because of reduced 1α-hydroxylase activity in the kidney) with increased parathyroid hormone (PTH). The increased PTH may result from phosphate retention, which leads to a decrease in ionized calcium. The clinical consequences are:
• osteoporosis produced by hyperparathyroidism;
• osteomalacia caused by lack of vitamin D; and
• ectopic calcification.

Hypocalcaemia rarely leads to tetany because acidosis and hypoproteinaemia reduce protein binding and increase ionized levels of calcium.

Plasma *uric acid* is often raised (but clinical gout is rare).

Haematological investigations usually reveal a *normochromic normocytic anaemia* which responds to parenteral erythropoietin. Gastrointestinal blood loss, iron, vitamin B_{12} or folate deficiency, decreased red cell survival, hyperparathyroidism and aluminium toxicity may also contribute to anaemia, and should

be considered if there is a failed response to erythropoietin.

Urinalysis should be performed to exclude urinary infection and look for cellular casts indicating active renal inflammation.

Renal ultrasound identifies obstruction or renal scars, and defines renal size. *Plain abdominal X-ray* also defines the renal outline, and excludes renal tract calcification. If renal size is normal, and the cause of renal disease unknown, *renal biopsy* should be considered.

Management

There are two main aims:
1 slowing the decline in renal function; and
2 preventing or treating complications (bone disease, cardiovascular disease, endocrine effects, anaemia, socioeconomic).

Regardless of the cause of renal disease, once renal function is compromised, a steady progressive fall in GFR is usually observed.

Risk factors for progression of renal disease are:
• persistent activity of underlying disease;
• uncontrolled hypertension;
• infection; and
• nephrotoxins (drugs).

Pathophysiology

Possible mechanisms of progression of renal failure include:
• increased glomerular pressure (as a result of increased systemic blood pressure, or efferent arteriolar constriction as a consequence of increased angiotensin II levels);
• glomerular protein leakage; and
• lipid abnormalities.

Hypertension in chronic renal failure

Progression in chronic renal failure is attenuated by treatment of hypertension. Thiazide diuretics, β-blockers, angiotensin-converting enzyme inhibitors and calcium antagonists are all effective in patients with early renal damage. Angiotensin-converting enzyme inhibitors and calcium-channel blockers do not modify glucose or lipid metabolism, have a favourable effect on left ventricular hypertrophy and have a potentially nephroprotective effect by reducing increased renal vascular resistance. Angiotensin-converting enzyme inhibitors have the additional advantage of producing a fall in proteinuria in patients with both diabetic and non-diabetic renal disease. They should be introduced with caution as they can reduce renal blood flow and precipitate acute renal failure, particularly in the presence of renal artery stenosis (p. 275).

Dietary protein restriction

Protein is often restricted to 0.6 g/kg/day once GFR falls below 50 ml/min, although there is little evidence that this retards progression of renal failure.

Complications

Bone disease

Hypocalcaemia from decreased renal 1,25-$(OH)_2D_3$ synthesis, hyperphosphataemia and resistance to peripheral actions of PTH all contribute to renal bone disease. Treatment is by dietary phosphate restriction with or without phosphate binders (calcium carbonate providing calcium has not become elevated as a result of tertiary hyperparathyroidism, p. 180), and early use of low-dose 1α-hydroxylated vitamin D derivatives.

Cardiovascular disease

Cardiovascular disease is the most common cause of mortality in patients with chronic renal failure. It is likely to reflect an increased incidence of hypertension, lipid abnormalities, glucose intolerance and haemodynamic abnormalities, including left ventricular hypertrophy. Of these, hypertension is probably the most susceptible to treatment.

Anaemia

Circulating erythropoietin levels are inappropriately low. Parenteral recombinant erythropoietin increases haemoglobin, improves exercise tolerance and reduces the need for blood transfusion. In patients with predialysis advanced renal failure erythropoietin corrects anaemia and improves well-being, without affecting the rate of decline in renal function.

Dose-dependent hypertension occurs in 35% of patients and can usually be controlled with hypotensive agents, although hypertensive encephalopathy can develop suddenly.

Sexual dysfunction

Decreased libido and impotence are common. Hyperprolactinaemia is present in at least one-third of patients, resulting in an inhibitory effect on gonadotrophin secretion. Prolactin levels may be reduced by bromocriptine, although side-effects are common (nausea, headache, drowsiness, postural hypotension).

End-stage renal disease requires replacement of renal function by the following.
• *Haemodialysis*. Diffusion of solutes occurs between blood and dialysate which flow in opposite directions, separated by a semipermeable membrane. The most common problems are cardiovascular instability during dialysis, and difficulty establishing vascular access. This is achieved by:

    (a) arteriovenous fistula, typically at the wrist with arterialization of the cephalic vein;

    (b) double-lumen jugular, subclavian or femoral line;

    (c) synthetic graft (usually Goretex) looping subcutaneously between an artery and vein in the forearm or leg; or

    (d) Scribner shunt—arteriovenous Teflon shunt between artery and vein, usually at the wrist or ankle (rarely used now).

• Continuous ambulatory peritoneal dialysis. Patients instil up to 2 l of isotonic or hypertonic glucose solution into the peritoneal cavity via a permanent indwelling Silastic catheter. The fluid equilibrates, across the 2 m^2 of peritoneal membrane, with blood in peritoneal capillaries. After several hours the fluid containing toxic waste products is drained out. This procedure is repeated three or four times daily. Excess fluid is removed by hypertonic solutions. The major complication is peritonitis, usually caused by *Staphylococcus epidermidis* or *S. aureus*.

• *Renal transplantation* is the treatment of choice in most patients, but is limited by supply of donor organs.

GLOMERULUS

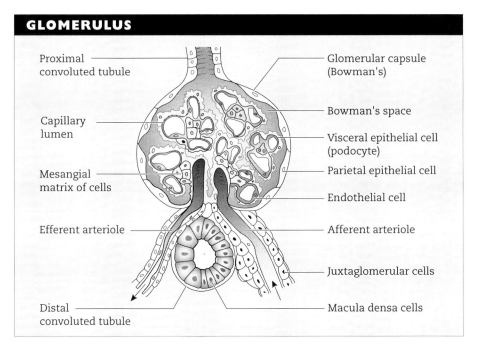

Proximal convoluted tubule

Capillary lumen

Mesangial matrix of cells

Efferent arteriole

Distal convoluted tubule

Glomerular capsule (Bowman's)

Bowman's space

Visceral epithelial cell (podocyte)

Parietal epithelial cell

Endothelial cell

Afferent arteriole

Juxtaglomerular cells

Macula densa cells

Fig. 12.1 Glomerulus.

Assessment of dialysis adequacy
Plasma urea and creatinine are poor predictors of outcome in dialysis patients—low predialysis urea, not high, has been found to be associated with increased mortality. This is because when protein intake is deficient or muscle mass is reduced, predialysis urea and creatinine may remain low even in the presence of inadequate dialysis. Assessment of dialysis adequacy is now achieved by the use of kinetic measurements—often referred to as *urea kinetic modelling*. Two parameters, *urea clearance* corrected for volume of distribution (Kt/V urea, where Kt = urea clearance and V = volume of distribution) and *protein catabolic rate* have been found in several studies to be useful predictors of outcome.

Glomerulonephritis

This describes a number of disorders that affect one or more of the glomerular components in both kidneys (Fig. 12.1). Patients present with one or more features of renal disease—hypertension, haematuria, proteinuria,

nephrotic syndrome and various degrees of renal failure.

The classification of glomerulonephritis is based on histology and immunofluorescence of renal tissue. Contraindications to renal biopsy include:
- one functioning kidney;
- small kidneys;
- hypertension; and
- bleeding disorders.

Confusion arises because renal biopsy findings do not necessarily correlate with clinical features, although they are sometimes useful in guiding management and predicting outcome.

Histological changes are described as:
- *focal*—affecting < 50% of glomeruli;
- *diffuse*—affecting > 50% of glomeruli;
- *segmental*—affecting part of the glomerulus;
- *global*—affecting all of the glomerular tuft;
- *proliferative*—an increase in glomerular cells (mesangial, epithelial and endothelial) with leucocytic infiltration;
- *crescent*—a crescent-shaped proliferation of epithelial cells and mononuclear cells in

Bowman's capsule. It occurs in any severe form of glomerular injury;
- *membranous*—thickening of the glomerular capillary wall; and
- *sclerosis*—capillary collapse with loss of the lumen.

IgA-related glomerulonephritis

Granular mesangial deposition of immunoglobulin A (IgA, and usually C3) with variable segmental mesangial proliferation (measurement of serum immunoglobulins is usually unhelpful—20–50% have raised IgA).

Clinically
Usually presents with haematuria (often provoked by infection).

Aetiology
Unknown. It is associated with liver disease (particularly alcoholic cirrhosis), coeliac disease, seronegative arthritis, neoplasia, infection.

Prognosis
It is probably the most common form of glomerulonephritis. Approximately 20% progress to renal failure. There is no specific treatment, but control of hypertension which is commonly present slows the decline in renal function.

Henoch-Schönlein purpura
(See p. 126.)

Membranous nephropathy
Diffuse uniform thickening of glomerular capillary wall, usually without cellular proliferation.

Classification
- Stage I: small subepithelial electron-dense deposits (diffuse granular IgG staining).
- Stage II: outgrowth of basement membrane between subepithelial deposits (seen as 'spikes' on silver stain).
- Stage III: deposits incorporated into basement membrane which becomes less electron-dense.
- Stage IV: thickened vacuolated membrane, sclerosis.

Clinical manifestations
Proteinuria (often nephrotic), hypertension, haematuria, deteriorating renal function.

Aetiology
Idiopathic, drugs (penicillamine, gold), neoplasia, SLE, infections (hepatitis B, malaria), diabetes.

Prognosis
The course of idiopathic membranous nephropathy is highly variable. Approximately 25% undergo complete spontaneous remission, 25% have a partial remission with stable impaired renal function, 25% have persistent nephrotic syndrome with stable renal function and 25% progress to end-stage renal disease. Poor prognosis is suggested by heavy proteinuria, hypertension, elevated creatinine at presentation, and stage IV lesion. Deterioration in renal function can be halted or reversed by a regimen of alternating steroids and chlorambucil (Ponticelli regimen, *N Engl J Med* 1992; **327**: 599–603).

Membranoproliferative (mesangiocapillary) glomerulonephritis

Mesangial expansion (caused by increased matrix and mesangial cells), and thickened capillary loops (caused by extension of matrix and mesangial cells between GBM and endothelium giving the characteristic double contour).

Classification
- Type I: subendothelial immune deposits (stain for C3 and Ig—most common type).
- Type II: linear dense deposits along GBM (linear C3, occasional Ig).

Aetiology
Secondary causes include:
- infection, whether bacterial (infective endocarditis, 'shunt nephritis', leprosy), viral (hepatitis B) or protozoal (schistosomiasis);
- neoplasia;
- SLE; and
- cryoglobulinaemia.

Nephritic factor occurs in >60% type I and 10–20% type II mesangiocapillary glomerulonephritis. It is an IgG autoantibody which binds to and stabilizes C3 convertase (C3bBb), permanently activating the alternative pathway and depleting C3. It is associated with partial lipodystrophy.

Clinical features
Proteinuria and haematuria, with variable degree of renal failure.

Prognosis
There is no evidence to support the use of immunosuppressive therapy. Half progress to renal failure in 10 years.

Minimal-change nephropathy
Normal light microscopy, with negative immunofluorescence. There is podocyte foot process fusion on electron microscopy (a relative non-specific consequence of proteinuria).

Clinical features
Accounts for over 75% of childhood and 30% of adult cases of nephrotic syndrome.

Aetiology
It is associated with allergy and malignancy (Hodgkin's).

Prognosis
The majority respond to steroids. Cyclophosphamide is beneficial if relapsing. Cyclosporin may also be of benefit.

Focal glomerulosclerosis
Segmental sclerosis affecting some glomeruli (focal). Granular IgM and C3 may be present in areas of sclerosis.

Aetiology
Idiopathic—focal glomerulosclerosis accounts for 10–20% of adult and childhood nephrotic syndrome. It is also associated with reflux nephropathy, focal proliferative glomerulonephritis, drugs (heroin, analgesic abuse), diabetes mellitus, hyperfiltration in a remnant kidney, human immunodeficiency virus (HIV) infection, sickle-cell disease, malignancy, Alport syndrome.

Clinical features
Proteinuria, often with hypertension and renal impairment.

Prognosis
There is a poor response to treatment—cyclosporin may be of benefit.

Systemic vasculitis
There is necrotizing inflammation of blood-vessel walls. Any organ system can be involved.

Renal involvement is usually seen in Wegener's granulomatosis and microscopic polyangiitis. Typically, there is a focal proliferative glomerulonephritis, often with necrosis and crescent formation. Granulomatous inflammation of upper and lower airway is usually present in Wegener's granulomatosis.

Vasculitis has been classified according to clinical features, size of vessel, and the presence of antibodies against neutrophil cytoplasm antigens (ANCA—most commonly directed against neutrophil proteases, including proteinase-3 and myeloperoxidase) (Table 12.2).

Renal lesion
Focal proliferation with necrosis and epithelial cell crescent formation. Immunofluorescence usually negative or sparse granular Ig and C3. Presents with rapidly progressive glomerulonephritis.

Prognosis
Remission occurs in over 90% of patients using oral cyclophosphamide (2 mg/kg/day) and prednisolone (60 mg/day). Steroids can be reduced and cyclophosphamide changed to azathioprine once remission has been induced. Relapse occurs in one-third of patients during the first year. Intravenous immunoglobulin and monoclonal anti-T-cell antibody therapy may be effective in patients with vasculitis refractory to further increases in immunosuppression.

Antiglomerular basement membrane disease
(Goodpasture disease)
Proliferative glomerulonephritis—usually severe glomerular inflammation with crescents and

CLASSIFICATION OF VASCULITIS

	ANCA+	ANCA±	ANCA−
Small vessel	Wegener's granulomatosis Microscopic polyangiitis	Henoch–Schönlein purpura	
Medium vessel	Churg–Strauss	Polyarteritis nodosa	
Large vessel			Takayasu's arteritis Giant-cell arteritis

ANCA, antibodies against neutrophil cytoplasm antigens.

Table 12.2 Classification of vasculitis.

necrosis. Immunofluorescence reveals linear IgG along GBM (may also occur in SLE and diabetes).

Aetiology
Anti-GBM antibodies recognize a restricted epitope on type IV collagen. They bind with high affinity to basement membrane in glomeruli, alveoli, the eye and ear.
NB Anti-GMB antibodies do not bind to Alport GBM in which type IV collagen is abnormal (p. 196), but may develop following transplantation of a normal kidney into a patient with Alport syndrome.

Clinical features
There is an acute renal failure caused by a rapidly progressive glomerulonephritis. Pulmonary haemorrhage (in smokers) causes breathlessness and haemoptysis. Chest X-ray shows pulmonary shadowing and transfer factor (T_{LCO}) is increased by the presence of haemoglobin in alveoli. The combination is known as Goodpasture syndrome, and anti-GBM disease (Goodpasture disease) is a common cause. The other major cause is systemic vasculitis (see above).

Prognosis
The disease usually responds to plasma exchange (to remove the autoantibody) combined with steroids and cytotoxic therapy (usually cyclophosphamide). Recovery of renal function is rare once anuria or dialysis dependence has occurred.

CLASSIFICATION OF RENAL DISEASE IN SLE

Class	Description
I	Normal (extremely rare)
II	Mesangial changes
	IIa Deposits by immunofluorescence and electron microscopy
	IIb Hypercellularity as well
III	Proliferative glomerulonephritis (< 50%)
IV	Proliferative glomerulonephritis (> 50%)
V	Membranous glomerulonephritis

Table 12.3 World Health Organization classification of renal disease in systemic lupus erythematosus (SLE).

Systemic lupus erythematosus
Renal involvement is common in SLE (p. 122) —over 90% of patients have abnormalities on renal biopsy. The World Health Organization (WHO) classification is shown in Table 12.3.

Clinical features
There can be almost any manifestation of renal disease, including hypertension, haematuria, proteinuria, nephrotic syndrome, acute renal failure and end-stage renal disease.

Prognosis
The prognosis differs according to WHO classification. It is good in class II, but poor in classes III and IV. The significance of membranous change

(class V) is unclear. Steroids in combination with azathioprine or cyclophosphamide can slow progressive renal damage. Plasma exchange may provide additional benefits.

Post-streptococcal glomerulonephritis

Diffuse proliferative glomerulonephritis with granular deposits of C3 and IgG.

Clinical features

Oliguria, oedema, hypertension, haematuria and renal impairment follow 2–3 weeks after infection with a nephritogenic strain of group A β-haemolytic streptococci.

Investigations

Throat or skin cultures may show group A streptococci if penicillin has not been given. Antibodies against streptococcal antigens provide evidence of recent infection, e.g. anti-streptolysin (ASO), antideoxyribonuclease-B (ADNase B). Hypocomplementaemia occurs with low C3 and CH_{50}.

Prognosis

Spontaneous recovery is usual. The disease is now very rare.

Fluid and electrolytes

Salt and water

Plasma sodium concentration and extracellular fluid volume vary independently of each other so alterations in plasma sodium reflect alterations in either sodium or water.

SERUM SODIUM DECREASED

(hyponatraemia = plasma sodium < 130 mmol/l)

Aetiology

Too little sodium or too much water, or both.

Clinical features

In salt depletion there is thirst, dry tongue, reduced tissue turgor and postural hypotension. In severe depletion mental confusion, hypotension and shock occur. None of these features are present if water excess because of inappropriate antidiuretic hormone (ADH) or psychogenic polydypsia is the cause.

Investigation

Check serum osmolality and urine sodium.
If:
1 Serum osmolality is decreased and urine sodium is increased:
   • excess renal sodium loss (renal failure, Addison's disease, p. 150); and
   • inappropriate ADH secretion (NB Some drugs such as chlorpropamide and carbamazepine can have an ADH-like action on the kidney).
2 Serum osmolality is decreased and urine sodium is decreased:
   • extrarenal loss of sodium (e.g. gastrointestinal tract, burns);
   • fluid retention associated with cardiac failure, hepatic failure or nephrotic syndrome; and
   • psychogenic polydipsia.
3 Serum osmolality is normal:
   • usually spurious, e.g. in severe hyperlipidaemia when the amount of sodium in the aqueous phase of plasma is normal, but its concentration is expressed in terms of the volume of the aqueous and lipid phase.

Management

Salt depletion is corrected with NaCl, either orally (slow sodium tablets) or as intravenous normal saline (0.9%, 150 mmol/l each of Na^+ and Cl^-). Water excess in inappropriate ADH secretion and psychogenic polydysia is treated by water restriction (< 600 ml/24 h).

SERUM SODIUM INCREASED

(hypernatraemia)

Aetiology

Too much sodium or too little water.

Investigation

Check urine sodium (normal 10–20 mmol/l) and whether urine osmolality is low (< 300 mosmol/l), or high (> 800 mosmol/l).
If:
1 Urine osmolality decreased and urine sodium increased:

- excess sodium load, either iatrogenic or endocrine (e.g. Conn syndrome, Cushing syndrome);
- previous renal loss of water and sodium (e.g. osmotic diuresis resulting from glucose).

2 Urine osmolality decreased and urine sodium decreased:
- diabetes insipidus (p. 147).

3 Urine osmolality increased and urine sodium decreased:
- previous and continuing extrarenal loss of sodium and water (e.g. from sweat, gastrointestinal tract).

4 Urine osmolality increased and urine sodium increased or normal:
- previous and continuing extrarenal loss of water but not sodium (e.g. from lungs during febrile illness).

Management

Patients with hypernatraemia need water which can be given orally or as intravenous 5% dextrose. The underlying cause should be determined and treated.

Serum potassium

Around 98% of potassium is intracellular (in contrast to sodium which is predominantly extracellular). Normal potassium intake = 60–200 mmol/day.

SERUM POTASSIUM DECREASED
(hypokalaemia)
Aetiology
- Gastrointestinal losses: diarrhoea and/or vomiting (colonic tumours, particularly villous adenomas, may secrete large amounts of potassium), laxative abuse.
- Renal loss:
  (a) diuretic therapy (thiazides, loop diuretics);
  (b) mineralocorticoid excess. Renin secreted by the juxtaglomerular apparatus in the kidney converts angiotensinogen to angiotensin. Angiotensin stimulates aldosterone secretion from the adrenal cortex which causes urinary sodium retention and potassium loss. Causes include Conn syndrome, Cushing syndrome, corticosteroid therapy,

ectopic adrenocorticotrophic hormone (ACTH, tumours), Bartter's syndrome (renal potassium loss associated with juxtaglomerular cell hyperplasia and hyperreninaemia);
  (c) osmotic diuresis (e.g. uncontrolled diabetes); and
  (d) renal tubular acidosis (renal tubular defect associated with potassium loss and an inability to acidify urine—causes hyperchloraemic, hypokalaemic acidosis (p. 205)).
- Shift to intracellular compartment (e.g. insulin therapy, familial periodic paralysis).
- Poor intake (including eating disorders, which may be associated with laxative or diuretic abuse).

Clinical features
Weakness and lethargy. The electrocardiogram (ECG) shows flat T and prominent U waves.

Management
Treat the underlying cause.
- Give oral potassium as potassium chloride.
- Where oral administration is not possible (e.g. diabetic ketoacidosis), potassium is given intravenously: 2 g/l (26 mmol/l) intravenous solution.

SERUM POTASSIUM INCREASED
(hyperkalaemia)
Aetiology
- Potassium retention:
  (a) renal failure (prerenal, renal, postrenal);
  (b) decreased mineralocorticoids: Addison's disease, spironolactone (aldosterone antagonist), angiotensin-converting enzyme inhibitors (e.g. captopril, enalapril); and
  (c) potassium-retaining diuretics (e.g. amiloride).
- Increased supply of potassium—potassium is predominantly intracellular, and released following cell destruction, e.g. haemolysis, trauma, cytotoxic therapy.

Clinical features
Severe hyperkalaemia (> 6–7 mmol/l) may be associated with life-threatening ECG abnormalities.

Management

Stop oral or intravenous intake.

Ion exchange resins, e.g. calcium resonium 15 g 6-hourly orally (or rectally).

In emergency states, intravenous calcium (10 ml 10% calcium gluconate) antagonizes the cardiac effects of hyperkalaemia. Intravenous dextrose and insulin (e.g. 100 ml of 50% dextrose with 20 units of soluble insulin) moves potassium into the intracellular compartment. Dialysis may be required.

Metabolic acidosis

Aetiology

• Exogenous acids (e.g. poisoning by salicylate, methanol, ethylene glycol).
• Accumulation of endogenous acids such as lactic acid (tissue hypoperfusion in cardiac arrest or shock) or acetoacetic acid in diabetic ketoacidosis.
• Loss of alkali (e.g. gastrointestinal loss in severe diarrhoea, biliary or enteric fistulae; or renal loss in proximal tubular acidosis).
• Failure of renal elimination of acid (renal failure and distal tubular acidosis).

Management

Treat the underlying cause.

The value of correcting acidosis in diabetic ketoacidosis or salicylate poisoning remains doubtful. In chronic renal failure acidosis is corrected by dialysing against a bicarbonate-based dialysis fluid (acetate which is converted to bicarbonate in liver and muscle can also be used).

Bicarbonate deficit can be calculated as the measured serum bicarbonate below normal standard bicarbonate × 30% body weight in kilograms. Bicarbonate can be replaced as 8.4% sodium bicarbonate solution (contains 1 mmol/ml). This should be rapid (give 50–100 ml) following sustained cardiac arrest as arrhythmias are difficult to revert in the presence of acidosis.

In *distal renal tubular acidosis (type 1)* there is a failure of hydrogen ion secretion in the distal tubule. Urine pH remains inappropriately high despite severe systemic acidosis. It may be inherited as an autosomal dominant trait or occur as a result of damage to the renal medulla from pyelonephritis, obstructive uropathy, medullary sponge kidney or ischaemia. In all, 70% of patients have nephrocalcinosis, and osteomalacia (or rickets in children) is common. Treatment is with oral bicarbonate, often with potassium supplements.

Proximal renal tubular acidosis (type 2) is less common. It is caused by a defect of proximal tubular bicarbonate reabsorption.

Metabolic alkalosis

Aetiology

• Excess intake of alkali, e.g. milk-alkali syndrome, massive blood transfusion (citrate is metabolized to bicarbonate), overtreatment of metabolic acidosis.
• Loss of gastric acid, e.g. pyloric stenosis.
• Increased renal losses of acid with bicarbonate generation, as in hyperaldosteronism, elevated corticosteroids or severe hypokalaemia.

Management

Identify and treat the underlying cause.

Hypercalcaemia

Aetiology

Hyperparathyroidism
• Primary (parathyroid adenoma or hyperplasia).
• Secondary (increased PTH secretion occurs in response to hypocalcaemia (e.g. in renal failure, malabsorption)—by definition the calcium is normal).
• Tertiary hyperparathyroidism: if secondary hyperparathyroidism gets 'out of control' an autonomous parathyroid adenoma develops, causing elevation of both PTH and serum calcium.

Malignancy
• Bone metastases (commonly breast, lung, prostate, kidney, thyroid).
• Multiple myeloma, leukaemia, Hodgkin's.
• Secretion of a PTH-like factor.

Sarcoid
Increased sensitivity to vitamin D—hypercalcaemia often precipitated by exposure to sunlight.

Drugs
- Excess vitamin D.
- Calcium-containing antacids (milk-alkali syndrome).
- Rarely, thiazides.

Endocrine (rare)
Thyrotoxicosis, adrenal insufficiency.

Hypocalcaemia
Aetiology
Hypoparathyroidism
- Idiopathic.
- Post-thyroid or parathyroid surgery.
- Pseudohypoparathyroidism (reduced sensitivity to PTH).

Inadequate dietary intake of vitamin D or calcium
(rarely, vitamin D resistance)
Malabsorption
Renal disease
Acute pancreatitis

Hypomagnesaemia
Magnesium is the second most abundant intracellular cation. Normal requirement is 150 mg/day. Normal intake is 300–400 mg/day.

Aetiology
Occurs in starvation, enteral nutrition, prolonged diarrhoea, enteric fistulae and drugs (diuretics, aminoglycosides, amphotericin, carbenicillin). Usually associated with hypocalcaemia.

Reduced calcium and magnesium are often found in the seriously ill where nutrition has been inaccurately estimated.

Clinical features are paraesthesia, cramp, tetany, apathy.

Hyperphosphataemia
Aetiology
- Reduced loss:

(a) renal failure;
(b) hypoparathyroidism.
- Increased load:
(a) phosphate enemas or laxatives;
(b) excessive vitamin D intake.

Hypophosphataemia
Aetiology
- Increased loss:
(a) diuretic therapy;
(b) hypoparathyroidism;
(c) renal tubular defects (e.g. Fanconi syndrome—glycosuria, aminoaciduria, phosphaturia, renal tubular acidosis).
- Decreased absorption:
(a) malabsorption;
(b) phosphate-binding agents (e.g. antacids such as aluminium hydroxide, calcium carbonate);
(c) vitamin D deficiency or resistance;
(d) malnutrition.
- Intracellular shift:
(a) diabetes mellitus;
(b) 'refeeding syndrome' (after starvation or severe illness).

Uric acid
Levels of uric acid are labile and show day-to-day and seasonal variation in the same person. They are also increased by stress and fasting.

Serum uric acid increased
Causes:
- Primary gout.
- 25% of relatives with primary gout.
- Diuretics (particularly thiazides).
- Small doses of aspirin (up to 2 g/day).
- Renal failure (the level does not correlate with the degree of renal failure—serum creatinine should be used for this).
- Increased destruction of nucleoproteins, usually in mycloproliferative disorders—particularly at the start of cytotoxic therapy or radiotherapy.
- Psoriasis (one-third of patients).
- Uric acid production can be inhibited by xanthine oxidase inhibitors (e.g. allopurinol).

Liver Disease

The most common liver disease is acute viral hepatitis. Drug jaundice, gallstones, biliary tract obstruction and carcinomatous secondary deposits are fairly common.

Acute hepatitis

This refers to inflammation of the liver with little or no fibrosis and little or no nodular regeneration. There may be minor distortion of lobular architecture. If there is extensive fibrosis with nodular regeneration (and hence distortion of architecture) the condition is called cirrhosis. These diagnoses are made histologically and there may or may not be clinical evidence of previous hepatic disease.

Inflammation with necrosis of liver cells results from:
• *Infection*, most commonly acute infectious hepatitis A, but also with the viruses of hepatitis B, C and E, infectious mononucleosis, cytomegalovirus (CMV) and yellow fever, and associated with septicaemia and leptospirosis. Amoebic hepatitis is common on a worldwide basis, and usually presents as a hepatic abscess or amoeboma.
• *Chemical poisons* and *drugs* are less frequent causes of acute hepatitis. Toxic chemicals include carbon tetrachloride, vinyl chloride, and ethylene glycol and similar solvents (glue sniffing). Toxic drugs include alcohol (ethanol and methanol), halothane (after repeated exposures), isoniazid and rifampicin, paracetamol, methotrexate, chlorpromazine and the monoamine oxidase inhibitors.
• *Pregnancy* (rare).

If the patient recovers this is usually complete but, rarely, progressive necrosis may affect almost the entire liver (fulminant hepatic failure or acute massive necrosis) causing hepatic coma (p. 212) and death.

Viral hepatitis
The clinical features of acute hepatitis A, B, C and E are similar, although they differ in severity, time course and progression to chronic liver disease.

Hepatitis A
Hepatitis A (infectious hepatitis) is a single-stranded RNA picornavirus of the enterovirus family which is excreted in the stool towards the end of the incubation period and disappears as the illness develops. Anti-hepatitis A virus immunoglobulin M (IgM) appears at the onset of the illness, and indicates recent infection. The disease is endemic but small epidemics may occur in schools or institutions. Spread is usually via the faecal–oral route by food products such as shellfish. The young (5–14 years) are chiefly involved.

Clinical presentation
After an incubation period of 2–6 weeks there is gradual onset of influenza-like illness with fever, malaise, anorexia, nausea, vomiting and upper abdominal discomfort associated with tender enlargement of the liver and, less commonly, the spleen. In smokers, there may be a distaste for cigarettes. After 3–4 days the urine becomes characteristically dark and the stools pale—evidence of cholestasis. Symptoms usually become less severe as jaundice appears, although pruritus may develop. Jaundice and symptoms tend to improve after 1–2 weeks and recovery is usually complete, although mild symptoms continue for 3–4 months in a few

patients. Recurrent hepatitis A is extremely rare, and immunity probably lifelong.

Diagnosis
Diagnosis depends on detecting anti-hepatitis A virus IgM in serum.

Differential diagnosis
• Obstructive jaundice, either in the early cholestatic phase, or in the rare case where cholestatic jaundice persists after other clinical and biochemical evidence of liver cell damage has settled. It is dangerous to diagnose infective hepatitis in patients over 40 years old—a safeguard against misdiagnosing major bile duct obstruction.
• Drug jaundice (p. 216).
• Glandular fever.
• Yellow fever (travellers).
• Acute alcoholic hepatitis may present with enlargement and tenderness of the liver and, sometimes, obstructive jaundice. There are usually other signs of alcoholism.
• Wilson disease must not be overlooked (pp. 102 and 215).

Management
If hospitalized, the patient should be isolated. Virus is present in stools for 1–2 weeks before the onset of jaundice, and for 1 week after. Symptomatic treatment only is required in the active disease state. No dietary restriction, other than alcohol, is necessary. Liver function tests usually return completely to normal in 1–3 months.

Recovery is the rule in virtually every case. Occasionally, jaundice may be prolonged by intrahepatic cholestasis, and corticosteroids can be used to reduce the jaundice rapidly, particularly if associated with pruritus.

Fulminant hepatic failure is rare but has a mortality of about 50%. Management should be in a specialized centre where liver transplantation can be considered.

Prophylaxis
Active immunization with inactivated virus is recommended for travellers to endemic areas.

Passive immunization with pooled human immunoglobulin gives partial, short-lived immunity, but is effective immediately after the injection.

Hepatitis B
Hepatitis B is a double-stranded DNA hepadnavirus. It is spread by infected blood and serum and also occurs in saliva, semen and vaginal secretions. Transmission occurs through percutaneous exposure (contaminated needles), sexual contact and maternal–neonatal infection. It is most frequently seen in drug addicts and homosexuals. Haemodialysis patients are screened.

Clinical features
After a long incubation period of 6 weeks to 6 months, there is a gradual onset of lethargy, anorexia, abdominal discomfort, jaundice and hepatomegaly. It is often asymptomatic in infants. Occasionally, a serum sickness-like illness occurs with polyarthritis, skin rashes and glomerulonephritis. Cholestatic hepatitis is very rare, about 1% develop fulminant hepatic failure. Chronic hepatitis, cirrhosis and primary liver cancer occur.

Diagnosis
Hepatitis B virus has three different antigens: a surface antigen (HepB$_s$Ag), a core antigen (HepB$_c$Ag) and an internal component (HepB$_e$Ag). HepB$_s$Ag appears in the blood about 6 weeks after acute infection and has usually gone by 3 months. HepB$_e$Ag occurs at a similar time and denotes high infectivity. HepB$_c$Ag is usually found only in the liver. The development of antibodies to HepB$_s$Ag usually follows acute infection and indicates immunity. In about 5% antibodies do not appear and HepB$_s$Ag persists in the blood (carrier state).

Hepatitis D virus (Delta virus) is an incomplete RNA virus that depends on the hepatitis B virus to replicate. It can cause an aggressive chronic hepatitis in HepB$_s$Ag-positive patients. Chronic infection is usually associated with progressive liver disease.

Management
In most cases spontaneous recovery occurs and treatment is supportive, as for hepatitis A. The carrier state is usually asymptomatic but is

associated with chronic hepatitis and hepato-cellular carcinoma. Infection during childhood is more likely to lead to chronicity than in adult life. Carriers respond to α-interferon plus a reverse transcriptase inhibitor (e.g. lamivudine) by losing HepB$_e$Ag and hepatitis B virus DNA from serum.

Immunization
Immunization using recombinant HepB$_s$Ag is advised for high-risk groups, including health workers who have contact with blood, patients with chronic renal failure, intravenous drug abusers, homosexual men and prostitutes. Three doses are given at 0, 1 and 6 months, and antibody status is checked 2–4 months thereafter. Booster is recommended every 5 years.

Hepatitis B immune globulin (HBIg) can be given with the vaccine to those accidentally infected.

Hepatitis C
Hepatitis C is a single-stranded RNA flavivirus. It predominantly affects intravenous drug abusers, and patients who have received multiple blood transfusions. It accounts for 20% acute hepatitis, 70% of chronic hepatitis, nearly half the cases of end-stage cirrhosis, 60% of primary liver cancer and 30% of liver transplants in the UK. Testing of blood products for hepatitis C has now virtually eradicated post-transfusion hepatitis.

Clinical features
Frequently asymptomatic—fewer than 10% of adults become jaundiced. Acute hepatitis following blood transfusion has been virtually eradicated by the introduction of testing of blood products for hepatitis B and C. The incubation period varies from 2 to 26 weeks. Slow progression (10–20 years) to chronic active hepatitis occurs in about 50% of cases and cirrhosis in about 15%.

Diagnosis
Antibody detection: first-generation enzyme-linked immunosorbent assay (ELISA) using recombinant antigen C100 were relatively non-specific. Newer assays using putative core antigens are more specific, although false

positives still occur. The mean time from infection to antibody detection is 12 weeks. Hepatitis C virus RNA determination is essential for monitoring hepatitis C infection.

Management
Forty per cent of patients with chronic infection respond to α-interferon plus ribarvirin, with a sustained fall in transaminase levels. All patients with chronic hepatitis C virus should be vaccinated against hepatitis A, which is reported to cause fulminant hepatic failure in hepatitis C virus carriers, and against hepatitis B because they are likely to share common risk factors.

Hepatitis E
Hepatitis E virus is an RNA calicivirus. Transmission is faecal–oral by water contamination from a bovine faecal reservoir. It is prevalent in the developing world, where it is the most common cause of self-limiting hepatitis in adults.

Clinical features
It is generally more severe than hepatitis A. The incubation period is 20–40 days. Progression to chronic liver disease does not occur. Like hepatitis A virus, it can cause a fulminant hepatitis. Pregnant women who develop acute hepatitis E infection have a high risk of liver failure, with a mortality of around 5%.

Hepatitis G
Hepatitis G is a positive stranded RNA flavivirus. There is no evidence at present that it causes acute or chronic liver disease.

Autoimmune hepatitis
These are classified according to the presence or absence of autoantibodies.

Type 1 autoimmune hepatitis is the most common type, with a female : male ratio of 8 : 1. It is characterized by the presence of antinuclear antibody (50–70%), or smooth muscle cell antibody (50–80%). Antimitochondrial antibodies are present in 20%. It affects all age groups and is associated with human leucocyte antigen (HLA) DR3 and DR4. IgG concentrations and serum aminotransferases are elevated. Liver histology reveals plasma cell infiltrates, liver cell rosettes and piecemeal necrosis. An association with hepatitis C virus infection has been reported in some studies.

Type II autoimmune hepatitis typically affects girls aged 2–14 years, although 20–30% of cases occur in adults. Onset is often acute, with rapid progression to liver failure. It is characterized by the presence of antibodies to liver/kidney microsome type 1 (anti-LKM1) in the absence of antinuclear or antismooth muscle cell antibodies. It has been further classified according to the absence or presence of hepatitis C virus infection.

Type III autoimmune hepatitis is characterized by antibodies to soluble liver antigen (SLA). These are identical to antibodies to liverpancreas (anti-LP), and have been designated anti-SLA/LP.

Management

Immunosuppressive therapy improves survival in the majority of cases. Eighty per cent of patients respond to steroids, alone or in combination with azathioprine. In patients who fail to respond, orthotopic liver transplantation is the treatment of choice.

Alcoholic hepatitis

Moderate alcohol consumption is associated with a reduction in mortality compared with either abstinence or heavy drinking. Drinking in excess of 3 units of alcohol daily may increase mortality, but sensitivity to alcohol varies between individuals (8 g or 10 ml = 1 unit of ethanol is present in half a pint of 3.6% beer, a glass of wine or a single measure of spirits). A 125 ml glass of 12.5% wine contains 1.6 units of alcohol. The clinical features of alcoholic liver disease vary from no clinical evidence at all, through nausea, episodes of right abdominal pain associated with tender hepatomegaly, fever and polymorphic leucocytosis, to cirrhosis with portal hypertension and fulminant hepatic failure. Marked jaundice is not always present.

The pathological spectrum includes fatty liver, alcoholic hepatitis, cirrhosis and hepatocellular carcinoma. Alcoholic hepatitis is characterized by liver cell damage, inflammatory cell infiltration and fibrosis. Injured hepatocytes are swollen, with pale granular cytoplasm ('ballooning degeneration'). In some cells Mallory's bodies are seen by haematoxylin and eosin stain as purple-red aggregates of material, predominantly around the nucleus. The γ-glutamyltransferase, which reflects levels of microsomal enzyme induction, and the mean corpuscular volume (MCV) may be the best indices of persistent ethanol ingestion.

The only effective treatment is total abstinence from alcohol, if necessary with the help of a support group. Nutritional deficiencies are common. Vitamin B preparations and dietary supplementation are usually given.

TRIALS BOX 13.1

Doll *et al.* studied mortality prospectively in 12 321 male doctors with various drinking patterns. Moderate alcohol consumption (1 or 2 units/day) was associated with lower all-cause mortality than consumption of no or substantial amounts. Alcohol consumption reduced ischaemic heart disease, irrespective of amount. *Br Med J* 1994; **309**: 911–918.

Fuchs *et al.* followed 85 709 women aged 34–59 prospectively over a 12-year period. Light-to-moderate alcohol consumption (1.5–3.0 g/day) was associated with a reduced mortality rate, principally because of a decreased risk of death from cardiovascular disease. Heavier drinking was associated with an increased risk of death from other causes, particularly breast cancer and cirrhosis. *N Engl J Med* 1995; **332**: 1245–1250.

Grønbæk *et al.* examined the relationship between intake of different types of alcohol and death using pooled cohort studies of 13 064 men and 11 459 women aged 20–98 years. J-shaped relations were found between total alcohol intake and mortality at various levels of wine intake. They found that wine intake may have a beneficial effect on all cause mortality that is additive to that of alcohol. This effect may be attibutable to a reduction in death from both coronary heart disease and cancer. *Ann Intern Med* 2000; **133**: 411–419.

Chronic liver disease

Chronic hepatitis and cirrhosis are pathological diagnoses, and therefore imply liver biopsy in all suspected cases.

Chronic hepatitis

The International Association for the Study of the Liver (*Hepatology* 1994; **19**: 1513–1520) and the World Congress of Gastroenterology (*Am J Gastroenterol* 1994; **89**: S177–S181) have published guidelines for the revised classification of chronic hepatitis. It is proposed that the terms chronic persistent hepatitis, chronic lobular hepatitis and chronic active hepatitis should be replaced by a description of the aetiology (commonly, hepatitis B, C or D; drug-induced; α_1-antitrypsin; Wilson disease), the grade of necrosis and inflammation in portal or periportal and lobular regions, and the stage of fibrosis or cirrhosis.

Cirrhosis

Cirrhosis is a pathological diagnosis. It is characterized by widespread fibrosis with nodular regeneration. Its presence implies previous or continuing hepatic cell damage. Liver function tests are normal in inactive disease (p. 39).

Identified causes include viral hepatitis B and C, alcoholic hepatitis, haemochromatosis, hepatolenticular disease, α_1-antitrypsin deficiency, chronic severe heart failure and a few drugs (isoniazid, methyldopa).

Classification

Micronodular (portal cirrhosis) is characterized by regular thick fibrotic bands joining the portal tracts to hepatic veins, and with small regenerative nodules. The liver is initially large with a smooth edge but subsequently shrinks with progressive fibrosis. It is often alcoholic in origin.

Macronodular (postnecrotic cirrhosis) is less common and characterized by coarse, irregular bands of fibrosis and loss of normal architecture and large regenerative nodules. It is believed usually to follow viral hepatitis with widespread necrosis. The liver is enlarged and very irregular as a result of large nodules.

Biliary cirrhosis is less common and is characterized by fibrosis around distended intrahepatic ducts. It may follow chronic cholangitis and biliary obstruction, or be idiopathic (primary).

Primary biliary cirrhosis

There is progressive damage to intrahepatic bile ducts. It chiefly (90%) affects women between 40 and 60 years of age, and presents with features of cholestasis: pruritus, jaundice with pale stools, dark urine and steatorrhoea, pigmentation and xanthelasma.

Osteodystrophy results from a combination of osteomalacia secondary to impaired vitamin D absorption and osteoporosis. The liver and spleen are usually palpable. Antimitochondrial antibodies are present in 95% of patients and this helps with the differential diagnosis from drug cholestasis, sclerosing cholangitis, carcinoma of the bile duct and biliary cirrhosis from chronic obstruction.

Histology shows progression from granulomatous changes around the bile ducts through bile duct proliferation to fibrosis and finally cirrhosis.

Management

The anion exchange resin cholestyramine, which binds bile acids in the gut, relieves pruritus.

Supplementary fat-soluble vitamins are given. The role of oestrogens in preventing osteoporosis in women with primary biliary cirrhosis is unclear. The bile acid ursodeoxycholic acid slows disease progression, leading to an improvement in both liver biochemistry and long-term survival. In patients with decompensated liver disease, liver transplantation should be considered. Five-year survival rates of over 70% post liver transplant have been reported.

Immunosuppressive agents are of little benefit. Prednisolone may promote further bone loss, and azathioprine is of doubtful value.

Primary sclerosing cholangitis

This condition is diagnosed by endoscopic retrograde cholangiography or MRI. Inflammatory bowel disease coexists in 70% of cases. The radiological picture may be mimicked by bacterial and parasitic cholangitis, polycystic liver disease and cholangiocarcinoma, which is a recognized complication.

Management

Immunosuppression increases the risk of secondary bacterial cholangitis, although this may be required for coexistent inflammatory bowel disease. Endoscopic stenting of strictures carries the same risk. Assessment for liver transplantation is recommended if cirrhosis is present.

Other rare causes of cirrhosis include autoimmune hepatitis, haemochromatosis and Wilson disease. Cardiac cirrhosis may occur in chronic cardiac failure. Centrilobular congestion leads to necrosis and fibrosis, but nodular regeneration is not marked.

NB Schistosomiasis causes periportal fibrosis and is not a form of cirrhosis. Liver involvement is more common (50%) in *Schistosoma mansoni* (bowel) infections than in *S. haematobium* (bladder) as a result of the portal rather than the systemic drainage of the primary infected area in the former. The schistosomes cause a granulomatous fibrosis in the portal tracts and enlargement of the liver. In severe cases the liver shrinks and extensive fibrosis develops leading to portal hypertension. There is little or no hepatocellular failure because the disease is presinusoidal. Late spread may occur to the lungs (cor pulmonale) and to the spinal cord (paraplegia).

Clinical features of chronic liver disease relate mostly to the development of hepatocellular failure and complications of portal hypertension.

Hepatocellular failure

Marked jaundice is uncommon. The oestrogen effects of gynaecomastia, spider naevi, liver palms and testicular atrophy may be present. In alcoholics, other features of alcoholism may be present (wasting, polyneuropathy, Korsakoff's psychosis, dementia, delirium tremens and Wernicke's encephalopathy, p. 186). Pigmentation, fetor hepaticus, clubbing, white nails, cyanosis and peripheral oedema may occur.

Encephalopathy (hepatic coma or precoma) may be absent or may completely dominate the picture. Precoma is characterized by irritable confusion, drowsiness, flapping tremor, fetor and other signs of hepatocellular failure. Exaggerated reflexes and upgoing plantar responses may be present. Constructional apraxia may be demonstrated in inability to draw or copy a star. In the electroencephalogram (EEG), δ waves (3–4 c/s) are characteristic. (They also occur in hypoglycaemia, uraemia, carbon dioxide retention and cerebral abscess.)

Acute liver failure

There are two main clinical situations in which hepatocellular failure may be precipitated, and in which there are different management objectives.

1 A previously healthy person with a serious hepatitic illness, such as paracetamol overdose (50%) or viral (C, B, A in that order) hepatitis (40%). This can also occur with other drugs and with chemical poisoning. This is less common. The history is usually less than 8 weeks and there is no evidence of chronic liver disease. The object is to support the patient to give time for the liver to recover.

2 A person with previously 'compensated' chronic liver disease, often alcoholic, with an acute precipitating cause:
  • excess protein in the bowel, e.g. after gastrointestinal haemorrhage;
  • acute alcoholic intoxication;
  • intercurrent infection, particularly Gram-negative septicaemia;
  • drugs, especially sedatives, and morphine or other alkaloids;
  • trauma, including minor or major surgical procedures and paracentesis; and
  • electrolyte imbalance (potassium and/or sodium depletion), usually from the diuretics used to treat oedema and ascites.

The underlying damage to the liver is not treatable.

Fulminant hepatic failure refers to hepatic encephalopathy occurring within weeks of the onset of other symptoms of acute liver failure. Profound hypotension and multiple organ failure are common. Cerebral oedema and sepsis are the most common causes of death.

Management

Preferably, this should be in a specialist unit.

• *Assess the conscious level.* Grade as follows (this is also a guide to prognosis):

Grade 1 drowsy, poor concentration

Grade 2 confused and disorientated

Grade 3 very drowsy, responding only to forceful, simple command, often aggressive and incoherent

Grade 4 unrousable, either responding only to painful stimuli (4a), or to none (4b).

NB In alcoholic liver disease, conscious level may also be affected by delirium tremens, thiamine (and other B vitamins) deficiency, epilepsy and acute alcohol intoxication. Monitor intracranial pressure and consider hourly mannitol (100 ml of 20%) until there is a diuresis.

• *Establish venous access* and consider nasogastric tube and central line.

• *Identify any site of bleeding* by fibroscopy, and treat as appropriate: gastric or duodenal ulceration (p. 217); variceal bleeding (p. 214).

• *Correction and maintenance of fluid and electrolyte balance.* Sodium restriction may be required despite hyponatraemia, which may be dilutional. Hypokalaemia is treated with standard oral potassium preparations. Diuretics (spironolactone followed, if necessary, by loop diuretics) are given for ascites (p. 214). The blood glucose may be very low, and should be maintained with dextrose infusions (up to 300 g/day).

• *Infection* is common. Use prophylactic broad-spectrum antibiotics and antifungal treatment. Take blood cultures and send ascitic fluid for bacteriological examination, including tuberculosis. In patients with septicaemia, half have Gram-negative infection and half staphylococcal. Treat the infection immediately, and then modify the antibiotic therapy as indicated by microbiological results, remembering that altered liver function may influence drug choice and dosage.

• *Minimize the protein load.* Identify any site of bleeding (see above). In those not bleeding, reduce the risk of gastrointestinal bleeding with sucralfate or parenteral H_2-blocker. Ensure a low protein intake (20–30 g/day), and

a high carbohydrate diet. Lactulose 50 ml t.d.s. produces osmotic diarrhoea to remove protein and blood (if present) from the bowel, and prevents proliferation of ammonia-producing organisms. Selective intestinal decontamination by the administration of non-absorbable antibiotics (e.g. neomycin) may reduce the risk of spontaneous bacterial peritonitis. $MgSO_4$ enema, 80 ml of 50%, 12-hourly may be added.

• *Correction of coagulation defects* is not usually needed in the absence of clinically significant bleeding. Use fresh frozen plasma or blood, and platelet infusion if the platelet count is low. Add Vitamin K, 10 mg intravenously, in case there is any cholestatic element.

• *Sedation* may be required. Short-acting benzodiazepines (e.g. oxazepam) are suitable.

• *Inotropic support* may be indicated.

• Support *respiration.* Early elective ventilation may be needed to maintain Pao_2.

• *Renal failure* may require dialysis.

• Give *B vitamins* parenterally. Thiamine deficiency is common in alcoholics.

• *Orthotopic liver transplantation* is becoming more widely available for all forms of liver failure. Consider referral: if there is Grade 2 or worse encephalopathy, if there is persistent hypotension (systolic blood pressure (SBP), < 100), hyponatraemia or thrombocytopenia, or if the international normalized ratio (INR) is > 3 or factor V < 20%.

NB A reduced level of consciousness in hepatocellular failure may be caused by septicaemia, hypoglycaemia, raised intracranial pressure from cerebral oedema, subdural haematoma or epilepsy. Prolonged administration of N-acetylcysteine may be of benefit in acute liver failure caused by paracetamol overdose (pp. 207 and 316) and other causes.

Portal hypertension

Cirrhosis accounts for 80% of the portal hypertension seen in the UK. The other postsinusoidal causes (which have poor hepatic function) are exceedingly rare and result from cardiac failure, constrictive pericarditis and hepatic vein thrombosis (Budd–Chiari syndrome, below). Presinusoidal obstruction causes portal hypertension with normal hepatic function in schistosomiasis (granulomatous portal tract fibrosis), and in obstruction to the portal vein by tumours or following venous thrombosis with umbilical sepsis.

Collateral circulation may be evident in the oesophagus (varices), anus (anorectal varices rather than haemorrhoids) and at the umbilicus where a venous hum may be heard. Tests of liver cell function are usually slightly abnormal although not always so, and there may be hypersplenism.

Haematemesis is the most common presenting symptom and may be precipitated by non-steroidal anti-inflammatory drugs, including aspirin. Bleeding is often from peptic ulceration or erosions in the alcoholic, and H_2-blockade or proton pump inhibitors are then useful.

Management of bleeding varices

The mortality is 30–50%, even in experienced hands. The initial aim is to replace blood and correct coagulation defects. Treat hepatic encephalopathy (p. 213). Endoscopic techniques remain the mainstay of treatment because 50% of patients even with florid varices are bleeding from a gastric ulcer. Therapeutic options are as follow.

• Injection sclerotherapy controls bleeding in up to 95% of cases, although rebleeding is common, and sclerotherapy has no influence on the mortality rate at 6 weeks. Complications include oesophageal ulceration and stricture formation.

• Variceal banding ligation is as effective as sclerotherapy in controlling acute bleeding.

• Intravenous vasopressin or terlipressin reduce splanchnic blood flow and can be used prior to more definitive treatment. It causes coronary artery constriction and may precipitate myocardial ischaemia and infarction.

• Octreotide, a synthetic somatic analogue, also reduces collateral splanchnic blood flow, and when combined with sclerotherapy is more effective than sclerotherapy alone in controlling acute bleeding.

• Balloon tamponade with a Sengstaken–Blakemore or Linton tube is now only used during transfer to a specialist centre, or when the above measures have failed.

• Non-selective β-blockers with isosorbide mononitrate reduce portal pressure and are effective in preventing first bleed from varices, and as secondary prophylaxis after variceal bleeding.

• Surgical oesophageal transection or portosystemic shunting can be considered in patients with recurrent or intractable variceal bleeding.

Management of ascites

Ascites is caused by a combination of factors, including portal hypertension, hypoalbuminaemia and secondary hyperaldosteronism. Management involves:

• sodium restriction;

• diuretics—aldosterone antagonists (e.g. spironolactone), alone or in combination with loop diuretics in patients with marked sodium retention;

• paracentesis is safe and effective, although expansion of plasma volume with albumin is required if large quantities of ascitic fluid are removed;

• peritoneovenous shunting or ultrafiltration and reinfusion of ascitic fluid are rarely employed in the setting of refractory ascites.

Spontaneous infection of ascites is common in cirrhotic patients. Most episodes respond to intravenous cephalosporins or oral quinolones (e.g. ciprofloxacin), but the overall prognosis is poor—30% die in hospital following an episode.

Budd–Chiari syndrome

This results from obstruction of the hepatic veins. Causes are:

• hepatic venous thrombosis, usually in association with a hypercoagulable state such as the antiphospholipid syndrome;

• occlusion of the hepatic veins by tumour, abscess or cyst; and

• webs of the suprahepatic segment of the inferior vena cava (IVC).

Patients present acutely with tender hepatomegaly (without hepatojugular reflux), resistant ascites and hepatic failure. Chronic onset is associated with weight loss, upper gut bleeding and spider naevi. All patients have abnormal liver function tests, but the pattern is variable and similar to other chronic liver diseases. Only half have the diagnostic liver scintiscan finding of maximum uptake in the caudate lobe (which drains directly into the IVC) with decreased uptake in the rest of the liver. Liver biopsy shows congestion around the hepatic venules. Laparotomy may produce abrupt deterioration. Treatment is surgical by side-to-side portocaval shunting or orthotopic liver transplantation. If there is a web, surgical correction may be attempted by transatrial membranectomy.

Rare cirrhoses

Idiopathic haemochromatosis
(bronzed diabetes)
An autosomal recessive disorder of iron metabolism characterized by increased iron absorption and deposition, chiefly in the liver, pancreas, heart, synovial membranes and pituitary. *HFE*, the gene for hereditary haemochromatosis, has been mapped to chromosome 6 (6p21.3). The HFE protein is expressed in crypt enterocytes of the duodenum where it is thought to modulate the uptake of transferrin-bound iron from plasma.

First-degree male relatives should be screened with serum iron and transferrin saturation. Females may present postmenopausally because continuous menstruation until then reduces the iron load.

Clinical presentation
It occurs almost entirely in men over the age of 30 years who present with:
• diabetes mellitus;
• skin pigmentation (caused by melanin rather than iron);
• hepatomegaly (large, regular, firm); portal hypertension and hepatocellular failure are not common;
• progressive pyrophosphate polyarthropathy (40%) and chondrocalcinosis;

• arrhythmias (30%) and cardiac failure (15%);
• testicular atrophy, loss of body hair and loss of libido; and
• osteoarthritis of the first and second metacarpophalangeal joints.

Diagnosis
The serum iron is raised so that the serum iron-binding capacity is nearly saturated. The serum ferritin is raised. The patient is not anaemic or polycythaemic. The glucose tolerance test is usually abnormal.

Biopsy of most tissues (skin, marrow, testes) shows excess iron deposits but diagnosis is usually made on liver biopsy, which shows iron staining of the liver with perilobular fibrosis.

Treatment
Deplete the body of the excess iron (up to 50 g) by weekly venesection of 500 ml (which contains 250 mg iron). This is continued until a normal serum iron is established and/or the patient becomes anaemic (in about 2 years). Maintenance venesection will be required (about 500 ml every 3 months, depending on the serum iron).

Treat appropriately the diabetes, hypogonadism, heart failure and arrhythmias, hepatic cell failure and portal hypertension. High alcohol intake must be stopped. The arthropathy and testicular function do not improve but other features do.
NB Primary hepatic carcinoma occurs in up to 20% of cases, whether treated or not. Alphafetoprotein is a suitable screen.

Overload of the tissues with iron can follow either repeated blood transfusions (about 100 units), as for instance in thalassaemia or, rarely, after excessive iron ingestion. If the iron is in the reticuloendothelial cells only, the patients tend not to develop serious sequelae and the condition is called haemosiderosis.

Hepatolenticular degeneration
(Wilson disease, p. 102)
Wilson disease is an autosomal recessive disorder of copper transport, resulting in copper accumulation and toxicity to the liver and brain,

caused by mutations in a putative adenosine triphosphatase (ATPase) gene, with six putative metal binding regions similar to those found in prokaryotic heavy metal transporters. Neurological manifestations (p. 102) and signs of cirrhosis appear during adolescence or early adult life. Low ceruloplasmin is found in the serum. The Kayser–Fleischer ring is a deep copper-coloured ring at the periphery of the cornea, which is thought to represent copper deposits. Hypercalciuria and nephrocalcinosis are not uncommon in patients with Wilson disease.

Drug jaundice

Drugs are responsible for up to 10% of all patients admitted with jaundice.

Hypersensitivity reactions
These are the most common cause of drug jaundice. They are dose-independent.

Cholestasis
Clinically and biochemically this is an obstructive jaundice. Histologically, there are bile plugs in the canaliculi and there may be an inflammatory infiltrate of eosinophils in the portal tracts.
    The classical example is chlorpromazine jaundice, which occurs 3–6 weeks after starting the drug. The prognosis is excellent if the drug is discontinued (and never given again).
    Other drugs producing cholestasis are other phenothiazines, carbimazole, erythromycin estolate (but not the stearate), sulphonylureas, sulphonamides, rifampicin and nitrofurantoin. Occasionally, there may be a more generalized reaction with fever, rash, lymphadenopathy and eosinophilia.

Acute hepatitis syndrome
Occasionally with acute necrosis. This is much less common, but much more serious (mortality up to 20%). It occurs 2–3 weeks after starting the drug, and is caused by halothane (after multiple exposure), monoamine oxidase inhibitors, methyldopa (which more commonly gives haemolytic jaundice) and the antituberculous drugs, ethionamide and pyrazinamide (p. 249).

Direct hepatotoxicity
In some cases this is dose-dependent, although individual susceptibility is extremely variable.
    The mechanisms are:
• cholestasis (without inflammatory infiltrate or necrosis). Chiefly as a result of C17-substituted testosterone derivatives, i.e. anabolic and androgenic steroids, including methyltestosterone and most contraceptive pills; and
• necrosis resulting from organic solvents, e.g. methotrexate, 6-mercaptopurine, azathioprine.

Haemolytic jaundice
This is a rare complication of therapy. It may occur with methyldopa (which more commonly gives a positive Coombs' reaction without jaundice), and the 8-aminoquinolines (e.g. primaquine) in patients with glucose-6-phosphate dehydrogenase deficiency.

Gastroenterology

Symptoms arising in the gastrointestinal tract are extremely common, usually caused by acute gastroenteritis or food poisoning. In clinics most are a result of disturbances in motility and over one-third may have irritable bowel syndrome. Peptic ulcer, hiatus hernia, appendicitis, diverticulitis, haemorrhoids, ulcerative colitis and carcinoma of the colon are common. Carcinoma of the stomach and carcinoma of the oesophagus are less common.

Gastric and duodenal ulceration

Peptic ulcer affects 1–2% of adults, and is a chronic disorder characterized by frequent recurrences.

Aetiology

Infection with *Helicobacter pylori* and the use of anti-inflammatory drugs, both steroidal and non-steroidal (including aspirin), are the most common precipitating factors. Smoking increases the rate of ulcer recurrence, and slows ulcer healing. Rarely, ulceration is associated with Zollinger–Ellison syndrome (p. 223), multiple endocrine neoplasia (MEN) Type I syndrome (p. 152), hyperparathyroidism (p. 180) or stress (e.g. extensive burns—Curling's ulcer).

Helicobacter pylori colonizes the mucus layer overlying gastric epithelium. Infection is often asymptomatic, although a chronic superficial gastritis invariably affects the underlying mucosa. *H. pylori* infection is associated with peptic ulceration, and an increased incidence of gastric cancer. Production of urease and cytotoxins, and disruption of the gastric mucosal barrier, is thought to contribute to disease production.

There is an association between *H. pylori* infection and the development of B-cell gastric lymphomas of mucosa-associated lymphoid tissue (MALTomas). Tumour regression following eradication of *H. pylori* has been reported.

Clinical presentation

It is usually impossible, on the basis of history and examination alone, to differentiate between duodenal ulceration, benign ulceration of the stomach and carcinoma of the stomach, but carcinoma is much less common.

Patients with duodenal ulceration classically present with a history of periodic epigastric pain, often waking at 1–3 a.m., relieved by food, milk or alkalis.

Gastric ulcer pain may be epigastric, or occur anywhere in the anterior upper abdomen. Anorexia, vomiting and weight loss are more frequent and severe in carcinomatous ulcers of the stomach than in benign peptic ulceration. Food occasionally precipitates pain immediately (as it may in reflux oesophagitis).

Examination

The patient characteristically puts the hand over the upper abdomen or may point to the epigastrium with a forefinger when asked where the pain is, and this is the point of maximum tenderness. The presence of an epigastric mass suggests a carcinoma. A gastric splash (or succussion) indicates the rare pyloric obstruction caused by benign duodenal stricture or to carcinoma of the pyloric antrum.

Complications

- Bleeding (p. 223).
- Perforation (usually duodenal ulceration).

EFFECTIVE *H. PYLORI* TREATMENTS

Dual treatments
Ranitidine bismuth citrate + clarithromycin for 14 days
Effective and easy to take with few side-effects

Triple treatments
Bismuth compound + tetracycline (or amoxicillin) + metronidazole for 7–14 days
Cheap and effective, but may cause side-effects

Proton pump inhibitor + 2 antibiotics (choose from metronidazole, amoxicillin, clarithromycin)
    for 7 days
Few side-effects, effectiveness limited by primary or induced resistance to
clarithromycin or metronidazole

Ranitidine bismuth citrate + clarithromycin + metronidazole for 7 days
Additional antimicrobial action of bismuth may help prevent resistance

Quadruple treatments
Proton-pump inhibitor + colloidal bismuth subcitrate + tetracycline + metronidazole for 7 days
Highest cure rate, but most complicated regimen

Table 14.1 Treatments that have been shown to be effective in eradicating H. pylori.

• Pyloric stenosis. This presents with recurrent vomiting of food ingested up to 24 h previously with immediate relief. Visible gastric peristalsis may be seen. Conservative management with gastric aspiration and intravenous fluids may sometimes allow time for a benign active ulcer to heal and relieve the obstruction. Surgery is usually required either on the first or subsequent admission. These patients may vomit profusely and become dehydrated and alkalotic. Fluid and electrolyte replacement is obligatory and particularly so prior to surgery.

Investigation
Endoscopy with biopsy in experienced hands is important in establishing the diagnosis, and allows identification of *H. pylori* infection. Duodenal ulcers are virtually always benign.

Gastric carcinomas are more common on the greater curve and in the antrum, but lesser curve ulcers may, nevertheless, be malignant. The size of the ulcer is no guide to whether a carcinoma is present. Carcinomas may have a rolled edge. Biopsy can give histological confirmation. Repeat endoscopy after 4 weeks of treatment should show healing of a gastric ulcer. If this has not occurred the presence of a carcinoma becomes more likely.

Barium meal should be performed if dysphagia is present.

H. pylori is rich in the enzyme urease which hydrolyses urea to NH_4 and CO_2. This observation is utilized in the urea breath test that measures the amount of $^{14}CO_2$ released after a dose of ^{14}C-labelled urea. Infection can also be detected by testing for antibodies in the serum by enzyme-linked immunosorbent assay (ELISA), and a stool antigen test.

Management
Antacids and diet often ameliorate symptoms, but do not hasten healing. The patient should stop smoking.

Patients with proven *H. pylori* infection are given eradication therapy. A number of regimens have been shown to be effective (Table 14.1). Cure rates are typically over 80%. Poor compliance and resistance against metronidazole and clarithromycin are causes of treatment failure.

H_2-receptor antagonists reduce gastric acid output. Maintenance treatment prevents ulcer relapse. In patients with a history of bleeding duodenal ulcer, long-term treatment with H_2-antagonists appears safe and effective in preventing recurrent haemorrhage.

H^+, K^+-ATPase (proton pump) inhibitors, cause a profound reduction in gastric acidity. Long-term treatment has been associated with the development of atrophic gastritis.

Misoprostol, a synthetic prostaglandin analogue, is effective in reducing gastrointestinal damage induced by non-steroidal anti-inflammatory drugs.

Indications for surgery

Duodenal ulcer

Acute indications include:

• perforation;

• pyloric obstruction; and

• persistent haemorrhage.

Failed medical management (a common indication in the past) is now rare.

Gastric ulcer

• Acute indication: persistent haemorrhage.

• Non-acute indications:

(a) carcinoma;

(b) failed medical treatment, either if there is a possibility of carcinoma or for persistent symptoms.

Gastric carcinoma

Gastric carcinoma is the eighth leading cause of cancer mortality worldwide. It is associated with *Helicobacter pylori* infection. It affects mainly the pylorus and antrum. Symptoms are those of a gastric ulcer in the early stages but pyloric obstruction or dysphagia may occur. Occasionally, the patient complains of no more than weight loss.

The prognosis is poor, with 5-year survival rates of 10%. Curative resection with removal of the primary tumour and regional lymph nodes is the most effective treatment, but only 40% of patients are potential candidates.

Hiatus hernia and gastro-oesophageal reflux

Aetiology

Weakness of the diaphragmatic sphincter allows the lower oesophagus and cardia of the stomach to rise into the thorax. Gastro-oesophageal reflux may occur in the presence or absence of a hiatus hernia, and is aggravated by smoking or alcohol.

Symptoms

Retrosternal burning pain, usually episodic, with acid regurgitation into throat and flatulence that may give relief; worse on lying flat or bending. It is relieved by milk and antacids. Bleeding may give positive occult blood tests and anaemia. Peptic oesophagitis may lead to ulceration and/or stricture.

Investigations

If persistent and symptoms severe or if associated with dysphagia (to exclude benign or malignant stricture) or weight loss (to exclude oesophageal or gastric carcinoma), barium swallow or endoscopy will reveal the hernia and the presence of gastric acid reflux.

Management

• Weight reduction and stop smoking. Avoid clothes that constrict and increase intra-abdominal pressure, and avoid foods that induce symptoms if recognized. Sleep propped up (raise head of the bed).

• Antacids for symptoms. Metoclopramide increases oesophageal sphincter contraction, and increases gastric emptying. It is a dopamine antagonist and may induce acute dystonic reactions which respond to procyclidine. A course of an H_2-receptor antagonist or a proton-pump inhibitor usually relieves symptoms if severe.

• Surgery for hiatus hernia is very rarely indicated in the absence of stricture formation as it is a major procedure and the results are uncertain.

In *Barrett's oesophagus* reflux is associated with columnar metaplasia of the normal stratified squamous epithelium of the lower oesophagus. It may predispose to carcinoma of the oesophagus and gastric cardia.

Inflammatory bowel disease
(ulcerative colitis and Crohn disease)

Aetiology
The aetiology of ulcerative colitis and Crohn disease remains unknown. A genetic predisposition is suggested by the increased incidence in first-degree relatives, higher prevalence in monozygotic vs. dizygotic twins and migrant studies. The incidence is highest in white people, and lowest in Asians. Antineutrophil cytoplasm antibodies (p. 124) are found in 50–70% of patients with ulcerative colitis, and 20–40% of patients with Crohn disease. Their significance is unclear.

Ulcerative colitis
Clinical features
Ulcerative colitis usually presents in the 20–40-year age group, but may occur at any age. First presentation over 65 years is uncommon but carries a greater mortality. At presentation 30% have disease confined to the rectum, and 20% have extensive disease. Intermittent diarrhoea with mucus and blood in the stool, associated with fever and remissions to near normal, are the most frequent symptoms.

Three patterns may be distinguished:

1 The disease may occasionally present as a single, short, mild episode of diarrhoea that appears to settle rapidly but may relapse at any time.

2 Usually, the history is of months or years of general ill health, with continuous or intermittent diarrhoea. In these cases the disease is usually restricted to the rectum and descending colon, and then usually termed proctocolitis. General symptoms may be mild or severe. Secondary complications are frequent.

3 Approximately one-fifth present with a severe acute episode of bloody diarrhoea with constitutional symptoms of fever and toxaemia and abdominal discomfort from toxic mega-colon which may proceed to perforation.

Diagnosis
This is suggested by the clinical picture and may be confirmed, except in the very ill, by sigmoidoscopy with biopsy and barium examination.

Sigmoidoscopy
The rectal mucosa is always abnormal in *ulcerative colitis*; it is a distal disease (proctitis) with a variable extension proximally up the large bowel. Abnormal appearances, in order of severity, are:
- granular mucosa with loss of normal vascular pattern;
- presence of pus and blood; and
- visible ulceration with contact bleeding at the rim of the sigmoidoscope.

Radiology
Barium enema shows loss of normal haustral pattern with shortening of the large intestine. The bowel takes on the appearance of a smooth tube (hosepipe appearance). Undermined ulcers and pseudopolypi may be seen. Stricture formation or carcinoma produces fixed areas of narrowing.

Plain abdominal film will show acute dilatation when present, and bowel gas may outline mucosal ulceration. Barium enema examination in such circumstances may produce perforation.

Differential diagnosis
- Carcinoma of the colon, which may present with bloody diarrhoea.
- Infective enteritis. The acute case may resemble *Campylobacter* enteritis or bacillary dysentery, and the chronic case amoebic colitis (these should be excluded by stool examination).
- Antibiotic-associated pseudomembranous colitis (PMC) follows within 3 weeks of taking antibiotics. It is caused by toxins of *Clostridium difficile* when it colonizes the colon following

antibiotic-induced suppression of the normal bacterial flora of the gut. On sigmoidoscopy, characteristically there are patchy yellowish areas of necrotic mucosa. Histology shows mucosal destruction with characteristic exudation of fibrin and inflammatory cells in the cross-sectional shape of a mushroom. *C. difficile* and its toxin may be found in the stool. The condition responds to oral metronidazole or vancomycin.

• Very rarely, acute ischaemic colitis may occur and affect the rectosigmoid junction (but not the rectum).

• Irritable bowel syndrome.

Crohn disease

Crohn disease of the large bowel may resemble ulcerative colitis. The diagnosis of Crohn disease is favoured by little blood loss, a normal rectal mucosa on sigmoidoscopy, the presence of perianal sepsis and the radiological differences.

Clinical features

Crohn disease usually starts in the teens and early 20s. There is a second peak of colonic Crohn disease in the elderly. The terminal ileum is most frequently diseased but any part of the alimentary tract may be involved. The colon is involved in 10–20% of cases. It usually presents (80–90%) as intermittent abdominal pain with diarrhoea and abdominal distension in a young thin person. Less commonly it presents as an 'acute abdomen' with signs of acute appendicitis with or without a palpable mass. A mass in the right iliac fossa from terminal ileitis must be differentiated from a caecal carcinoma and an appendix abscess. Amoebic abscess and ileocaecal tuberculosis are less common causes.

The granulomatous inflammatory process affects short lengths of the intestine, leaving normal bowel between—skip lesions. The wall is thickened and the lumen narrowed. Mucosal ulceration and regional lymphadenopathy are present. The characteristic microscopic features are of submucosal inflammation, less marked than in ulcerative colitis. There are

numerous fissures down to the submucosa with or without chronic granulation tissue, consisting of non-caseating granulomas not unlike those found in sarcoid.

Radiology

Barium enema. The terminal ileum is most commonly involved and may produce incompetence of the ileocaecal valve. Mucosal ulceration may be deep and 'spikes' of barium may enter deep into the bowel wall (rose thorn). Lesions may be multiple with normal bowel between (skip lesions). Coarse cobblestone appearance of the mucosa appears early. Later in the disease fibrosis produces narrowing of the intestine (string sign) with some proximal dilatation.

Small-bowel enema. There may be mucosal ulceration, luminal narrowing or pooling of barium in irregular clumps at the site of an inflammatory mass.

Indium-labelled white cell scanning is helpful in localizing active inflammatory bowel disease.

Histology

In *ulcerative colitis* histology shows superficial inflammation with chronic inflammatory cells infiltrating the lamina propria with crypt abscesses, with little involvement of the muscularis mucosa and with reduction of goblet cells.

In *Crohn disease* the characteristic microscopic features are of submucosal inflammation, less marked than in ulcerative colitis. There are numerous fissures down to the submucosa with or without chronic granulation tissue consisting of non-caseating granulomas not unlike those found in sarcoid.

Complications

Fever, anaemia and weight loss. Hypoalbuminaemia results from loss of protein, and in small-bowel disease malabsorption. Clubbing is fairly common. Occasionally, uveitis (5%), arthritis (5%) and skin rashes (erythema nodosum and pyoderma gangrenosum) occur.

Fistulae, perianal sepsis and intestinal sepsis may complicate Crohn disease. Renal stones occur in 5–10%.

The benefit of colonoscopy surveillance for colorectal carcinoma in ulcerative colitis remains unclear. The risk is greater if the entire colon is involved, if the history is prolonged (10% after 10 years), if the first attack was severe and if the first attack occurred at a young age. Medical treatment appears to lessen the risk of carcinoma. In Crohn disease there is an increased risk of both colorectal and small-bowel cancer.

Medical management of inflammatory bowel disease

• Attention to nutritional deficiencies (p. 185) and electrolyte imbalance is essential.
• *Aminosalicylates* are of value in inducing and maintaining remission in colitis. Their value in small-bowel Crohn disease is less clear. Sulfasalazine is a combination of 5-aminosalicylic acid (5-ASA) and sulfapyridine, which acts as a carrier to deliver 5-ASA to its site of action in the colon. Mesalazine is 5-ASA by itself, and olsalazine is two linked molecules of 5-ASA that separate in the lower bowel. These newer aminosalicylates lack sulphonamide-related side-effects, and may be of more benefit in treating Crohn disease. Mesalazine suppositories can be useful for localized rectal disease.
• *Corticosteroids* are of benefit in moderate to severe active ulcerative colitis and Crohn disease. Side-effects and dependence limit their long-term use. Enemas or suppositories are used for localized rectal disease.
• *Azathioprine* and *6-mercaptopurine* are of value as a steroid-sparing agent in both ulcerative colitis and Crohn disease.
• *Methotrexate* has also been used for its steroid-sparing effect. Long-term benefits are unclear.
• *Cyclosporin A* has successfully healed refractory fistulas in Crohn disease. Variable responses of active colitis to cyclosporin A have been reported.
• *Antibiotics: metronidazole* has been used in Crohn disease, particularly for perianal disease. *Ciprofloxacin* may also be of value.

• *Elemental diets* may be of benefit in Crohn disease.
• *Monoclonal antibodies which inhibit tumour necrosis factor-α.* Infliximab has been used for the treatment of severe, active Crohn disease refractory to steroids or immunosuppressive therapy, and for treatment of refractory fistulas in Crohn disease.
• Smoking aggravates Crohn disease, but can improve the clinical course of ulcerative colitis. *Nicotine* may be of value in maintaining remission in ulcerative colitis.

Surgery in inflammatory bowel disease

In *ulcerative colitis*, surgery (proctocolectomy, or total colectomy with ileoanal anastomosis) is indicated if there is:
• severe haemorrhage;
• perforation;
• acute toxaemia with dilatation of the colon which fails to respond within 24–48 h to high-dose steroids; and
• prophylactic colectomy should be performed if regular colonoscopy shows high-grade dysplasia or carcinoma.

In *Crohn disease* surgery is used for relief of acute emergencies (obstruction), abscesses and fistulae. Surgery eventually becomes necessary in about 30% of cases. Resection of diseased intestine and bypass operations may become necessary for severe, chronic ill health, but these are not curative. Fistula formation may result and recurrence is the rule. Intestinal obstruction is best managed conservatively in the first instance with gastric aspiration and intravenous feeding to allow time for the acute inflammation to resolve.

Endocrine tumours of the gut

All are very rare.

Apudomas

Amine precursor uptake and decarboxylation (APUD) cells: these are the hormone-secreting cells found chiefly along the length of the gastrointestinal tract. They have molecular and functional similarities with each other and may form various kinds of functioning tumour. They secrete a number of hormones including gastrin, cholecystokinin, secretin, glucagon and vasoactive intestinal peptide (VIP).

Zollinger–Ellison syndrome

This rare disorder is characterized by multiple recurrent duodenal and jejunal ulceration associated with a very high plasma gastrin level (> 300 mg/l with the patient off H_2-receptor blockade), gross gastric acid hypersecretion and the presence of a gastrin-secreting adenoma (which may be malignant), usually in the pancreas but sometimes in the stomach wall.

Diarrhoea sometimes with steatorrhoea may be a feature (lipase is inactivated by the low pH). The volume of gastric secretion is enormous (7–10 l/24 h) and acid secretion persistently raised (and raised little further by pentagastrin). Normal fasting gastrin is < 100 pg/ml. In Zollinger–Ellison syndrome there is a rise in serum gastrin level > 200 pg/ml after infusion of secretin 2 units/kg.

The presence of an adenoma may be associated with adenomas of other endocrine glands, i.e. adrenals, parathyroids and anterior pituitary (p. 144).

Treatment is by removal of the tumour, which is usually benign. If it cannot be found, give either long-term proton pump inhibitor or H_2-blockade.

Other endocrine tumours of the gut

These are very rare indeed but are sometimes discussed in examinations.

Insulinoma

A tumour of the pancreatic islet β cells which produces episodic hypoglycaemic attacks which may present as epilepsy or abnormal behaviour. Fasting produces prolonged hypoglycaemia with high insulin levels in the serum. In all, 10% are malignant and 5% are multiple.

Glucagonoma

A tumour of the α cells which produces a syndrome of mild diabetes with diarrhoea, weight loss, anaemia, glossitis and a migratory necrolytic rash.

Vipoma

A variant of the Zollinger–Ellison syndrome with severe watery diarrhoea, hypokalaemia with or without achlorhydria caused by a pancreatic tumour producing a VIP. Abdominal pain and flushing are typical features. Vipomectomy may be curative.
- *Benign tumours* account for 40% of cases.
- *Malignant tumours* account for 60% of cases. Two-thirds have metastasized at diagnosis.

Gastrointestinal haemorrhage

Upper gut
Aetiology
Acute
- Duodenal ulcer (30%). Duodenal ulcers and duodenitis are more common in men.
- Gastric ulcer (20%). Gastric ulcers are more common in women.
- Gastric erosions (20%).
- Mallory–Weiss (mucosal tears) and oesophagitis (10%).
- Oesophageal varices (5%). Up to 50% in France and parts of USA.
- Others (10%).

Half the patients are over 60 years old. Bleeding from gastric ulcers is rare under the age of 50 years, as is bleeding from duodenal ulcers in females. Melaena as a presenting symptom suggests less severe bleeding than haematemesis. The concurrent use of non-steroidal anti-inflammatory drugs or aspirin with selective serotonin reuptake inhibitors (SSRIs) greatly increases the risk of upper gastrointestinal bleeding.

Oesophagitis, oesophageal ulcer, gastric ulcer and malignancy are more common in elderly people. Mallory–Weiss syndrome, gastritis and duodenal ulcer are more common in young people. Oesophageal varices, oesophageal ulcer and gastrointestinal malignancy are associated with increased risks of death. Mallory–Weiss syndrome, oesophagitis, gastritis and duodenitis, which tend to be associated, have significantly lower risks of death.

Clinical presentation

Haematemesis is a reliable indication of bleeding above the duodenojejunal flexure, and bright red rectal bleeding of the lower colon or rectum. The colour of altered blood passed per rectum is related to transit time more than to the site of bleeding.

Faintness, weakness, sweating, palpitation and nausea often precede the evidence of bleeding. The patient is pale and sweating, and has tachycardia and hypotension.

Chronic

Bleeding from hiatus hernia and gastric carcinoma is usually insidious (but not always).

Management

- Admit to hospital (trivial bleeding can quickly progress to exsanguination).
- Establish venous access. Take blood for grouping and cross-matching, creatinine, urea and electrolytes, liver function tests including the prothrombin time and full blood count with platelets.
- Treat shock if present with transfusion of blood (or colloid if blood is not yet available) and monitor by frequent pulse and blood pressure. Conventionally, give blood when the pulse is over 100 beats/min or the systolic arterial blood pressure under 100 mmHg and the haemoglobin under 10 g/dl if the trends are adverse. If the patient has cardiac disease or is elderly, or if the bleeding is continuous and severe, a central venous pressure monitor should be inserted as a guide to further transfusion and rebleeding. A central venous pressure of 5–10 cm of saline should be maintained. Oxygen should be given. The urine output should be monitored in shocked patients.
- Sedate the patient if anxious. Diazepam probably causes less hypotension than morphine or diamorphine.
- When bleeding has stopped (steady pulse, blood pressure and central venous pressure), assess progress with repeat haemoglobin.

Variceal bleeding (p. 214).

Investigation (for site and cause of bleeding)

Within 24 h, as soon as the patient's condition allows, upper gastrointestinal endoscopy should be performed; this shows the site of bleeding in up to 90% of cases. Local diathermy or injection of a sclerosant may arrest bleeding. Selective angiography may show the site of active bleeding if not previously determined, particularly when angiodysplasia must be excluded. If bleeding is sufficiently fast (2 ml/min) a labelled red blood cell isotope scan or selective angiography may help to locate bleeding, e.g. from a Meckel's diverticulum.

If bleeding continues or recurs, surgery may be necessary (see below). If bleeding has stopped, the patient should be given oral iron and a normal diet. Parenteral H_2-blockade is usually given early and may reduce blood loss. Patients should be advised not to smoke.

Indications for surgery (in haemorrhage from peptic ulcer)

Although there are no absolute indications, surgery is indicated if bleeding does not stop spontaneously or the patient rebleeds in hospital (the central venous pressure may be the first indication of this, but slower continuous bleeds are indicated by a persistently low haemoglobin). The overall mortality is worse in older patients (10% in the over-60s) than in the young (2% in the under-60s). Bleeds from gastric ulcers (mortality up to 20% in the over-60s) carry twice the mortality of bleeds from duodenal ulcers. Also the operative risk for gastric ulcer surgery is less than for duodenal ulcers.

Hence the tendency is to operate early in older patients, particularly if bleeding from a gastric ulcer. Supplies of compatible blood may be a controlling factor.

Lower gut

Acute loss may occur from haemorrhoids, fissures, ulcerative colitis and Crohn disease, ischaemic colitis, colonic and caecal carcinoma and diverticular disease. Patients with chronic and occult bleeding usually present with lethargy and iron-deficiency anaemia and diagnosis is confirmed by positive faecal occult blood tests. Any of the causes of upper or lower gut bleeding given above may be responsible. Other very rare causes include polyps and vascular abnormalities, such as arteriovenous malformations, angiodysplasia of the ascending colon, Peutz–Jeghers syndrome (small intestinal polyposis and blotchy pigmentation around the mouth) and Rendu–Osler–Weber (hereditary (autosomal dominant) haemorrhagic telangiectasia in which thin-walled dilatated blood vessels rupture causing gastrointestinal bleeding, epistaxis, haemoptysis or haematuria) syndromes. Meckel's diverticulum, polyps and endometriosis may also present with bleeding.

Steatorrhoea and malabsorption

Malabsorption signifies impaired ability to absorb one or more of the normally absorbed dietary constituents, including protein, carbohydrates, fats, minerals and vitamins.

Steatorrhoea signifies malabsorption of fat, and is defined as a faecal fat excretion of more than 18 mmol/day (6 g/day) on a normal fat intake (50–100 g). Apart from the occasions when the cause of steatorrhoea is obvious (such as obstructive jaundice), the diagnostic problem revolves around the differentiation between enteropathy (commonly gluten-induced) and other causes of steatorrhoea.

Diarrhoea is not necessarily a presenting symptom and malabsorption may present with one or more of its complications (e.g. anaemia, weight loss, osteomalacia).

Gluten-sensitive enteropathy
(Coeliac disease)
Aetiology
There is mucosal sensitivity to wheat gluten (in particular α-gliadin, a polypeptide in gluten) and to barley and rye, and occasionally oats (although not rice or maize). IgA α-gliadin antibodies are present in 80–90% of patients with coeliac disease. It is associated with human leucocyte antigen (HLA) B8, A1, DR3, DR7, DQW2 and antibodies to reticulin may be present. There is an increased incidence in near relatives and there is a high incidence of gut lymphoma and carcinoma.

NB Virtually all patients with dermatitis herpetiformis have gluten-sensitive enteropathy.

Clinical presentation
There is usually a history of intermittent or chronic increased bowel frequency, classically with pale, bulky, offensive, frothy, greasy stools that flush only with difficulty. There may be a history of intermittent abdominal colic, flatus and abdominal distension. Depending on the severity and duration of the disease, there may be weakness and weight loss. If the malabsorption started in childhood, the patient may be short compared with unaffected siblings or parents. Children may present with irritability, failure to gain weight or failure to thrive.

The malabsorption involves not only fat and the fat-soluble vitamins but also minerals and water-soluble vitamins (Table 14.2).

Examination
In addition to the features mentioned above there may be:
• evidence of weight loss;
• pigmented, scaly and bruised skin; and
• distended abdomen with increased bowel sounds.
NB The anaemia has many causes including anorexia, blood loss, mucosal damage, folate deficiency and bacterial overgrowth.

Clubbing may occur. Signs of subacute combined degeneration of the cord are very rare.

Other causes of malabsorption
Bile salt deficiency
Patients present with obstructive jaundice usually secondary to carcinoma of the head of the pancreas or to gallstones (which may sometimes be seen on plain abdominal X-ray) or, rarely, in primary biliary cirrhosis or bile duct stricture.

Pancreatic enzyme deficiency
This is usually caused by chronic pancreatitis or carcinoma affecting the pancreatic ducts (also, rarely, cystic fibrosis, pancreatic calculi and benign pancreatic cystadenoma). The differentiation between chronic pancreatitis and carcinoma may be very difficult at presentation.

VITAMIN AND MINERAL DEFICIENCIES

Vitamin B$_{12}$	To produce megaloblastic anaemia (p. 301)
Iron	To produce iron-deficiency anaemia (p. 299)
Vitamin D and calcium	Resulting in osteomalacia with bone tenderness and muscle weakness. Tetany may occur
	Children may develop rickets
Vitamin B group	Glossitis and angular stomatitis
Vitamin K	Deficient prothrombin formation to produce bruising and epistaxis
Associated impairment of amino-acid absorption	May produce hypoproteinaemia and oedema
Potassium	May produce weakness

Table 14.2 Vitamin and mineral deficiency following malabsorption.

Tests for malabsorption, glucose tolerance, serum bilirubin and barium meal are of little help.

Imaging
• Straight abdominal X-ray can demonstrate the presence of calcification of the pancreas or of gallstones, which favour chronic pancreatitis.
• Ultrasound, which can be difficult to interpret, shows changes in pancreatic size and shape, and calcification. The biliary tract, neighbouring structures and fluid collections can be shown. Endoscopic ultrasound allows more detailed study.
• Computed tomography (CT) scan, unlike standard ultrasound, is not affected by bowel gas. It may show gallstones and dilatated ducts from partial obstruction at the sphincter of Oddi.
• Magnetic resonance imaging (MRI) endoscopic retrograde cholangiopancreatography (ERCP). It can give information about bile duct and vascular structure and help define tumours and cystic lesions.

Duodenal fibroscopy with ERCP can show duct anatomy, ectasia or stricture, and calculi. Carcinoembryonic antigen (CEA) studies are useful only for assessing completeness of resection of a CEA-producing tumour.

Tests of exocrine pancreatic function
These are rarely used clinically because they are difficult to perform.

Stimulation tests. The duodenum is intubated, and duodenal contents aspirated before and after a stimulus (e.g. secretin, cholecystikinin). The fluid is analysed for pancreatic enzymes and bicarbonate.

Bentiromide test. Bentiromide is a synthetic peptide that releases para-aminobenzoic acid (PABA) when cleaved by pancreatic chymotrypsin. PABA is absorbed and excreted in urine. The patient is given bentiromide and urinary PABA measured in a 6-h urine sample. A reduction in PABA excretion indicates pancreatic dysfunction.

Symptoms of pancreatic malabsorption are improved by a low-fat diet (40 g/day), replacing minerals and vitamins, and giving pancreatic supplements (e.g. Nutrizym, Creon, Pancrex V Forte), preferably with H$_2$-blockade. Avoid alcohol.

Other intestinal disease
Postsurgical. Incomplete food mixing may follow gastrectomy or gastroenterostomy and there may be a diminished area for absorption following small bowel resection.

Abnormal intestinal organisms. Bacterial overgrowth can be distinguished from ileal disease using the early (40 min) peak in breath hydrogen after lactulose (10 g) (p. 227) or glucose (50 g).

The normal bacterial count in jejunal juice is $< 10^3$–10^5 organisms/ml. The organisms

(*Escherichia coli* and *Bacteroides*) break down dietary tryptophan to produce indoxylsulphate (indican) which is excreted in the urine. Overgrowth can be detected by urinary indican excretion of more than 80 mg/24 h.

An aetiological role of the cultured organisms in malabsorption is difficult to prove but the steatorrhoea may respond to antibiotic therapy (e.g. tetracycline or erythromycin). There may be a close association between bacterial overgrowth and stasis from blind loops, diverticula and strictures. It may occur after gastrectomy as a result of reduced acid and pepsin, and in diabetic autonomic nephropathy.

In the radioactive bile acid breath test, ^{14}C glycine-labelled bile salt is given orally, and anaerobic bacteria in the intestine deconjugate the bile acid. The released ^{14}C amino acid is transported to the liver and metabolized to $^{14}CO_2$ which can be detected in the breath.

Crohn disease (p. 221).

Rare causes

The following are very uncommon but well recognized:

Zollinger–Ellison syndrome (p. 223).

Disaccharidase deficiency. Malabsorption of lactose, maltose and sucrose may occur in isolation caused by primary enzyme deficiency, or as part of a general malabsorption picture in any disease that damages the intestinal brush border. The most important is isolated lactase deficiency that presents, usually in children, with milk intolerance and malabsorption. Patients have abdominal pain, diarrhoea, distension and borborygmi (i.e. symptoms of bacterial fermentation of unabsorbed sugars) after 50 g lactose by mouth and the blood glucose rises by < 1.1 mmol/l over the following 2 h. The diagnosis is confirmed by the absence of lactase activity in the jejunal mucosa on biopsy. Management consists of withdrawal of milk and milk products from the diet.

Other intrinsic disease of the intestinal wall caused by tuberculosis, Hodgkin disease, lymphosarcoma, diffuse systemic sclerosis, amyloidosis and Whipple disease (intestinal lipodystrophy), associated with the organism *Tropheryma whippeli.*

Tropical sprue is a disorder that produces steatorrhoea and occurs almost exclusively in Europeans in or from the tropics, especially in India and the Far East. The aetiology is unknown. The most common associated deficiency is folic acid. The disease frequently remits spontaneously on return from the tropics. In some cases that do not remit, a course of parenteral folic acid, metronidazole or oral tetracycline may be curative.

Very rarely, malabsorption is associated with diabetes, cardiac failure and giardiasis.

Investigation of malabsorption

In a patient with a characteristic history, the investigation with the greatest likelihood of achieving a diagnosis is jejunal biopsy. However, tests of absorption may quantitate the degree of malabsorption and help with the differential diagnosis between pancreatic and intestinal disease.

Using the hydrogen breath test, after an oral dose of lactose (2 g/kg up to 50 g, in 250 ml water), normal subjects show no rise in breath hydrogen over the following 3 h because they absorb the disaccharide completely. If, because it is not absorbed higher up the gut, the disaccharide reaches the colon, the anaerobic bacteria there ferment it so that hydrogen can be detected in the breath at about 90 min. The hydrogen breath test can also be used to assess small-bowel transit time using lactulose.

NB Intestinal malabsorption tends to give a total malabsorption. Pancreatic malabsorption (p. 231) is much less common and tends to affect the absorption only of fat and proteins and to leave the absorption of sugars, minerals and water-soluble vitamins relatively unaffected.

Blood tests
• Anaemia is common and may be iron-deficient, megaloblastic or both (dimorphic).
• Serum and red cell folate, iron and transferrin may be low.

• Serum albumin may be reduced and the prothrombin time prolonged.

• Serum calcium, phosphate and magnesium may be low and the serum alkaline phosphatase increased (osteomalacia pattern).

Tests of absorption
Faecal fat excretion. The diagnosis of steatorrhoea is made formally by measuring faecal fat excretion over 3–5 days on a normal diet of 50–100 g of fat in 24 h (upper limit of normal 6 g/24 h—18 mmol/24 h). This is now rarely required and has been replaced by the radioactive triolein breath test. Triolein is a triglyceride that is hydrolysed by pancreatic lipase and absorbed in the small intestine. It releases CO_2 upon metabolism. ^{14}C-triolein is given to the patient and the amount of exhaled ^{14}C (as $^{14}CO_2$) is measured. Values less than 3.5 % suggest fat malabsorption.

Radiology
A small intestinal barium meal with a flocculable contrast medium may show flocculation and segmentation of barium—evidence of excess mucus secretion. Of more significance are widening of the small intestinal calibre and increased distance between adjacent loops of bowel, indicating thickening of the intestinal wall. All these changes are non-specific and the main purpose of the barium meal is to detect diverticula, fistulae or Crohn disease.

The bones may show evidence of osteomalacia and/or osteoporosis, and even of hyperparathyroidism (secondary or tertiary) if very severe and prolonged.

Jejunal biopsy
In gluten-induced enteropathy, dissecting microscopic examination usually reveals flattening of the mucosa, with partial or total villous atrophy.

Management of gluten-induced enteropathy
Gluten-free diet. In adults the response may take several months. Repeat biopsy is performed and the diagnosis is confirmed by a return to normal appearances.

NB There may be a predisposition to malignancy—lymphomas and gut carcinoma (particularly oesophagus)—in gluten-induced enteropathy and there is some evidence that gluten-free diets may reduce the incidence of these. Hence the diet is continued for life.

Replace vitamins and minerals as indicated, and, if necessary, parenterally.

Diverticular disease

Diverticula occur anywhere in the alimentary tract but chiefly in the colon—diverticulosis. They are caused by a weakening of the colonic wall and increased intracolonic pressure. They affect chiefly the descending and sigmoid colon. It is a disorder of middle and old age (5% of the population over 50 years in the UK), more common in women than men and is usually discovered incidentally during barium enema performed to exclude colonic carcinoma.

Clinical features
Inflamed diverticula produce diverticulitis with:
• pain, discomfort and tenderness in the left iliac fossa (there may be a mass from pericolic abscess)—'appendicitis of the left side';
• change in bowel habit with constipation and/or diarrhoea sometimes alternating (NB exclude carcinoma);
• rectal bleeding, which may be acute and sometimes massive and the first symptom;
• subacute obstruction;
• frequency of micturition and cystitis, resulting from vesicocolic fistula; and
• perforation with peritonitis or fistulae.

Management
Acute diverticulitis may be extremely painful and require rest in bed, analgesia and antibiotics (e.g. cefotaxime and metronidazole). Occasionally surgery is required, particularly colostomy and resection for obstruction.

Dietary fibre
Diverticulosis is rare in communities which take a fibre-rich diet, where there is also far less carcinoma of the colon and appendicitis. A

diet high in dietary fibre results in bulkier stools and rapid intestinal transit times. The soft stool prevents straining which may help to prevent diverticulosis. In the established disease added dietary fibre (2 teaspoonsful to 2 tablespoonsful daily) reduces symptoms in most patients. Fibrerich diets also decrease serum cholesterol and increase faecal excretion of bile salts and their relative absence from western diets has been suggested as a possible contributory factor in coronary artery atheroma and gallstones.

Irritable bowel syndrome

Clinical presentation
Irritable bowel syndrome is one of the most common bowel disorders, affecting about 20% of adults in the industrialized world, more often female than male. It is associated with abnormal gut motility. Patients present with different combinations of various characteristic symptoms: e.g. colicky abdominal pain eased by bowel movement often loose with pencil-like stools at the onset of pain, alternating constipation/diarrhoea, bloating and a sense of incomplete evacuation. Examination is usually normal although there may be tenderness in the left iliac fossa. There may be symptoms unrelated to the gastrointestinal tract, including lethargy, urinary symptoms and dyspareunia. About 50% of patients have symptoms of anxiety and/or depression.

The cause of the disturbed gastrointestinal function is unknown, but increased sensitivity to distension of the bowel and abnormalities of motility are found in some patients.

Investigation
Diagnosis is usually made from the pattern of symptoms and signs on history and examination, but exclusion of more serious disease is necessary, particularly in patients over 45 (where weight loss, rectal bleeding and new signs and symptoms may point to carcinoma of the colon).

If the history is typical, the examination and sigmoidoscopy normal, and blood count, erythrocyte sedimentation rate, C-reactive protein and serum proteins normal and at least three faecal occult blood examinations negative, serious alternative diagnoses are effectively excluded. If there are changes in bowel habit, flexible sigmoidoscopy or barium enema can exclude carcinoma and demonstrate diverticula.

Treatment
There is no uniformly successful treatment. Antispasmodics may be tried, e.g. hyoscine (Buscopan) 10–20 mg t.d.s. before meals. If a cause of anxiety (e.g. cancer) can be identified and treated, symptoms may be markedly reduced. 5-HT$_3$ antagonists (e.g. ondansetron) or antidepressants (tricyclics and SSRIs) can help with abdominal pain and discomfort, urgency and stool frequency in patients with diarrhoea-predominant symptoms (but not those with constipation/bloating). Occasionally, specific foods (cereal, dairy, fructose) may produce symptoms of irritable bowel syndrome, and these should be excluded from the diet. Dietary bran makes symptoms worse in 50% of patients, but ispaghula husk, a gluten-free fibre (e.g. Fybogel), is indicated when there is associated constipation.

Ischaemic colitis

Clinical features
This is a disorder of middle and old age that often presents as an acute abdomen with the sudden onset of pain followed by bloody diarrhoea, sometimes copious.

Diagnosis
If subacute, it must be distinguished from the bleeding of diverticular disease and of ulcerative colitis. Any part of the colon can be affected although, because it has the most precarious blood supply, the splenic flexure is usually involved. If the colon looks normal on sigmoidoscopy, ulcerative colitis is virtually excluded, although large-bowel Crohn disease or diverticular disease is not. Barium enema shows mucosal oedema with characteristic

'thumb-printing', as if a thumb had been pressed along the outside of the affected colon.

Prognosis

In mild cases there may be complete recovery but colonic strictures can develop later. In colonic gangrene, surgical resection is necessary. The differential diagnosis includes *Campylobacter* enteritis, and diverticular disease, in which bleeding can be torrential. Pseudo-membranous colitis does not usually cause bloody diarrhoea.

Pancreas

Carcinoma

A total of 75% of tumours occur in the head of the pancreas. It is more common in men and in cigarette smokers.

Clinical presentation

Patients present with one or more of the following features.
• Anorexia and weight loss.
• Indigestion or epigastric pain often indistinguishable from duodenal or gastric ulceration. Back pain suggests pancreatic disease (and posterior ulcers).
• Obstructive jaundice. Intermittent jaundice suggests a gallstone in the bile duct (rarely, carcinoma of the ampulla of Vater).
• About 20% of patients have diabetes, usually of short duration, and some present with it. In the elderly, sudden onset or worsening of diabetes may indicate malignancy.

Investigation

Ultrasound or CT scan may show the tumour.
ERCP may confirm the diagnosis and allows palliative stenting of the obstructed common bile duct to relieve pruritus and jaundice.

Management

Ampullary carcinoma presents early with obstructive jaundice and can be resected.
Carcinoma of the head and body of the pancreas is usually fatal within 1 year.

Islet cell tumours
See Zollinger–Ellison syndrome and insulinoma (p. 223).

Acute pancreatitis

Aetiology

About 90% are associated with gall bladder disease (especially gallstones) and alcoholism. It is uncommon after cholecystectomy.

Clinical presentation

There may be a previous history of cholecystitis as biliary colic associated with gallstones. Pancreatitis occurs occasionally in association with mumps, drugs (e.g. thiazides) or severe hypertriglyceridaemia.

Abdominal pain, often very severe, occurs suddenly, usually in the epigastrium or across the upper abdomen with radiation to the back or shoulder. It spreads to involve the entire abdomen, which is tender with guarding and rebound tenderness. Hypotension with sweating and cyanosis occurs in severe attacks. There may be bruising around the umbilicus or in the flanks.

Differential diagnosis

It presents initially as an 'acute abdomen' and resembles:
• cholecystitis;
• acute myocardial infarction, dissecting aortic aneurysm, mesenteric vascular occlusion; and
• intestinal perforation, particularly duodenal ulcer (although shock is not often a feature of a perforated duodenal ulcer).

Investigation

The serum amylase is very high (> 1000 units/ml) within 24 h of onset. The level falls rapidly. Posterior duodenal ulcers can also cause very high amylase levels but not usually above 1000 units. Peritoneal fluid also has high amylase levels.

Straight abdominal X-ray may show gallstones, pancreatic calcification (indicating previous inflammation) and a distended loop of jejunum or transverse colon if they are close to the inflamed pancreas. Check serum calcium (which may fall as a result of the formation of calcium soaps). There is usually a leucocytosis.

Management
• If the diagnosis is definite, conservative management is preferred by most clinicians.
• Relieve pain with pentazocine or pethidine.
• Gastric aspiration and intravenous rehydration.
• Maintain the circulating volume.
• Monitor the blood glucose.
• If shock is present, give plasma expanders (e.g. dextran, plasma) while monitoring the central venous pressure, and give oxygen.
   Other measures are of less certain value.
• Propantheline 15–30 mg 6-hourly to block the vagus and relax the sphincter of Oddi.
• H_2-blockade.
• Antibiotics to prevent infection.
• Calcium if the serum level falls.
• In very severe cases, peritoneal lavage and parenteral nutrition may be tried.

Prognosis
Complete recovery occurs in over 95% of patients and recurrence is uncommon. Pancreatic abscess or pseudocyst may complicate acute pancreatitis. Patients should be investigated to exclude gallstones ($< 5\%$). Alcohol should be avoided if it is a possible cause.

Chronic pancreatitis
Aetiology
• Alcoholism after a mean interval of 18 years in men and 11 years in women, but also increased in people with modest alcohol consumption e.g. 20 g/day.
• Gallstones in most cases.
• More common in those on a high fat, high protein diet.
Also: pancreatic malformations, hyperparathyroidism.

Clinical presentation
• Recurrent, although mild, attacks that resemble acute pancreatitis.
• Malabsorption and steatorrhoea from pancreatic insufficiency (p. 225).

• Anorexia and weight loss.
• Diabetes mellitus when the islet cells are involved.
• Obstructive jaundice, which may be intermittent.
• In association with cystic fibrosis and haemochromatosis.

Investigation
The serum amylase is unhelpful in chronic pancreatitis although it is sometimes slightly raised, and isotope scanning of the pancreas is of little value.

   Investigate for malabsorption and exocrine pancreatic function (p. 225), diabetes mellitus (p. 153) and obstructive jaundice (p. 38), if relevant.

Treatment
• There is no specific therapy for chronic pancreatitis.
• Treat pancreatic malabsorption with low-fat diet (45 g/day), fat-soluble vitamins, calcium and pancreatic enzymes (e.g. Pancrex V, Creon) plus H_2-blockade.
• Treat diabetes mellitus (p. 153).
• Remove gallstones if present.
• Treat recurrent attacks and consider sphincterotomy or pancreatectomy.
• Alcohol is forbidden.
• Chronic severe pain is common and may lead to opiate addiction.

Gall bladder

Acute cholecystitis
Clinical features
The history is of fever, occasionally with rigors, abdominal pain, usually right subcostal with acute pain on palpation over the gall bladder region. The disease is more common in obese females over 50, but may occur in young adults. Gallstones are present in over 90% of cases. Occasionally, acute cholecystitis may be difficult to distinguish from a high appendix and right basal pneumonia and even perforated peptic ulcer, pancreatitis and myocardial infarction.

Management

The acute inflammation usually settles with bed rest, analgesia (pethidine) and antibiotics. Penicillin and co-trimoxazole are both secreted in the bile but one-third of biliary coliforms are now ampicillin-resistant. Cefotaxime is probably the antibiotic of choice. The gall bladder is removed 2–3 months later, after the inflammation has settled, although some surgeons elect to operate within 48 h because this is technically easier.

Rarely, an empyema develops or the gall bladder perforates.

Chronic cholecystitis

Clinical presentation

Recurrent episodes of cholecystitis are usually associated with gallstones. The attacks are often less severe than classical acute cholecystitis, and may resemble peptic ulceration and peptic oesophagitis. Myocardial ischaemia may be confused if the site of the pain is high.

Gallstones

Cholelithiasis is twice as common in women as men. There is an increased incidence in women taking oral contraceptives. The incidence rises with age. Stones occur in 10% of women over 40, classically in the fair, fat, fertile, female of 40–50 years on a low-fibre diet. They are usually cholesterol or mixed. Rarely, they are pigment stones associated with haemolytic anaemia.

Clinical features

Most stones produce no symptoms, but they may cause:

- flatulence upwards;
- biliary colic;
- acute cholecystitis;
- chronic cholecystitis; and
- obstructive jaundice, which may be intermittent, giving attacks of fever, jaundice and upper abdominal pain—Charcot's triad. Gall bladder empyema from bile duct obstruction is uncommon.

Gallstones are associated with acute and chronic pancreatitis and their presence indicates a higher risk of gall bladder carcinoma, although this is still extremely rare.

Investigation

Straight abdominal X-ray and ultrasonography with acoustic shadow will reveal many stones. Cholecystogram will confirm and reveal the rest but contrast medium will not concentrate in the gall bladder if the bilirubin is above 35 μmol/l and intravenous cholangiography then becomes necessary, although it only shows stones in the biliary tree.

Although surgeons may explore the bile duct at surgery, stones are sometimes missed and may later produce symptoms. Operative cholangiography and/or fibreoptic examination of the bile duct make this less likely.

Management

If causing symptoms, the gall bladder and stones should be removed. It is at this stage that pigment stones are detected and indicate investigation for haemolysis. In elderly patients or if surgery is contraindicated, sphincterotomy via ERCP may release the stones if they are in the common bile duct. Ursodeoxycholic acid may dissolve radiolucent stones if the stones are < 2 cm in diameter, and if the gall bladder is functioning. The stones may recur after treatment. Rowachol (a monoterpene mixture including menthol) has been proposed as an adjuvant to bile acid therapy.

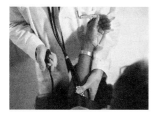

Respiratory Disease

The most common respiratory diseases are infections of the upper respiratory tract, e.g. the common cold. The most common diseases of the lower respiratory tract are bronchitis (acute and chronic), asthma and carcinoma of the bronchus.

Chronic obstructive pulmonary disease (COPD)

Definitions

The WHO-sponsored 'Global initiative for chronic obstructive lung disease' (http://www.goldcopd.com) defines COPD as 'a disease state characterized by airflow limitation that is not fully reversible. The airflow limitation is usually both progressive and associated with an abnormal inflammatory response of the lungs to noxious particles or gases.'

A diagnosis of COPD should be considered in any patient who has symptoms of cough, sputum production or dyspnoea, and/or a history of exposure to risk factors for the disease. It covers many previously used labels, including the following.

• *Chronic bronchitis*—daily cough with sputum for at least 3 months a year for at least 2 consecutive years.

• *Emphysema*—enlargement of the air spaces distal to the terminal (smallest) bronchioles with destructive changes in the alveolar wall. In centrilobular emphysema, damage is limited to the central part of the lobule around the respiratory bronchiole, whereas in panacinar emphysema, there is destruction and distension of the whole lobule. If the air spaces are > 1 cm in diameter, they are called bullae.

• *Chronic obstructive airways disease.*
• *Chronic airflow limitation.*

Poorly reversible airflow limitation may also occur in bronchiectasis, cystic fibrosis, tuberculosis, and some cases of chronic asthma.

Pathogenesis

There is chronic inflammation throughout the airways and pulmonary vasculature. In the trachea, bronchi and bronchioles > 2–4 mm in internal diameter, inflammatory cells infiltrate the surface epithelium and there is hypersecretion from enlarged mucus secreting glands and increased numbers of goblet cells. In the small bronchi and bronchioles that have an internal diameter < 2 mm, chronic inflammation is associated with remodelling of the airway wall, with increased collagen and scar tissue, narrowing the lumen and producing fixed airways obstruction.

Destruction of the lung parenchyma typically occurs as centrilobular emphysema. In mild cases lesions usually involve upper lung regions, but in advanced disease they may appear diffusely throughout the entire lung. Vascular changes occur early. Intimal thickening of the vessel wall is followed by smooth-muscle proliferation and an inflammatory cell infiltrate. These pathological changes lead to characteristic physiological changes. Mucus hypersecretion and ciliary dysfunction cause a chronic productive cough. Airflow limitation, hyperinflation and gas exchange abnormalities cause breathlessness. Pulmonary hypertension and cor pulmonale are late features.

Aetiological factors

• *Tobacco smoking.* The increased mortality risk from bronchitis has an approximately

straight-line relationship with numbers of cigarettes smoked per day (increased risk $= ^1/_2 \times$ cigarettes smoked per day).
• *Atmospheric pollution.*
• α_1-*Antitrypsin deficiency* is a recessive disorder that accounts for about 5% of all patients with emphysema (and about 20% of neonatal cholestasis). Five per cent of homozygotes tend to develop emphysema by the age of 40 years and heterozygotes are at risk. The emphysema is predominantly of the lower zones and is much worse in smokers.
• There is a relationship to lower social class and industrial environment.

Smoking tobacco (from Action on Smoking and Health, ASH)
• Causes 110 000 deaths in UK, 70% male, and 17% of all premature deaths.
• Fifty per cent of all teenagers currently smoking will die from it if they continue.
• In the 50 years from 1950, 6×10^6 have died from smoking.
• Those who die under 70 years old will lose 23 years of life.
   Most die from one of three diseases: carcinoma of the bronchus; CHD; COPD.

Clinical presentation
Initially, the patient has a productive morning cough and an increased frequency of lower respiratory tract infections producing purulent sputum. The organisms responsible are usually *Haemophilus influenzae*, *Streptococcus pneumoniae* and the respiratory viruses. Over the years there is slowly progressive dyspnoea with wheezing, exacerbated in the acute infective episodes. There is clinical emphysema with hyperinflation of the lungs. Respiratory failure (p. 238) and chronic right heart failure (cor pulmonale) are long-term complications.

Investigation
Ventilatory function tests. The diagnosis of COPD is established by spirometry, which shows a forced expiratory volume in 1 s (FEV_1) $< 80\%$ of predicted value, and a FEV_1 : forced vital capacity (FVC) ratio $< 70\%$.

The peak expiratory flow rate (PEFR) is reduced. The airways obstruction is only partially reversible by bronchodilator (or other) therapy.

Chest X-ray. This may be normal. Abnormalities correlate with the presence of emphysema and are caused by:
• overinflation with a low, flat, poorly moving diaphragm and a large retrosternal window on lateral X-ray;
• vascular changes with loss of peripheral vascular markings but enlarged hilar vessels—the heart is narrow until cor pulmonale develops; and
• bullae if present.
   The chest X-ray is an important investigation because it excludes other disease (carcinoma, tuberculosis, pneumonia, pneumothorax).

Arterial blood gas estimations. These may be normal. In later stages the P_{O_2} falls and the P_{CO_2} rises, particularly with exacerbations.

Electrocardiogram (ECG). This records the presence and progression of cor pulmonale (right atrial and ventricular hypertrophy).

Sputum for bacterial culture and sensitivity. This is useful in acute infective episodes when infections other than *Haemophilus influenzae* or *Streptococcus pneumoniae* may be present.

Haemoglobin estimation may show secondary polycythaemia.

Management
Management should include assessment and reduction of risk factors in addition to the management of stable COPD and exacerbations. There should be a stepwise increase in treatment according to disease severity, which can be classified as follows.
Stage 0 (at risk): normal spirometry; chronic cough/sputum
Stage 1 (mild): FEV_1 : $FVC < 70\%$; $FEV_1 = 80\%$ predicted, with or without symptoms

Stage 2 (moderate): $FEV_1 : FVC < 70\%$; $30\% < FEV_1 < 80\%$ predicted, with or without symptoms

Stage 3 (severe): $FEV_1 : FVC < 70\%$; $FEV_1 < 30\%$ or $FEV_1 < 50\%$ predicted + respiratory failure or clinical signs of right heart failure.

Patients benefit from rehabilitation and exercise programmes. Education can help patients to cope and achieve certain goals, including stopping smoking.

None of the available medications for COPD has been shown to modify long-term decline in lung function.

Bronchodilators are used to prevent or reduce symptoms: the β_2-agonists, e.g. salbutamol (Ventolin), terbutaline (Bricanyl), the anticholinergic ipratropium (Atrovent) or a combination of these drugs are given by metered aerosol or nebulizer on an as required or regular basis. Theophylline may also help.

Regular treatment with inhaled steroids can benefit symptomatic patients with a documented spirometric response to steroids, or who have repeated exacerbations requiring treatment with antibiotics or oral steroids. Chronic treatment with systemic steroids should be avoided. Long-term home oxygen (> 15 h/day) increases survival in patients with chronic respiratory failure. Patients should receive annual influenza vaccination.

Exacerbations are treated with inhaled bronchodilators, theophylline and systemic steroids are effective treatments. Although a cause is often not identified, infection is a common trigger and patients with signs of infection are given antibiotics—amoxicillin or a macrolide (erythromycin or clarithromycin). Bacterial sensitivities are useful if clinical improvement has not occurred.

Non-invasive intermittent positive pressure ventilation (NIPPV) can decrease the need for intubation and mechanical ventilation.

Asthma

Asthma affects 5–7% of the population of Europe and North America. It is characterized by recurrent shortness of breath, wheeze or cough caused by reversible narrowing of the airway lumen. The principal cause of increased airways resistance is contraction of smooth-muscle cells as a result of hypersensitivity to many different stimuli such as cold air, smoke, exercise and emotion, as well as antigens. Thickening of the airways by oedema and cellular infiltrates, as well as blockage of airways by mucus and secretions, also contributes. Wheeze is not an essential feature.

Asthma is sometimes classified into extrinsic and intrinsic, although treatment is the same.

Clinical features
Acute attacks
These may be fairly abrupt in onset and brief in duration (hours), or longer (a week or two), remittent and less severe. Longer severe attacks are called 'status asthmaticus' (p. 236). In an attack the patient feels tightness in the chest and both inspiratory and expiratory effort difficult. There may be a cough that is initially dry but later becomes productive, particularly if there is infection. The patient usually sits up with an overinflated chest, an audible expiratory wheeze and a fixed shoulder girdle using the accessory muscles of respiration. The respiratory rate may be little altered but the pulse is invariably rapid. Acute attacks are precipitated by specific allergens (e.g. pollens or house dust mite), exertion, excitement, cold air, a respiratory infection or β-blockers.

Recurrent asthma
Mild asthmatics (particularly with extrinsic asthma) usually have normal respiratory function between attacks, but those with long-standing severe asthma tend to develop emphysema and some degree of dyspnoea and persistent airways obstruction between acute attacks.

Investigation
Investigation includes chest X-ray (for regional collapse, pneumonia, pneumothorax) and measurement of ventilatory function (FEV_1 or PEFR, preferably at several times in a day on several days at home) and the response to

bronchodilators. Variability through the day, especially with a 'morning dip' in PEFR, is characteristic. Skin hypersensitivity tests performed by pricking standard allergens into the skin can help the patient recognize and avoid environmental precipitants. Bronchial reactivity may be more precise but should be tested only in carefully controlled conditions. Adrenaline (0.5 ml of 1 : 1000) must be available in case of acute anaphylactic reactions (p. 239).

Management of chronic asthma

The patient should be asked about precipitant factors, including the relationship of attacks to upper respiratory tract infection, season (grass pollen and fungal spores), cold, exercise, food, house dust (contains the mite *Dermatophagoides*), smoke, emotion and drugs (e.g. aspirin, non-steroidal anti-inflammatory drugs, β-blockers). Patients should be trained to use a peak flow meter reliably and to document waking and end-of-day values at home. Increasing morning dips provide an early warning of deterioration.

Most patients and almost all extrinsic asthmatics respond to simple therapy and may be controlled by:
• removing known allergies, e.g. feather pillows, cats;
• inhaled short-acting β₂-agonists, e.g. salbutamol, as required—the response is a guide to severity;
• inhaled corticosteroids in a regular regimen;
• inhaled sodium cromoglicate (Intal), 2–4 Spincaps/day or aerosol for children;
• inhaled antimuscarinic preparations e.g. ipratropium (Atrovent);
• theophylline preparations, given as a slow-release preparation at night to control overnight symptoms;
• leukotriene receptor antagonists, e.g. montelukast, are used as add-on therapies in the prophylaxis of moderate asthma not controlled by the above therapies;
• oral steroids may be required for exacerbations; and
• hyposensitization is of value in only a small number of patients who demonstrate specific allergies.

The British Thoracic Society (*Br Med J* 1993; **306**: 776–782, updated in *Thorax* 1997; **52** (Suppl 1): 52–58) has established guidelines for the 'stepped, guided self-management' of asthma. The patient is trained to assess the severity of the asthma in five steps and to use a cumulative drug regimen prescribed for each step, stepping up if necessary to achieve control, and stepping down when control is good.
Step 1. Occasional, as required use of relief inhaled short-acting β₂-agonist bronchdilators: no more often than once a day.
Step 2. Step 1 (as required inhaled bronchodilators) + regular inhaled anti-inflammatory agents: steroids (e.g. inhaled low-dose beclometasone 200 μg b.d. or fluticasone 100 μg b.d. and/or cromoglicate or nedocromil).
Step 3. High-dose inhaled corticosteroids. (e.g. inhaled beclometasone 500 μg b.d. (or low-dose corticosteroid + long-acting inhaled β₂-agonist).
Step 4. High-dose inhaled corticosteroids + regular bronchodilators.
Step 5. Addition of a single daily dose of prednisolone 30 mg.

The patient should establish the 'best PEFR' value so that future values can be evaluated. If there is a day-on-day drop in PEFR, or values fall below 60% of best, a course of oral corticosteroids can be given whatever the 'Step'.
NB When metered aerosols are used, always check inhaler technique. A number of simple inhalers are available: spacers, discs, rotahalers, breath-actuated aerosols. In some patients the PEFR tends to fall for a few days before an acute attack and prophylactic therapy with steroids may then abate it.

Acute severe asthma

Status asthmaticus is defined as an asthma attack of over 24 h duration. This is not a clinically useful definition because of those who die in an acute asthma attack half are dead within 24 h. Moreover, death is frequently sudden and sometimes unexpected, as the patient may not appear severely ill. It is this lack of recognition of severity plus inadequate early treatment that is so dangerous. Most patients have some degree of respiratory failure at presentation.

TRIALS BOX 15.1

The **National Heart, Lung, and Blood Institute's Asthma Clinical Research Network** compared regular with as-needed use of a β-agonist (albuterol) in mild asthma. Regular use provided neither beneficial nor deleterious effects, and as-needed use was recommended. *N Engl J Med* 1996; **335**: 841–847.

A **meta-analysis of increased dose of inhaled steroid or addition of salmeterol in symptomatic asthma (MIASMA)** examined the benefits of adding salmeterol compared with

increasing dose of inhaled corticosteroids in a systematic review of randomized, double blind, clinical trials. The authors concluded that addition of salmeterol in symptomatic patients aged 12 and over on low to moderate doses of inhaled steroid gives improved lung function and increased number of days and nights without symptoms or need for rescue treatment with no increase in exacerbations of any severity. *Br Med J* 2000; **320**: 1368–1373.

British Thoracic Society guidelines report an increased risk of death associated with the following features:

Clinical
- Respiratory rate $\geq$ 30 breaths/min
- Diastolic blood pressure < 60 mmHg
- Age $\geq$ 60 years
- Atrial fibrillation
- Underlying disease, confusion, multilobar involvement

Laboratory
- Urea $\geq$ 7 mmol/l
- Albumin $\leq$ 35 mmol/l
- $Pao_2 \leq$ 8 kPa
- White blood cells $\leq 4000 \times 10^9/l$ or $\geq 20 \times 10^9/l$
- Bacteraemia

Clinical presentation

Inability to speak or difficulty in maintaining speech is one criterion of severity. It also implies inability to drink and therefore dehydration. Hypoxaemia is usually then present.

A severe attack is indicated by tachycardia over 110 beats/min, a tachypnoea over 25 breaths/min, a peak flow rate < 50% of predicted values, a heart rate > 110 beats/min, and arterial hypotension.

Very severe, life-threatening airways obstruction is indicated by absence of wheeze (because of poor ventilation), PEFR < 33% of best (PEFRs can usually not be obtained), bradycardia or hypotension, and confusion, drowsiness and exhaustion. Cyanosis is also

ominous and tends to occur at a lower Po_2 than in the chronic bronchitic (because the bronchitic tends to have polycythaemia).

NB The clinical signs of drowsiness, cyanosis, bradycardia or hypotension are those of a very severe attack and vigorous treatment is essential before they are apparent.

Investigation

A chest X-ray is mandatory to exclude a pneumothorax. Arterial blood gases provide the most useful guide to the severity of the attack and to the success of treatment. The following values indicate a very severe attack: $Sao_2 < 92\%$, $Pao_2 < 8$ kPa, $Paco_2 > 5.0$ kPa, pH < 7.36.

Management

Sedation may depress respiration further and is contraindicated.
- *Continuous high-flow oxygen* should invariably be given in high concentration, e.g. 40–60%. It is not necessary to give controlled (e.g. 28%) oxygen unless there is evidence of chronic respiratory failure.
- *Bronchodilators*: β$_2$-agonists (e.g. salbutamol, terbutaline) plus ipratropium by oxygen-driven nebulizer or intravenous infusion.
- *Corticosteroids*. Hydrocortisone is given early and in large doses intravenously, e.g. 200 mg 6-hourly. The patient is transferred to oral prednisolone (e.g. 40–60 mg/day) when he or she can swallow and this is subsequently withdrawn gradually.

• If life-threatening features are present, amino-phylline 250 mg intravenously over 20 min.
NB Too rapid infusion may cause circulatory collapse. This is dangerous in patients already on oral preparations, including theophylline-containing cough mixtures, because of toxicity: check blood theophylline levels first. Children are particularly at risk.
• *Intravenous fluids* are required both to make up the initial dehydration and for as long as oral fluids are not taken. Monitor urine output.
• *Bacterial infection* is a rare trigger but *anti-biotics* are given if it is present or strongly sus-pected. The usual organisms are *Strepcococcus pneumoniae* or *Haemophilus influenzae* (p. 239).
• *Mechanical ventilation* may be necessary. Persistent or increasing elevation of arterial P_{CO_2}, especially with accompanying exhaustion, indicates the need for artificial ventilation.
NB Check the chest X-ray for pneumothorax. Discharge from hospital after PEFR returns to > 75% of best with day variability < 25%, with early clinic follow-up.

Respiratory failure

Respiratory failure can be defined as a reduc-tion in arterial P_{O_2} below 8 kPa with a normal arterial P_{CO_2} (hypoxaemic repiratory failure), or with an increase in arterial P_{CO_2} above 6.6 kPa (hypercapnic respiratory failure).
NB The mean P_{O_2} is about 13 kPa. Normally values of P_{O_2} are about 1.3 kPa, lower in the elderly.

The P_{O_2} may fall while the P_{CO_2} remains nor-mal. This may occur with alveolar parenchymal lung disease: infiltrations, fibrosing alveolitis and 'pure' emphysema. Much more commonly, both arterial gas levels are abnormal. This occurs with ventilatory failure.

Acute
• Patients with normal lungs, with upper airways obstruction (e.g. croup and acute anaphylaxis) or mechanical failure (e.g. flail chest, drug overdosage) or sleep apnoea.
• Patients with abnormal lungs (e.g. asthma, chronic bronchitis).

Chronic
Usually in patients with abnormal lungs, espe-cially COPD. These patients are particularly likely to develop acute failure if infection occurs.

In restrictive disorders, lung expansion is limited by:
• lung disease, such as fibrosis collapse, oedema, consolidation;
• pleural disease, such as fibrosis, effusion or mesothelioma;
• chest-wall disease, such as costospinal rigid-ity and deformity, or abdominal splinting by obesity, ascites or pregnancy; and
• neuromuscular disease, such as muscular dystrophy, myasthenia or phrenic nerve paralysis.

Acute on chronic respiratory failure
This usually occurs on a background of COPD.

Clinical presentation
• Peripheral vasodilatation with headache, engorged veins in the fundi, warm hands and a bounding pulse, all caused by carbon dioxide retention.
• Varying degrees of agitated confusion, drowsiness and coma.
• Increasing cyanosis.
• Signs of right heart failure.
• Flapping tremor of the outstretched hands and papilloedema are late signs.
NB Unfortunately, the physical signs are a poor guide to the presence and degree of respiratory failure. It is therefore necessary to measure blood gases in all patients in whom the diagnosis is suspected.

Management
This consists of the measures used for chronic bronchitis as given above, with the addition of controlled oxygen therapy. The danger to life in this situation is hypoxia but, paradoxically, relief of hypoxia may make the situation worse because of the patient's reliance on hypoxic drive. Give oxygen at 24 or 28% by Ventimask (or other controlled technique) if the arterial P_{O_2} is low. Oxygen is not required unless the

P_{O_2} is < 6.7 kPa (50 mmHg). It is given continuously until the acute situation (including infection and heart failure) has recovered. The P_{CO_2} is monitored. Intravenous aminophylline (10 ml) very slowly and doxapram infusion may be valuable. For chronic failure (P_{O_2} < 7.3 kPa; P_{CO_2} > 6 kPa; FEV_1 < 1.5 l; FVC < 2 l), controlled oxygen can be given continuously at home, usually from an oxygen concentrator for not less than 15 h in 24, over several months with improvement in symptoms and an increase in life expectancy.

NB Sedatives are absolutely contraindicated.

Indications for respiratory support and mechanical ventilation

If the P_{CO_2} falls or rises only slightly (e.g. by 1.3 kPa (10 mmHg)), conservative therapy should be continued and reassessed periodically. If the P_{CO_2} rises, this indicates that the patient's ventilation is inadequate and is the prime indication for non-invasive positive pressure ventilation using a tight fitting mask, or if this fails mechanical positive-pressure ventilation. Patients should be ventilated before they become exhausted. The final decision to ventilate a patient is determined mainly on the basis of respiratory function before the acute illness: if very poor, it may not be possible to wean the patient off.

Acute anaphylaxis

This rare condition occurs in previously healthy people following exposure to allergens such as certain foods, e.g. peanuts, drug therapy, e.g. penicillin, or insect stings. Patients with known previous hypersensitivity or allergy should not be given immune serum, live vaccine or known allergens.

Clinical features range from mild with flushing of the face, pruritus and blotchy wheals, to severe with asthma, which may proceed to respiratory obstruction from oedema of the larynx (angioedema) and to hypotension.

Immediate treatment is with adrenaline (epinephrine) 0.5–1.0 ml of 1 : 1000 (1 mg/ml) solution, i.e. 500–1000 µg given intramuscu-

larly or subcutaneously and repeated every 15 min until improvement is observed to reverse the type 1 acute reaction. Most patients will wish to carry self-adminstration preassembled pens containing 300 µg for intramuscular injection. Oxygen, if available, is important early. Hydrocortisone takes several hours to act and is not the immediate therapy of choice. It is given (after the first injection of adrenaline (epinephrine)), in a dose of 200 mg intravenously, with chlorphenamine 10 mg slowly intravenously or intramuscularly.

Hereditary angioedema is a rare condition caused by C_1 esterase deficiency (autosomal dominant). It gives rise to erythema (but not wheals), patchy oedema and colicky abdominal pain. It responds to danazol prophylaxis and fresh frozen plasma to correct the deficiency during attacks.

Pneumonia

Community-acquired pneumonia affects approximately 12/1000 adults per year. One in 1000 require hospitalization, and mortality in these patients is around 10%.

Clinical presentation

Symptoms of cough, sputum, pleurisy and dyspnoea are less common in the elderly.

Clinical findings include fever (80%), tachypnoea (> 20 breaths/min), crackles (80%) and signs of consolidation (30%).

The most common organism in UK studies is *Streptococcus pneumoniae* (60–75%), followed by *Mycoplasma pneumoniae* (5–18%). *Haemophilus influenzae*, *Legionella* species, *Chlamydia psittaci* and *Staphylococcus aureus* account for most of the remainder. Gram-negative bacilli, *Coxiella burnetii* and anaerobes are rare.

Viruses (including influenza) account for up to 15%.

Investigations

Investigations are performed to establish the diagnosis and assess severity.

• *Chest X-ray* shows infiltrates. Computed tomographic (CT) scanning is more sensitive

and may be useful in detecting interstitial disease, cavitation or empyema.
- *Blood gases* to assess severity and guide oxygen treatment.
- *Blood count*—white cell count $\geq 15 \times 10^9/l$ suggests bacterial infection; white cell count $> 20 \times 10^9/l$ or $\leq 4 \times 10^9/l$ indicates poor prognosis. Haemoglobin for haemolysis.
- *Urea, electrolytes and liver function tests* for underlying or associated renal or hepatic disease.
- *Gram staining and culture of sputum*—but cough is unproductive in one-third of patients, and negative results are common, particularly if antibiotics have been given.
- *Blood culture.*
- *Pleural fluid*, if present, should be aspirated for culture.
- *Acute-phase serum* is usually taken for later microbiological analysis.

Management
- *Oxygen*—to maintain Pao_2 above 8 kPa.
- *Antibiotics*—the organism is usually unknown initially. Treatment is started immediately and should cover *Streptococcus pneumoniae*. In uncomplicated pneumonia, treatment is usually started with oral amoxicillin or a macrolide (erythromycin or clarithromycin). In severe pneumonia intravenous therapy is given, often using a combination of a macrolide (erythromycin) and a second- or third-generation cephalosporin (cefuroxime or cefotaxime).
- *Intravenous fluids* may be required.
- *Analgesia* for pleuritic pain.

Pneumococcal pneumonia is the most common bacterial pneumonia. *S. pneumoniae* is a Gram-positive diplococcus. It affects all ages, but is more common in the elderly, after splenectomy, in the immunosuppressed, alcoholics, patients with chronic heart failure, and those with pre-existing lung disease. It typically presents acutely with fever, pleuritic pain and rust-coloured sputum. It causes both lobar and bronchopneumonia. Treatment is with penicillin, or erythromycin in the penicillin-sensitive. A polysaccharide pneumococcal vaccine is available for those at high risk. It

should be given at least 2 weeks before splenectomy and before chemotherapy.

Staphylococcal pneumonia produces widespread infection with abscess formation. It may complicate influenzal pneumonia, and this makes it relatively common during epidemics of influenza. It also occurs in patients with underlying disease, which prevents a normal response to infection, e.g. chronic leukaemia, Hodgkin disease, cystic fibrosis. Flucloxacillin and fusidic acid are the drugs of choice. Lung abscess, empyema and subsequent bronchiectasis are relatively common complications.

Legionnaire's disease was first described in a group of American army veterans (legionnaires). The causative Gram-negative bacillus flourishes in the cooling waters of air conditioners and may colonize hot-water tanks kept at $< 60°C$. It begins as an influenza-like illness with fever, malaise and myalgia, and proceeds with cough (little sputum), dyspnoea and sometimes severe anorexia, marked confusion and coma. Diarrhoea and vomiting are common and renal failure may develop. Examination shows consolidation that usually affects both lung bases. X-ray changes may persist for more than 2 months after the acute illness. Erythromycin or ciprofloxacin are the antibiotics of choice, but the mortality remains high (20%).
NB Legionnaire's disease (and *Mycoplasma pneumoniae* or psittacosis) should be suspected in all patients who develop atypical pneumonia that does not respond to standard antibiotics.

Mycoplasma pneumonia is caused by *M. pneumoniae*, the only mycoplasma definitely pathogenic to humans. The clinical picture resembles bacterial pneumonia, although cough and sputum are absent in one-third of cases.
   Respiratory symptoms and signs and X-ray changes (patchy consolidation with small effusions) are usually preceded by several days of influenza-like symptoms. Polyarthritis occurs and may persist for months. Malaise and fatigue may persist long after the acute illness is over. The diagnosis is confirmed by a positive

Mycoplasma-specific immunoglobulin M (IgM) titre. Erythromycin or tetracycline are the antibiotics of choice.

Psittacosis pneumonia is caused by *Chlamydia psittaci*. It is transmitted in the excrement of infected birds (the bird need not be ill). Headache, fever and dry cough may be accompanied by a rash and splenomegaly. Hepatitis, encephalitis, renal failure and haemolysis also occur. Treatment is with tetracycline or erythromycin.

Viral pneumonia. The most common virus causing pneumonia in children in the UK and USA is the respiratory syncytial virus (RSV)—so called as it is a respiratory virus which produces syncytium formation when grown in tissue culture. Infection may be indistinguishable from acute bacterial bronchitis or bronchiolitis in children and infants. The presence of a skin rash supports the likelihood of RSV infection.

Acute viral pneumonia in adults is less common, but occurs during epidemics of influenza. Fever, headache and myalgia are followed after a few days by dry cough and chest pain. Treatment is largely symptomatic (paracetamol, rest, fluids). Influenza vaccines are available for those at high risk. The most common cause of pneumonia during influenza epidemics results from secondary bacterial infection, the most serious being staphylococcal pneumonia. The viruses of measles, chickenpox and herpes zoster may directly affect the lung. The diagnosis is confirmed by a rise in specific antibody titre.

Aspiration pneumonia. There are two main varieties, differentiated from each other by the type of fluid aspirated and the circumstances in which it occurs.

Aspiration of gastric contents may produce a severe chemical pneumonitis with considerable pulmonary oedema and bronchospasm (Mendelson syndrome). The acute respiratory distress and shock can be very rapidly fatal and very difficult to treat. It tends to occur in states of reduced consciousness such as general anaesthesia, drunks and when gastric lavage (for drug overdose) has been performed inexpertly.

Aspiration of bacteria from the oropharynx may follow dental anaesthesia and can occur in bulbar palsies. The bacteria, apart from *Bacteroides*, are nearly all penicillin-sensitive and amoxicillin (or ampicillin) with metronidazole are the antibiotics of choice until sensitivities of isolated organisms are known. Recurrent episodes occur in some oesophageal disorders, including hiatus hernia, stricture, achalasia of the cardia, and in patients with diverticula or pharyngeal pouch.

Recurrent bacterial pneumonia. In the absence of chronic bronchitis, recurrent pneumonia arouses suspicion of:
• bronchial carcinoma preventing drainage of infected areas of lung;
• bronchiectasis;
• cystic fibrosis;
• achalasia of the cardia, 25% of which present as chest disease, pharyngeal pouch and neuromuscular disease of the oesophagus, e.g. bulbar palsy, all producing aspiration; and
• hypogammaglobulinaemia and myeloma.

Opportunistic infection of the lungs occurs in patients immunosuppressed as a result of treatment, e.g. for myeloproliferative disorders or acquired immunodeficiency syndrome (AIDS, p. 328).

Lung abscess
Aetiology
• Aspiration (see above).
• Bronchial obstruction, usually by carcinoma or a foreign body (especially peanuts and teeth).
• Pneumonia partially resolved or treated, particularly when caused by the *Staphylococcus*, *Klebsiella* or *Pneumococcus* organisms.

Clinical features
There is a swinging fever and the patient is very ill. The sputum is foul and purulent and there is a high polymorph cell count. Clubbing may develop.

Investigation
Sputum is sent for Gram stain and culture, and blood for culture. Chest X-ray shows round lesions which usually have a fluid level,

and serial X-rays monitor progress. It may be necessary to proceed to bronchoscopy to exclude obstruction and to obtain a biopsy and sputum trap specimen.

Treatment

Antibiotic therapy is given according to sensitivities and continued until healing is complete. Repeated postural drainage is started. In resistant cases, repeated aspiration, antibiotic instillation and even surgical excision may be required.

Bronchiectasis

Bronchiectasis means dilatation of the airways. It only becomes of clinical significance when infection and/or haemoptysis occurs within these dilatated airways. Severe forms are now rare, especially in the young.

Aetiology

• Following acute childhood respiratory infection, particularly measles, whooping cough or pneumonia.
• Cystic fibrosis.
• Bronchial obstruction predisposes to bronchiectasis (e.g. peanuts).
• Tuberculosis has become less common as a cause.
• Congenital (rare): primary ciliary dyskinesia, e.g. Kartagener syndrome (bronchiectasis, sinusistis, situs inversus).

Clinical features

• Chronic cough, often postural.
• Sputum, often copious, especially with acute infections. Halitosis.
• Febrile episodes.
• Haemoptysis: may be the only symptom ('dry bronchiectasis') and is occasionally severe.
• Dyspnoea, coarse basal crepitations and wheeze.
• Cyanosis and clubbing.
• Loss of weight and cor pulmonale in advanced cases.

Management

Stop smoking.

The object is to get rid of chronic sepsis. Twice-daily postural drainage will help empty dilatated airways and decrease the frequency of further infections. Bronchodilators will often help improve clearance of sputum. Antibiotics, as for chronic bronchitis, are given for acute infections and exacerbations. Treatment is unnecessary in the absence of symptoms.

Surgery is virtually never indicated unless there is uncontrolled bleeding because the disease is seldom limited to one or two lung segments. Patients with severe disease may develop respiratory failure.

Pneumothorax

Aetiology
Spontaneous

This is the most common type and usually occurs in normal, tall, thin, young, male smokers following rupture of a small subpleural bulla. The history is of the sudden onset of one-sided pleuritic pain and/or dyspnoea. Dyspnoea rapidly increases in tension pneumothorax and the patient becomes cyanosed. The classical signs are of diminished movement on the affected side with deviation of the trachea to the other side. There is hyperresonance to percussion and reduced pulmonary sounds (breath sounds, tactile fremitus and vocal resonance). All pneumothoraces are best diagnosed by seeing a lung edge on X-ray; it is clearest on an expiratory film. It recurs in 25% within 5 years, usually in the first year. Conditions predisposing to pneumothorax include:
• emphysematous bullae;
• tuberculosis—often with a small effusion; and
• bronchial asthma.
Other rare causes include staphylococcal pneumonia, carcinoma, occupational lung disease and connective tissue disorders, e.g. Marfan and Ehlers–Danlos syndromes.

Management (of spontaneous pneumothorax)

Often no therapy is required if the pneumothorax is small and symptoms minor.

Spontaneous recovery occurs in 3–4 weeks. Indications for aspiration of air are:
• tension pneumothorax (an acute emergency);
• severe dyspnoea; and
• collapse of more than 50% of the total lung field on chest X-ray.

Aspirate using a 16-gauge cannula and three-way tap. If this fails, insert an intercostal catheter with a valve or water seal. When the lung is re-expanded, X-ray the chest. If the lung remains expanded for 24 h the tube may be removed and, if not, suction should be applied to the tube.

Rarely, a continuing air leak persists from the lung into the pleural space (bronchopleural fistula). Pleurodesis with talc, abrasion or tetracycline may be required. Surgical pleurectomy is performed in patients at risk, such as airline pilots and patients with contralateral disease.

Cystic fibrosis

This is an autosomal recessive disorder affecting 1 in 3000 live births that occurs equally in males and females and usually presents in early childhood. It is caused by mutations of the cystic fibrosis transmembrane conductance regulator (CFTR) gene located on chromosome 7. CFTR functions as a cyclic adenosine monophosphate (cAMP)-regulated chloride channel on the apical surface of airway and other epithelial cells. Abnormally thick secretions are produced by glandular tissue. It predominantly affects the pancreas and respiratory tract, leading to pancreatic insufficiency and lung damage from recurrent chest infections. Secondary bronchiectasis or lung abscess may result. Recurrent small haemoptyses and finger clubbing are common, and pneumothorax occurs. Persistent productive cough is associated initially with *Staphylococcus aureus*, *Haemophilus influenzae* and Gram-negative bacilli. Later, *Pseudomonas aeruginosa* predominates and is associated with a poor prognosis.

Other manifestations are meconium ileus (15% of newborns), diabetes mellitus (20%),

---

TRIAL BOX 15.2

Fuchs *et al.* compared inhaled recombinant human deoxyribonuclease (rhDNase) with placebo in patients with cystic fibrosis. Over a 24-week period rhDNase improved pulmonary function and reduced the frequency of respiratory exacerbations requiring intravenous antibiotics. *N Engl J Med* 1994; **331**: 637–642.

---

biliary obstruction (15%) and azoospermia (over 90% of males).

Most males are sterile and women subfertile. A high sodium concentration in the sweat (above 70 mmol/l) is characteristic.

Management
Pancreatic enzymes and fat-soluble vitamins
Clearance of pulmonary secretions and treatment of infections
• Chest physiotherapy with postural drainage.
• Bronchodilators.
• Inhaled recombinant human deoxyribonuclease 1 (rhDNase) reduces the viscoelasticity of sputum by digesting viscous extracellular DNA in mucus (it is expensive).
• Antibiotics—exacerbations are usually treated with two parenteral antibiotics (to reduce antibiotic resistance). Choice is guided by sensitivity of isolated organisms but usually includes an aminoglycoside with an antipseudomonal penicillin (e.g. ticarcillin), cephalosporin or quinolone. The benefits of maintenance antibiotic therapy have to be weighed against the risks of antibiotic resistance. Inhaled aminoglycosides may allow delivery of high concentrations to the lungs with less risk of toxicity.

Respiratory failure with or without cor pulmonale usually occurs in early adult life, when lung or heart–lung transplantation should be considered.

The social and emotional problems can be enormous and, for this reason, as well as the complexity of clinical management, the condition should be supervised from specialist centres.

TRIAL BOX 15.3

Suri *et al.* compared the effect of hypertonic saline, delivered by jet nebulizer, and alternate-day or daily recombinant human deoxyribonuclease in 48 children with cystic fibrosis in an open cross-over trial. Children treated with daily rhDNase showed a significantly greater increase in FEV_1 than hypertonic saline. They found no evidence of a difference between daily and alternate-day rhDNase. *Lancet* 2001; **358**: 1316–1321.

Carcinoma of the bronchus

Incidence
This causes about 40 000 deaths per year in the UK, half of them under 65 years of age. About 60% are squamous cell (epidermoid) and 25% small cell. They are 2–3 times more common in men than women. Five per cent are undifferentiated large cell tumours and about 10% are adenocarcinoma. Alveolar cell carcinoma, an adenocarcinoma, is very rare.

Aetiological factors
Cigarette smoking (p. 234). The increased mortality risk of carcinoma of the bronchus (squamous and small cell) has an approximately straight-line relationship with numbers of cigarettes smoked per day (increased risk of death = cigarettes smoked per day, numerically). Stopping smoking decreases the risk by one-half in 5 years, and to only twice that of life-long non-smokers in 15 years.

Other atmospheric pollution (coal smoke and diesel fumes) may prove to be aetiologically relevant, but quantitatively small compared with cigarettes.

Exposure to chromium, arsenic, radioactive materials or asbestos (which in addition produces interstitial fibrosis and mesothelioma) is associated with a higher incidence of bronchial carcinoma.

Clinical presentation
The patient is usually a cigarette smoker, sometimes with tobacco-stained fingertips.

Cough or the accentuation of an existing cough is the most common early symptom, and haemoptysis the next. Dyspnoea, central chest ache or pleuritic pain, or slowly resolving chest infection are common early manifestations. Occasionally, patients are identified following a routine chest X-ray. The patient may also present with inoperable disease.

• Metastatic deposits involving brain, bone, liver, skin, kidney, adrenal glands or other site.

• Symptoms from local extension e.g. superior vena cava obstruction (puffy, dusky head, neck and arms, a raised pulseless jugular venous pulse, headache, dilatated veins over the chest wall), cervical lymph glands, dysphagia from oesophageal involvement, cardiac arrhythmia or pleural effusion. The Pancoast syndrome consists of symptoms from local extension at the apex of the lung. There may be pain in the shoulder, upper back or arm, weakness and atrophy of the hand muscles from brachial plexus involvement, hoarseness from involvement of the recurrent superior laryngeal nerve, or a Horner syndrome (p. 8).

The presence of systemic and non-specific symptoms (anorexia, weight loss and fatigue) usually, but not always, implies late and possibly inoperable disease.

Blood and marrow
Anaemia (often normochromic or normocytic). Polycythaemia is uncommon.

Marrow infiltration is common in small cell carcinoma.

Neuromuscular
Dementia or focal neurological deficit (caused by cerebral secondaries or rarely cortical atrophy), cerebellar syndrome, mixed sensorimotor peripheral neuropathy, proximal myopathy, polymyositis (p. 128), and the myasthenic (Eaton–Lambert) syndrome (p. 116).

Skin, connective tissue, bone
Clubbing, hypertrophic pulmonary osteoarthropathy, dermatomyositis and acanthosis nigricans.

Endocrine
Syndromes caused by ectopic hormone pro-

TRIAL BOX 15.4

The **Non-small Cell Lung Cancer Collaborative Group** performed a systematic review and quantitative meta-analysis was therefore undertaken to evaluate the effect of cytotoxic chemotherapy on survival in patients with non-small cell lung cancer included data from 52 trials and 9387 patients. The results for modern regimens containing cisplatin favoured chemotherapy in all comparisons and reached conventional levels of significance

when used with radical radiotherapy and with supportive care. Trials comparing surgery with surgery plus chemotherapy gave a benefit of 5% at 5 years. Trials comparing radical radiotherapy with radical radiotherapy plus chemotherapy gave a benefit of 4% at 2 years, and trials comparing supportive care with supportive care plus chemotherapy gave a 10% improvement in survival at 1 year. *Cochrane Database Syst Rev* 2000; **2**: CD002139.

duction, the pituitary-like ones (adrenocorticotrophic hormone (ACTH), antidiuretic hormone (ADH), prolactin) usually from oat cell tumours, and parathyroid hormone from squamous cell tumours. Hypercalcaemia is usually caused by bone secondaries.

Cardiovascular
Atrial fibrillation (local extension) and migratory thrombophlebitis. Pericarditis.

Diagnosis
Chest X-ray:
• the tumour may be visible often as a unilaterally enlarged hilum or peripheral circular opacity, occasionally cavitated;
• collapse/consolidation caused by bronchial obstruction by the tumour; and
• effusion, raised hemidiaphragm of phrenic paralysis, and bone erosion suggest local extension.

Magnetic resonance imaging (MRI) or CT scan shows the tumour position better and demonstrates bronchial narrowing and mediastinal involvement. Positron emission tomography (PET) scan can be used for detecting metastatic spread. Exfoliative cytology may be diagnostic.

Fibreoptic bronchoscopy with biopsy is performed if possible to establish histological diagnosis and assess operability. The site of the tumour is a guide to operability (not less than 2 cm from the carina). CT-guided percutaneous needle biopsy is used for peripheral lesions.

Treatment
Patients are staged using a TNM (tumour, node, metastasis) classification. Surgery offers the only 'cure': 15–20% of all cases are resectable and only 30% of these survive 5 years. Surgery is contraindicated by metastasis (present in 60% at the time of presentation—chiefly in bone and liver), local spread and inadequate respiratory function. Radiotherapy is valuable for relief of distressing symptoms (major airway narrowing, haemoptysis, mediastinal compression, Pancoast syndrome and relief of pain produced by bony secondaries).

Small cell carcinoma may be palliated with chemotherapy, often using a combination of etoposide plus *cis*- or carboplatin (an alkylating agent, p. 313).

Bronchial adenoma

This rare tumour is usually benign but locally invasive. Ninety per cent are histologically 'carcinoid' tumours but only a few patients present with the carcinoid syndrome (p. 170). They usually present with cough and haemoptysis. The tumour may either occur anywhere within the thoracic cavity and appear as a well-circumscribed peripheral mass on chest X-ray or, more often, in the major bronchi and appear as a pedunculated intrabronchial mass seen bronchoscopically. The tumours are removed in view of the risk of neoplastic change.

Sarcoidosis

Sarcoidosis is characterized by a systemic non-caseating granulomatous infiltration that may involve any tissue. It most commonly affects the lungs, mediastinal lymph nodes and skin. The aetiology is not known, but acid-fast cell wall deficient mycobacterial forms have been grown from the blood during active disease.

Clinical presentation
Pulmonary sarcoid (90%)
In the UK, the annual incidence of clinical disease is 3–4/100 000. It occurs in young people of 20–40 years, and in females five times more commonly than males. Most commonly it presents as a subacute syndrome with fever, malaise and lassitude, erythema nodosum (sarcoid is the most common cause in the UK), polyarthralgia usually of the ankles and knees, and mediastinal hilar lymphadenopathy. Dyspnoea is not usually a feature of this acute form, which is self-limiting (2 months-2 years).

Less commonly and more seriously, it presents as a chronic insidious disease with respiratory symptoms of cough and progressive dyspnoea with malaise and fever leading to progressive pulmonary fibrosis.

Non-pulmonary sarcoid
Apart from erythema nodosum, this is relatively uncommon.
• Skin (70%). Erythema nodosum (not sarcoid tissue) in the acute syndrome; infiltration of scars: lupus pernio.
• Hypercalcaemia occurs in about 10% of patients with sarcoidosis and may be the presenting abnormality (p. 206). Hypercalciuria is even more common. This is probably because of an excessive sensitivity to vitamin D, and responds to steroids.
• Eyes (15%). Uveitis and keratoconjunctivitis sicca. Blindness may result.
• Parotitis (5%).
• Hepatosplenomegaly (12%).
• Generalized lymphadenopathy (30%).
•ᐧ Bone and joints, producing cystic lesions most commonly in the phalanges (4%).

• Nervous system, causing isolated cranial nerve lesions and peripheral neuropathy (3%).
• Heart: conduction defects and arrhythmias. Rare.
• Endocrine, producing diabetes insipidus from pituitary involvement (very rare).
• Renal damage from hypercalcaemia or an associated interstitial nephritis or glomerulonephritis.

Investigation
The chest X-ray shows symmetrical lobulated bilateral hilar and paratracheal gland enlargement (interbronchial rather than tracheobronchial) or, less commonly (40%), parenchymal mottling or diffuse fibrosis. CT scan will help distinguish gland enlargement from prominent pulmonary artery shadows.

'Blind' transbronchial lung biopsy at bronchoscopy often shows non-caseating epithelioid granulomas (60% in classical disease; 90% if pulmonary fibrosis is present).

Liver biopsy reveals granulomas in 70%.

The Mantoux test is usually negative (70%); a positive test is not uncommon but a strongly positive test is very unusual.

Hypercalcaemia (10%) returns to normal with steroids.

Polyclonal increase in γ-globulins is nonspecific but common.

Management
The differential diagnosis of bilateral hilar lymph node enlargement is from Hodgkin disease (and other reticuloses), and any deviation of the patient's syndrome from the usual pattern makes a definite diagnosis by biopsy imperative. Treatment, other than simple analgesics and non-steroidal anti-inflammatory agents, is usually unnecessary.

Indications for corticosteroids in sarcoidosis (e.g. prednisolone 20 mg/day, reducing after 1 month to the minimum dosage necessary to suppress activity for 1 year) include the following.
• Progressive lung disease, to try to prevent fibrosis. The indication is progressive pulmonary shadowing or increasing breathlessness. The effect of therapy is monitored by symptoms, chest X-rays and lung function

PROGNOSIS OF PULMONARY SARCOID

Chest X-ray appearance	Recovery stage	X-ray (%)	Clinical (%)
Bilateral hilar lymphadenopathy alone	I	75	90
Bilateral hilar lymphadenopathy with fine pulmonary reticular–nodular shadowing	II	50	60
Coarse reticular–nodular shadowing or fibrosis	III	30	30

Table 15.1 Prognosis of pulmonary sarcoid.

tests, including carbon monoxide transfer factor, T_{LCO}.
• Hypercalcaemia.
• When vital organs are threatened, e.g. eyes, nervous system, kidneys and heart.

Prognosis (of pulmonary sarcoid)
Complete clinical resolution in 3–4 months, and radiological resolution in 1–2 years, occurs in 70–80%. The chest X-ray remains abnormal in about half of all cases (Table 15.1). Clinical disability brought about by the disease is much less common and is related to:
• age—the younger, the better;
• presence of erythema nodosum where over 95% recover by 1 year;
• extent of extrapulmonary involvement—bone or chronic skin lesions indicate chronicity and the more widespread it is, the worse the prognosis; and
• extent of intrathoracic involvement.
NB In systemic sarcoidosis, the activity and clinical course of the disease in any one tissue (e.g. skin, eyes) is a guide to the activity in any tissue less easily observed (e.g. lungs).

Tuberculosis

Infection with the acid–alcohol-fast bacillus (AAFB) of *Mycobacterium tuberculosis* affects predominantly the lungs, lymph nodes and gut. Some features of the disease vary with the patient's sensitivity to tuberculin.

Primary tuberculosis

This is the syndrome produced by infection with *M. tuberculosis* in non-sensitive patients, i.e. in those who have not previously been infected. There is a mild inflammatory response at the site of infection (subpleural in the mid-zones of the lungs, in the pharynx or in the terminal ileum), followed by spread to the regional lymph nodes (hilar, cervical and mesenteric respectively)—the primary complex. One to two weeks following infection, with the onset of tuberculin sensitivity, the tissue reaction changes at both the focus and in the nodes, to the charateristic caseating granuloma. The combination of a focus with regional lymph node involvement is called the *primary complex*. Patients are usually symptomless. The complex heals with fibrosis and, frequently, calcifies without therapy. The enlarged lymph node may be obvious in the neck or cause obstruction to a bronchus with consequent collapse—consolidation. Blood dissemination of the organisms occurs rarely from the primary complex to cause widespread miliary disease, especially in infants.

Postprimary tuberculosis

This is the syndrome produced by infection with *M. tuberulosis* in the previously infected and therefore tuberculin-sensitive patient. Reactivation (or reinfection) is followed by an immediate brisk granulomatous response that tends to localize the disease and regional lymph node involvement is uncommon. As with primary tuberculosis, the lesion may:
• heal with fibrosis (and calcification);
• rupture into a bronchus giving tuberculous bronchopneumonia; or
• spread via the blood to produce miliary tuberculosis of liver, spleen, lungs, choroid, bone and/or meninges.

Presenting features

Symptoms occur relatively late and therefore in established disease. The earliest are non-specific, such as malaise, fatigue, anorexia and weight loss. Of more specific symptoms, the most common is cough, often with mucoid sputum. Other symptoms include repeated small haemoptysis, pleural pain, slight fever or, occasionally, exertional dyspnoea. Frequently, the diagnosis is made presymptomatically on routine chest radiography. Signs also occur late in the disease and are not very specific, e.g. crepitations (usually apical) and, later, signs of consolidation, pleural effusion or cavitation.

Diagnosis

Clinical suspicion should be particularly high in high-risk groups:
• the hostel-dwelling 'down-and-out', and the alcoholic;
• Pakistani and Indian immigrant (lymph node tuberculosis is common in Indian and Pakistani patients);
• diabetics;
• patients with AIDS;
• patients on immunosuppressive therapy (steroids or cytotoxic drugs); and
• occupations at risk—doctors and nurses.

Ideally, the diagnosis is made by repeated examination for AAFB in sputum and bronchial washing on direct smear or culture. Six to 12 specimens (or more) may be required. Sometimes the diagnosis can only be made radiologically where activity is suggested by:
• changing 'soft' shadows;
• progression of apical lesions;
• cavitation; and
• a strongly positive Heaf test.

It may be necessary to treat on clinical grounds alone and response to specific therapy in 2 weeks is taken as proof of diagnosis.
NB AAFB on smear may not be pathogenic mycobacteria, particularly in urine specimens.

Management

Isolate patients who are sputum-positive. Tuberculosis is notifiable in the UK. The British Thoracic Society Guidelines on Control and Prevention of Tuberculosis in the UK: Code of Practice 2000 (*Thorax* 2000; **55**: 887–901) reported that notified cases in England and Wales rose from 5085 in 1987 to 6087 in 1998, when 30% of patients were estimated to also be HIV infected. Of initial isolates 6.1% were resistant to isoniazid and 1.3% were multidrug resistant.

Close contacts should be screened with chest X-ray and/or Heaf testing depending on their age and bacille Calmette–Guérin (BCG) status. Contacts who have had BCG should have a chest X-ray if over 16, and be investigated if this is abnormal. Children under 16 should be Heaf tested, and investigated if this is strongly positive. Contacts who have not had BCG should be Heaf tested immediately, and if negative 6 weeks later. Heaf postive contacts should have a chest X-ray and investigated further if this is abnormal. If the chest X-ray is normal chemo-prophylaxis should be considered. In the UK the recommendation for chemoprophylaxis is for either isoniazid for 6 months or isoniazid and rifampicin for 3 months (Joint Tuberculosis Committee of the British Thoracic Society. Chemotherapy and management of tuberculosis in the United Kingdom: recommendations 1998. *Thorax* 1998; **53**: 536–548).

Start therapy if AAFB is detected in sputum. If the clinical suspicion of tuberculosis is high but the sputum smear is negative, collect sputum for culture and start therapy. For most UK patients with presumed sensitive organisms, British Thoracic Society guidelines recommend a 6-month regimen comprising rifampicin, isoniazid, pyrazinamide and ethambutol for the initial 2 months, followed by rifampicin and isoniazid for a further 4 months is recommended as standard. In cases where a positive culture for *M. tuberculosis* has been obtained but susceptibility results are outstanding after 2 months, treatment including pyrazinamide (and ethambutol) should be continued until full susceptibility is confirmed, even if this is for longer than 2 months. The fourth drug (ethambutol) can be omitted in patients with a low risk of resistance to isoniazid.

For tuberculous meningitis see p. 109.

Common antituberculosis drug doses and complications

The first four drugs are considered 'first-line'.

• Rifampicin 450–600 mg/day: abnormal liver function tests. Colours the urine pink.

• Isoniazid (INAH) 300 mg/day (with pyridoxine 10 mg): peripheral neuropathy and encephalopathy—these are extremely rare, occur in slow acetylators and respond to pyridoxine, often given prophylactically.

• Pyrazinamide 1.5–2.0 g/day: hepatotoxic (rare but severe).

• Ethambutol 15 mg/kg/day: optic neuritis with colour vision and acuity reduced.

• Thiacetazone 150 mg/day: gastrointestinal and skin rashes.

• Streptomycin 1 g/day by intramuscular injection: vertigo and nerve deafness. In the elderly and in the presence of raised blood urea, the dosage is reduced to 0.75 or 0.5 g/day to maintain blood levels of 1–2 μg/ml.

Second-line drug complications

• Ethionamide: nausea and vomiting; hepatotoxic.

• Cycloserine: neurotoxicity with confusion and depression.

• Para-aminosalicylic acid: nausea, vomiting and skin rash.

In developing countries, where cheapness is a priority, streptomycin, thiacetazone and isoniazid are more often used. For example, twice-weekly treatment with streptomycin (1 g) and high-dose isoniazid (15 mg/kg) with pyridoxine for 1 year is reasonably effective except where resistance is a problem. Isoniazid plus thiacetazone once daily is 80–95% effective.

Corticosteroids

Steroids are indicated for severely ill tuberculous patients at the onset of chemotherapy, for tuberculous meningitis, and in miliary tuberculosis to try and prevent fibrosis. The value of steroids other than when life is immediately threatened remains unproven and they probably do not affect long-term morbidity.

Occupational lung diseases

There are four main groups: dust diseases, asthma, extrinsic allergic alveolitis and irritant gases.

Dust diseases

These include the pneumoconioses, asthma and allergic alveolitis.

• coal pneumoconiosis;

• silicosis in rock drilling and crushing—also occurs in coal miners;

• asbestosis in insulation workers; this can produce fibrosis, carcinoma and pleural mesothelioma; and

• benign (no fibrosis).

These are radiographic diagnoses made in the light of the patient's known occupational hazards; the shadows are caused by the metals themselves, e.g. siderosis (iron) and stannosis (tin). All are rare.

Clinical features

In the early stages there are no symptoms but X-ray changes occur; later there is dyspnoea on exertion, cough, sputum and attacks of bronchitis. In coal miners, progressive massive fibrosis may occur and Caplan syndrome (rheumatoid arthritis and pulmonary nodules) occurs in association with rhematoid arthritis. The patients may eventually develop cor pulmonale.

Asthma

Occupational asthma can occur in response to precipitants of animal, vegetable, bacteriological or chemical origin. Some of the more common occupations are: animal laboratory workers (urinary proteins), grain and flour workers (mites and flour), sawmill operatives and carpenters (hardwoods), those who manufacture biological detergents (inhalation of *Bacillus subtilis* proteolytic enzymes), in the electronics industry (colophony in solder flux), paint sprayers and polyurethane workers (isocyanates), workers with epoxy resins or platinum salts and in the pharmaceutical industry. All these are recognized for compensation under industrial injuries legislation in the UK.

Extrinsic allergic alveolitis

Inhalation of organic dusts may give a diffuse allergic (type III precipitin-mediated) reaction in the alveoli and bronchioles.

Aetiology

Exposure to mouldy hay (*Micropolyspora faeni*) causes farmer's lung, to mouldy sugar cane causes bagassosis, to mushroom dust causes mushroom picker's lung, to bird droppings (containing avian serum proteins) causes bird fancier's lung, to contaminated malting barley (*Aspergillus clavatus*) causes malt worker's lung and to pituitary snuff (containing foreign serum protein) causes pituitary snuff-taker's lung. Precipitating antibodies against the offending antigen can be found in the patient's blood.

Clinical features

Acute (i.e. 4–6 h after exposure). Dyspnoea, dry cough, malaise, fever and limb pains occur, and examination shows fine inspiratory crepitations with little wheeze. The symptoms subside in 2–3 days.

Chronic. After repeated acute attacks fibrosis occurs with persistent inspiratory crepitations, respiratory failure and cor pulmonale.

Investigation

Chest X-ray shows a diffuse haze initially and later micronodular shadowing develops, progressing to honeycombing. Ventilatory function tests initially show a reversible restrictive defect with low T_{LCO} during the acute attacks. This becomes permanent as the chronic disorder develops. There is little or no obstruction. The Po_2 falls and Pco_2 is normal or reduced by the hyperventilation. There is no eosinophilia.

Treatment

Separate the patient and the allergen. Masks are of little use and positive-pressure helmets should be worn. High-dose steroids are tried in serious cases and should be continued only if there has been a measured response in lung function.

Obstructive sleep apnoea

The sleep apnoea syndrome is defined as absence of airflow in periods of at least 10 s occurring not less than 30 times per night's sleep.

There are repeated episodes of upper airways obstruction during sleep with hypoxaemia and sudden arousal. This results in poor sleep, snoring, excessive daytime sleepiness and observed apnoeas in sleep. It is associated with male gender, obesity and evening alcohol consumption. Diagnosis requires overnight sleep studies (observation in a sleep laboratory) where arterial oxygen saturation, body movements, rapid eye movement (REM) sleep, apnoeas, sleep stages and electroencephalogram (EEG) can be monitored. Management involves slimming and alcohol reduction, followed by continuous positive airways pressure (CPAP) if these fail.

Pulmonary embolism

Emboli usually arise in the veins of the pelvis or legs and, rarely, from the right atrium.

They occur more frequently:
* following surgery (classically, although not always about 10 days);
* following myocardial infarction;
* following a stroke;
* in disseminated malignancy;
* in prolonged bed rest associated with illness;
* during air flights over 3 h or 3000 miles, not necessarily economy class;
* following trauma, especially to the pelvis and legs (including caesarean section);
* in antiphospholipid syndrome (p. 124); and
* in hypercoagulable states—antithrombin III, protein C and S deficiencies. In factor V Leiden a single point mutation in the factor V gene causes resistance to activated protein C.

The risk may increase if other factors are present:

- advancing age;
- obesity;
- pregnancy and postpartum;
- treatment with oestrogens (oral contraceptive pill or hormone replacement therapy); or
- previous venous thrombosis or family history of it.

About 50% of those who die from pulmonary embolism have had premonitory signs and symptoms of small emboli (unexplained breathless attacks) or venous thrombosis in the previous weeks. A deep vein thrombosis should be regarded as potential pulmonary embolus and must be suspected, diagnosed and treated early.

Clinical features

The clinical features of deep venous thrombosis are:
- erythema and warmth of the affected leg (30%);
- swelling and tenderness (75%); and
- the thrombosed vein may be palpable.

Homan's sign is neither specific nor sensitive. Thromboses that extend above the knee are more likely to produce clinically recognizable and life-threatening pulmonary emboli.

NB Diagnosis is confirmed by Doppler ultrasound with vein compression or venography. Swelling of the calf also occurs in rupture of a Baker's cyst behind the knee. An effusion of the knee makes this more likely. The cyst can often be shown on ultrasound.

Clinical presentation (of pulmonary embolus)

This depends upon the size of the embolus. Multiple small acute emboli may remain undetected until up to 50% of the vascular bed is involved and present with effort dyspnoea.
- *Small.* Transient faints and dyspnoea, with slight pyrexia.
- *Medium.* Usually results in infarction and produces, in addition, haemoptysis, pleurisy and, occasionally, a pleural effusion.
- *Large.* (Affecting over 60% of the pulmonary bed.) Acute cor pulmonale with sudden dyspnoea and shock. There is a small-volume rapid pulse, with hypotension, cyanosis, peripheral vasoconstriction and a raised jugular venous pressure. There may be a gallop rhythm.

Investigation

Chest X-ray to demonstrate:
- pulmonary oligaemia of the affected segment (usually present but difficult to diagnose except in retrospect);
- the corresponding pulmonary artery is sometimes dilatated at the hilum;
- small areas of horizontal linear collapse, usually at the bases, with a raised diaphragm; and
- a small pleural effusion.

With larger emboli, the heart enlarges acutely and the superior vena cava distends.

Electrocardiogram changes usually occur only with larger emboli but are then common. The characteristic changes are as follows (see also p. 76):
- tachycardia;
- right ventricular 'strain' pattern (inverted T waves in leads $V1-4$);
- acute, often transient, right bundle branch block pattern;
- S_1, Q_3, T_3 pattern; and
- transient arrhythmias, e.g. atrial fibrillation.

Arterial blood gases

With larger emboli, a fall in Pao_2 and $Paco_2$ is common.

Lung perfusion scan is a useful non-traumatic investigation in doubtful cases and may show underperfusion of one or more parts of the lung that are radiologically normal (and ventilated normally on ventilation scan).

Combined ventilation and perfusion scans may be helpful in pre-existent lung disease in which ventilation and perfusion defects are usually matched. A normal scan virtually excludes pulmonary embolism.

Pulmonary angiography is the most precise for cases presenting difficulty in diagnosis. If available a high resolution CT pulmonary angiogram has a high accuracy rate for the evaluation of pulmonary embolism.

TRIALS BOX 15.5

Imperiale and Speroff performed a meta-analysis of methods to prevent venous thromboembolism following total hip replacement. Low-molecular-weight heparin was more effective than low-dose heparin. *J Am Med Assoc* 1994; **271**: 1780–1785.

Lensing *et al*. performed a meta-analysis of trials comparing the efficacy and safety of low-molecular-weight heparin vs. standard heparin in the initial treatment of deep venous thrombosis. Low-molecular-weight heparins were more effective and safer than standard heparin. *Arch Intern Med* 1995; **155**: 601–607.

Samama *et al*. studied the efficacy and safety of thromboprophylaxis in patients with acute medical illnesses who may be at risk for venous thromboembolism. 1102 hospitalized patients older than 40 years received enoxaparin 40 mg, 20 mg, or placebo subcutaneously once daily for 6–14 days. Prophylactic treatment with enoxaparin 40 mg/day subcutaneously safely and effectively reduced the risk of venous thromboembolism in patients with acute medical illnesses. *N Engl J Med* 1999; **34**: 793–800.

Eriksson *et al*. compared fondaparinux, a synthetic pentasaccharide, which acts as an antithrombotic agent with enoxaparin in 1711 consecutive patients undergoing surgery for fracture of the upper third of the femur. Fondaparinux was more effective than enoxaparin in preventing venous thromboembolism and equally safe. *N Engl J Med* 2001; **345**: 1298–1304.

D-DIMER is a fibrin degradation product formed by the enzymatic activity of plasmin on cross-linked fibrin polymers. Plasma levels can be measured and are raised in patients with pulmonary embolism or deep vein thrombosis. Negative test results rule out the likelihood of these diseases.

Treatment

Prophylaxis is given pre- and postoperatively, especially in lower abdomen and lower limb surgery, and in patients confined to bed or with predisposing disorders (e.g. cardiac failure). Aspirin with graduated-compression stockings are given to at-risk long-distance air travellers. Low-molecular-weight heparins are prepared by depolymerization of standard (unfractionated) heparin. They have a longer duration of action than standard heparin and, given as a once-daily subcutaneous dose, produce a more predictable anticoagulant response. They are safe and effective as low-dose prophylaxis, and can be used in weight-adjusted dosage for treatment of deep vein thrombosis without laboratory monitoring.

For established deep vein thrombosis or pulmonary embolism, patients are usually treated with heparin initially, followed by warfarin for a minimum of 3 months.

In massive pulmonary embolism, cardiac massage and correction of acidosis with urgent intravenous heparin may improve survival. With large emboli, oxygen in high concentration and thrombolytic therapy with urokinase or streptokinase may be valuable. The operative removal of large emboli with bypass surgery may be life-saving.

Placement of a vena caval filter should be considered when anticoagulation is hazardous or in patients who develop emboli despite adequate anticoagulation.

Hyperventilation syndrome

Breathlessness in the absence of abnormal clinical signs and increased by emotion (e.g. clinical examination and ward rounds) should never be described as psychogenic until the following diagnoses have been excluded:
- early pulmonary congestion of left ventricular failure;
- silent multiple pulmonary emboli (lung scan may be diagnostic);
- lymphangitis carcinomatosa;
- interstitial fibrotic pulmonary infiltrations;
- metabolic acidosis (e.g. uraemia, diabetic ketosis); and
- respiratory muscle weakness.

The chest X-ray may appear normal in all of these at the time of presentation.

Hyperventilation syndrome may be the presenting symptom of psychiatric disease and the patient should be asked about symptoms of anxiety, depression and enquiries made about personality previously. The breathlessness is usually episodic and not directly related in degree to exertion (often even occurring at rest). It is frequently described as an inability to take a deep breath or shortage of oxygen. There are associated symptoms of hypocapnia (tingling in the fingers, dizziness, headache, heaviness in the chest, cramp). Tetany may occur with carpopedal spasm. Spirometry usually gives a disorganized trace but the FEV_1 and FVC are normal when obtained.

Fibrosing alveolitis

Clinical features
The disease begins in middle age and presents with progressive dyspnoea and dry cough, usually without wheeze or sputum. The typical signs are clubbing, cyanosis and crepitations in the mid and lower lung fields. Polyarthritis is common. There is an association with autoimmune diseases, particularly rheumatoid arthritis.

Investigation
The arterial Po_2 is reduced and hyperventilation may cause a reduction in Pco_2. Spirometry (p. 54) demonstrates a restrictive pattern, i.e. a grossly reduced FVC with rapid initial exhalation of this small volume, thus giving a normal or high $FEV_1 : FVC$. The transfer factor is reduced.

Chest X-ray shows diffuse bilateral basal nodular–reticular shadowing that extends upwards as the disease progresses. The differential diagnosis of the chest X-ray includes other causes of diffuse pulmonary fibrosis and infiltration: occupational dust lung diseases, sarcoidosis, scleroderma, lymphangitis carcinomatosa, collagen diseases, miliary tuberculosis, radiation pneumonitis, drugs (busulfan and other cytotoxic drugs, nitrofurantoin,

paraquat), histoplasmosis, coccidioidomycosis and histiocytosis X. Clinically, the problem is less difficult. Lung biopsy, either open by thoracotomy or transbronchial via a bronchoscope, may be diagnostic. There is alveolitis with lymphocytic and plasma cell infiltration and diffuse pulmonary fibrosis.

Management
The disease is progressive and, although steroids are usually given, sometimes in combination with azathioprine or cyclophosphamide, response is variable. The patient eventually dies with severe hypoxia. Lung transplantation should be considered, although about 15% develop carcinoma of the lung.

Adult respiratory distress syndrome

Adult respiratory distress syndrome (ARDS) refers to acute progressive respiratory failure starting hours to days after a number of pulmonary or systemic insults. These include sepsis, trauma (lung contusion or non-thoracic), aspiration (gastric contents, toxins, smoke), shock from any cause, disseminated intravascular coagulation, and air and fat emboli. It can occur in association with pneumonia, and may be drug-induced (heroin, barbiturates). The pulmonary oedema is caused by capillary leakage rather than the elevated left atrial pressure of heart failure.

It is characterized by:
- arterial hypoxia;
- reduced thoracic compliance;
- normal pulmonary capillary wedge pressure; and
- diffuse infiltrates on chest X-ray.

Treatment should be aimed at the underlying condition, although in many cases the lung injury has already occurred. Ventilation with positive end-expiratory pressure is usually necessary. Neither steroids nor surfactant have been shown to be of benefit in sepsis-associated ARDS. Mortality is high (50–70%) and associated with sepsis, organ failure and age.

Cardiovascular Disease

Ischaemic heart disease

This presents as the tight or crushing central chest pain of angina or myocardial infarction. Less commonly, it presents as an arrhythmia or conduction defect, or heart failure.

Myocardial ischaemia is normally caused by atherosclerosis but cardiac pain is also produced by:

- aortic dissection;
- paroxysmal tachycardias; and
- severe anaemia, cardiomyopathy, coronary artery embolism and vasculitis are all rare causes.

Coronary artery disease

Examination of atherosclerotic plaques suggests an interaction between blood constituents and cellular elements of the arterial wall. Alteration of normal endothelial cell function may allow accumulation of macrophages, which form foam cells and provoke proliferation of smooth-muscle cells and connective tissue. Cholesterol crystals and other lipids accumulate at the base of plaques, which is covered by a fibrous cap. Plaque rupture leads to thrombosis.

Factors associated with coronary artery disease.

- *Sex*: it is more common in men than in women, particularly before the menopause.
- *Age*: there is a steady increase with age.
- *Smoking* is a powerful risk factor for coronary heart disease (CHD). Cessation is associated with significant reduction in risk, which decreases by half after 1 year, and approaches that of never-smokers after several years.
- *Hypertension*: the risk of coronary heart disease rises progressively with increasing blood pressure. Although most antihypertensive trials

have shown a lower than expected reduction in risk, this may reflect the short duration of the trials.

- *Obesity*: central adiposity is a better marker for CHD risk than the overall level of obesity.
- *Hyperlipidaemia*: CHD is associated with raised total cholesterol and low ratio of total cholesterol : high-density lipoprotein (HDL) cholesterol. Hypertriglyceridaemia appears to be associated more with risk of myocardial infarction than coronary atherosclerosis, possibly because it affects coagulation.
- *Diabetes mellitus*: hyperlipidaemia in diabetics is a powerful risk factor. Men with diabetes have 2–3 times and women 4–5 times the risk of CHD.
- *Alcohol*: the association between CHD and alcohol is J-shaped—the lowest risk is associated with moderate alcohol intake.

Angina pectoris

Diagnosis

The diagnosis of angina is clinical, based on the characteristic history:

- *site*—central chest;
- *character*—usually tight, heavy, crushing;
- *radiation*—to arms, epigastrium, jaw or back;
- *precipitation*—by effort or emotion, particularly after meals or in the cold; and
- *relief*—within minutes by rest or sublingual or buccal glyceryl trinitrate.

There are no specific physical signs. A noncardiac cause is favoured by continuation for several days, precipitation by changes in posture or deep breathing, the ability to continue normal activities, and lack of relief by rest. The more common alternatives in the differential diagnosis are oesophageal pain and musculoskeletal pain.

Unstable angina refers to:
• angina of effort of recent onset with no previous history;
• increased frequency and/or severity of pre-existing angina; and
• angina at rest.

Investigation
Electrocardiogram
The electrocardiogram (ECG) is usually normal between attacks, but may show evidence of old myocardial infarction, T-wave flattening or inversion, bundle branch block or signs of left ventricular hypertrophy. ST segment depression is usually seen during attacks, and may be provoked by exercise testing. A negative exercise test, in which there is no chest pain, no ST depression, no arrhymia and no sustained fall in blood pressure, indicates a very good prognosis. Radionuclide studies can be performed if the patient is physically unable to exercise. Images at rest are compared with images obtained after pharmacological stimulation of coronary flow to evaluate the presence of local ischaemia or infarction.

In unstable angina there is ST depression or T-wave change during typical anginal pain but without diagnostic elevation in cardiac enzymes. Nitrates can reverse ST segment elevation.

Coronary arteriography has a small morbidity and mortality (< 0.1%) that varies from centre to centre. It may supply unequivocal evidence of arterial narrowing, and define its site to guide revascularization procedures.

Management of stable and unstable angina
Risk factors should be identified and advice given about stopping smoking, losing weight and taking regular exercise. Treat hypertension and specific hyperlipidaemic syndromes. Anaemia should be investigated and treated.

Sublingual glyceryl trinitrate remains the mainstay of symptomatic treatment. The major side-effect is headache. It should be taken for pain, and prophylactically before known precipitating events. β-Blockers reduce morbidity as well as control symptoms in stable angina. Verapamil is the preferred alternative for those who cannot tolerate β-blockers. Treatment with oral nitrates and the other calcium-channel blockers provides effective control of symptoms, although there is no evidence that they reduce the risk of myocardial infarction or death. Nicorandil, a potassium-channel activator, can be useful. Low-dose aspirin (75 mg/day) reduces the risk of acute coronary events and myocardial infarction in patients with stable angina. Clopidogrel, an adenosine diphosphatase (ADP) receptor antagonist, may confer additional benefits, but increase the risk of bleeding (see Trials Box 16.1).

In unstable angina, low-dose aspirin, low-molecular-weight heparin and intravenous nitrates are given with, if necessary, β-blockade and/or calcium antagonists.

Medical management vs. revascularization
Coronary angiography should be considered if non-invasive testing reveals:
• ST- or T-wave changes at low levels of exercise (exercise testing, p. 78);
• blood pressure fall during exercise;
• significant left ventricular dysfunction (echocardiography, p. 78); or
• multiple or large transient perfusion defects (radionuclide studies, p. 78).

If angina persists, urgent angioplasty/stenting or cardiopulmonary bypass surgery is indicated.

Patients with unstable angina should be admitted to hospital and precipitating factors (anaemia, arrhythmia, fever) identified and treated. Anti-ischaemic drug therapy is escalated (nitrates and β-blockers with addition of calcium antagonist if symptoms persist) and heparin and aspirin given.

Myocardial infarction

A consensus document of the Joint European Society of Cardiology/American College of

TRIALS BOX 16.1

The **Atenolol Silent Ischemia Study (ASIST)** randomized 306 asymptomatic or minimally symptomatic outpatients with mild or no angina, abnormal exercise tests and ischaemia on ambulatory monitoring were randomized to receive either atenolol (100 mg/d) or placebo. Atenolol treatment reduced daily life ischaemia and was associated with reduced risk for adverse outcome in asymptomatic and mildly symptomatic patients compared with placebo. *Circulation* 1994; **90** (2): 762–768.

A **randomized, blinded, trial of clopidogrel versus aspirin in patients at risk of ischaemic events (CAPRIE)** assessed the relative efficacy of clopidogrel (75 mg once daily) and aspirin (325 mg once daily) in reducing the risk of a composite outcome cluster of ischaemic stroke, myocardial infarction or vascular death in patients with atherosclerotic vascular disease manifested as either recent ischaemic stroke, recent myocardial infarction or symptomatic peripheral arterial disease. Long-term administration of clopidogrel to patients with atherosclerotic vascular disease was more effective than aspirin in reducing the combined risk of ischaemic stroke, myocardial infarction or vascular death. The overall safety profile of clopidogrel was at least as good as that of medium-dose aspirin. *Lancet* 1996; **348**: 1329–1339.

The **fragmin in unstable coronary artery disease (FRIC) study** compared low-molecular-weight heparin with unfractionated heparin acutely and with placebo for 6 weeks in 1482 patients with unstable angina or non-Q-wave myocardial infarction. The results suggested that the low-molecular-weight heparin dalteparin administered by twice-daily subcutaneous injection may be an alternative to unfractionated heparin in the acute treatment of unstable angina or non-Q-wave myocardial infarction. Prolonged treatment with dalteparin at a lower once-daily dose in our study did not confer any additional benefit over aspirin (75–165 mg) alone. *Circulation* 1997; **96**: 61–68.

FRAX.I.S. (FRAxiparine in Ischaemic Syndrome) compared two treatment durations (6 days and 14 days) of a low-molecular-weight heparin with a 6-day treatment of unfractionated heparin in the initial management of 3468 patients with unstable angina or non-Q-wave myocardial infarction.

Treatment with nadroparin for 6 ± 2 days provided similar efficacy and safety to treatment with unfractionated heparin, for the same period, in the therapeutic management of acute unstable angina or non-Q-wave myocardial infarction. A prolonged regimen of nadroparin (14 days) did not provide any additional clinical benefit. *Eur Heart J* 1999; **20**: 1553–1562.

The **thrombolysis in myocardial infarction (TIMI) IIB trial** randomized 3910 patients with angina/non-Q-wave myocardial infarction to intravenous unfractionated heparin for ≥ 3 days followed by subcutaneous placebo injections or uninterrupted antithrombin therapy with enoxaparin during both the acute phase and outpatient phase. Enoxaparin was superior to unfractionated heparin for reducing a composite of death and serious cardiac ischemic events without causing a significant increase in the rate of major hemorrhage. No further relative decrease in events occurred with outpatient enoxaparin treatment, but there was an increase in the rate of major haemorrhage. *Circulation* 1999; **100**: 1593–1601.

The **Clopidogrel in Unstable Angina to Prevent Recurrent Events (CURE) Trial Investigators** studied the effects of clopidogrel in addition to aspirin in patients with acute coronary syndromes without ST-segment elevation. 12 562 patients were randomly assigned within 24 h after the onset of symptoms to receive clopidogrel (300 mg immediately, followed by 75 mg once daily, 6259 patients) or placebo (6303 patients) in addition to aspirin for 3–12 months. Clopidogrel had beneficial effects, but the risk of major bleeding was increased among patients treated with clopidogrel. *N Engl J Med* 2001; **345**: 494–502.

The **CURE Trial Investigators** studied 2658 patients with non-ST-elevation acute coronary syndrome undergoing percutaneous coronary intervention (PCI) in the CURE study. Patients were randomly assigned double-blind treatment with clopidogrel (*n* = 1313) or placebo (*n* = 1345). Patients were pretreated with aspirin and study drug for a median of 6 days before PCI during the initial hospital admission, and for a median of 10 days overall. Clopidogrel pretreatment followed by long-term therapy was beneficial in reducing major cardiovascular events, compared with placebo. *Lancet* 2001; **358**: 527–533.

TRIALS BOX 16.2

Revascularization for coronary artery disease
The **Randomized Intervention Treatment of Angina (RITA) study** compared the long-term results of percutaneous transluminal coronary angioplasty (PTCA) and coronary artery bypass grafting (CABG). Interim results after a mean follow-up of 2.5 years showed that both procedures were effective in relieving symptoms, although antianginal therapy was prescribed more widely following PTCA. Over 2 years, 38% of the PTCA group and 11% of the CABG group experienced a major cardiac event. *Lancet* 1993; **341**: 573–580.

Emory Angioplasty vs. Surgery Trial (EAST) compared PTCA and CABG in 392 patients followed over 3 years. CABG achieved a more complete revascularization and was associated with a reintervention rate of 13% at 3 years, compared with 54% in patients undergoing PTCA. *N Engl J Med* 1994; **331**: 1044–1050.

A follow-up study showed that long-term survival was not significantly different between angioplasty and surgery, and late (3–8 year) revascularization procedures were infrequent. Patients without treated diabetes had similar survival in both groups. *J Am Coll Cardiol* 2000; **35**: 1116–1121.

The **Coronary Angioplasty vs. Bypass Revascularization Investigation (CABRI) trial** compared PTCA and CABG in 1054 patients with symptomatic multivessel disease. Both treatments were effective in relieving angina at equivalent risk of myocardial infarction or death. However, patients undergoing PTCA were more likely to require intervention and to have clinically significant angina at 1 year. *Lancet* 1995; **346**: 1179–1184.

The **Bypass Angioplasty Revascularization Investigation (BARI) Investigators** compared angioplasty with coronary artery bypass surgery as initial treatment in 1829 patients with multivessel disease. Initial treatment by angioplasty did not compromise 5-year survival, although subsequent revascularization was required more often than in patients treated by surgery in the first instance. In diabetics 5-year survival was better in patients treated initially by surgery. *N Engl J Med* 1996; **335**: 217–225.

The **Arterial Revascularization Therapies Study Group** randomly assigned 1205 patients to undergo stent implantation or bypass surgery when a cardiac surgeon and an interventional cardiologist agreed that the same extent of revascularization could be achieved by either technique. One year after the procedure, coronary stenting for multivessel disease was less expensive than bypass surgery and offers the same degree of protection against death, stroke and myocardial infarction. However, stenting was associated with a greater need for repeated revascularization. *N Engl J Med* 2000; **344**: 1117–1124.

The **Stent In Small Arteries (SISA) Trial Investigators** assessed whether stents reduce angiographic restenosis in small coronary arteries compared with standard balloon angioplasty. Symptomatic patients needing dilatation of one native coronary vessel between 2.3 and 2.9 mm in size were assigned to angioplasty alone (*n* = 182) or stent implantation (*n* = 169). Stenting and standard coronary angioplasty were associated with equal restenosis rate in small coronary arteries, but with a lower in-hospital complication rate, stenting may be a superior strategy in small vessels. *Circulation* 2001; **104** (17): 2029–2033.

In the **Intracoronary Stenting or Angioplasty for Restenosis Reduction in Small Arteries (ISAR-SMART) Study** patients with symptomatic coronary artery disease with lesions situated in native coronary vessels between 2 and 2.8 mm in size were randomly assigned to be treated with either stenting (*n* = 204) or angioplasty (PTCA, *n* = 200). Stenting and PTCA were associated with equally favourable results when used for treating lesions in small coronary vessels. *Circulation* 2000; **102** (21): 2593–2598.

The **Total Occlusion Study of Canada (TOSCA)** randomized 410 patients with non-acute native coronary occlusions to PTCA or primary stenting with the heparin-coated Palmaz–Schatz stent. Primary stenting of broadly selected non-acute coronary occlusions was superior to PTCA alone, improving late patency and reducing restenosis and target-vessel revascularization. *Circulation* 1999; **100**: 236–242.

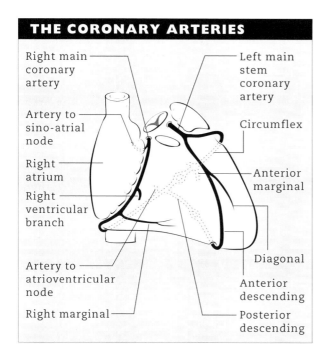

THE CORONARY ARTERIES

Right main coronary artery

Left main stem coronary artery

Artery to sino-atrial node

Circumflex

Right atrium

Right ventricular branch

Anterior marginal

Artery to atrioventricular node

Diagonal

Anterior descending

Right marginal

Posterior descending

Fig. 16.1 Anatomy of the coronary arteries. Note that the right coronary artery supplies both the SA and AV nodes.

Cardiology Committee for the Redefinition of Myocardial Infarction (Alpert *et al. J Am Coll Cardiol* 2000; **36**: 959–969) agreed the following definitions.

Criteria for an acute, evolving or recent myocardial infarction are as follow.
• Typical rise and gradual fall (troponin) or more rapid rise and fall (creative kinase, p. 259) of biochemical markers of myocardial necrosis with at least one of the following:
• ischaemic symptoms;
• development of pathological Q waves on the ECG;
• ECG changes indicative of ischaemia (ST segment elevation or depression);
• coronary artery intervention (e.g. coronary angioplasty); or
• pathological findings of an acute myocardial infarction.

Any one of the following criteria satisfies the diagnosis for *established myocardial infarction*.
• Development of new pathological Q waves on serial ECGs. The patient may or may not remember previous symptoms. Biochemical markers of myocardial necrosis may have norm-

alized, depending on the length of time that has passed since the infarct developed.
• Pathological findings of a healed or healing myocardial infarction.

Aetiology

The most common cause is thrombosis in association with an atheromatous plaque that has cracked or ruptured. Necrosis of muscle supplied by the vessel is followed by scarring.

Rare causes (consider in young patients without risk factors) are:
• coronary artery embolism—from thrombus in left atrium or ventricle, or mitral or aortic valve lesions;
• congenital abnormalities, such as anomalous origin of coronary artery from pulmonary artery;
• coronary artery vasculitis—consider Kawasaki disease in children; and
• dissecting aneurysm with coronary artery occlusion.

The size and location of the infarct depend on which artery is involved (Fig. 16.1), and the presence of any collateral supply. Occlusion of:

- left anterior descending affects the anterior wall of the left ventricle, and sometimes the septum;
- right coronary artery involves the inferior part of the left ventricle, as well as part of the septum and right ventricle; and
- left circumflex involves the lateral or posterior walls of the left ventricle.

The infarct may extend from endocardium to epicardium (transmural), or involve only the subendocardial region.

Symptoms

- Pain—onset, duration (over 20 min), character (often tight or compressing), site and radiation (usually chest going to arms or neck). Associated sweating, breathlessness, nausea and vomiting are common. There may be a previous history of angina or myocardial infarction.

NB Intensity is no guide to the extent of the infarct, especially in the elderly and in diabetics where pain may be absent. If there is interscapular pain associated with a 'myocardial infarction' syndrome, consider dissection of the thoracic aorta.
- Past history of hypertension, stroke, intermittent claudication, diabetes mellitus, hyperlipidaemia.
- Family history of cardiovascular disease, hyperlipidaemia.
- Smoking.

Examination

Once any distress has been alleviated by pain control there may be no signs. Examine:
- for evidence of associated diseases:
    (a) xanthelasmas and xanthomas of hyperlipidaemia;
    (b) evidence of diabetes, thyroid disease, diabetes mellitus, gout, cigarette smoking (smell and finger staining);
- pulse for small volume (low cardiac output), arrhythmia;
- blood pressure (hypotension usually indicates low cardiac output, hypertension may not be long-standing);
- jugular venous pressure (JVP) is usually normal—elevation suggests heart failure;

- listen to heart for:
    (a) fourth heart sound (common); third heart sound if there is heart failure
    (b) pericardial friction rub
    (c) mitral regurgitation (papillary muscle dysfunction or ventricular dilatation)
    (d) ventricular septal defect (VSD) caused by a ruptured septum is rare;
- listen to lungs for basal crackles of heart failure;
- fever is usual within the first few days.

Investigations

ECG

Serial ECGs typically show ST segment elevation and T-wave inversion in anterior or inferior leads, with the development of Q waves indicating full-thickness myocardial necrosis (see Figs 7.10 (p. 72) and 7.11 (p. 73)). Subendocardial myocardial infarction leads to ST segment and T-wave changes, but not Q waves. A normal ECG does not exclude myocardial infarction. Posterior infarction is rare and does not produce Q waves, but gives a tall R wave in V1.

Right ventricular infarction is usually associated with inferior infarction, and produces ST elevation which can be detected if right ventricular leads (V3R and V4R) are recorded by placing chest electrodes on the right side of the chest in positions equivalent to V3 and V4.

Cardiac enzymes

Creatine kinase (CK) and troponin T, both from cardiac muscle breakdown, are the markers of choice.

CK is formed by dimerization of two polypeptide chains, denoted B and M, giving rise to three different isoenzymes. The predominant isoenzyme in skeletal muscle is MM, whereas in brain it is BB. Cardiac muscle contains both MM and MB, and the MB isoenzyme is used in diagnosis of myocardial infarction, although it is also elevated in skeletal muscle disease and by muscle trauma.

Troponin T is cardiac specific.

Management

The early mortality (within 4 weeks) is

30–40%, chiefly within the first 2 h and usually from ventricular fibrillation.

Any patient suspected of having a myocardial infarction requires:
• pain relief—usually in the form of opiates plus antiemetics;
• oxygen;
• aspirin 300 mg to chew immediately; and
• specialist coronary care where facilities for defibrillation, resuscitation and administration of thrombolytic therapy are available.

Thrombolysis
Several studies in the late 1980s showed that intravenous streptokinase reduced mortality in patients reaching hospital with myocardial infarction from just over 10% to around 8%. ISIS-2 showed that aspirin gives additional benefit, and subsequent trials showed that alteplase had similar effects (see Trials Box 16.3).

Streptokinase 1 500 000 Units is given by intravenous infusion over 1 h. It is cheaper than alternatives but can cause allergic reactions. Because it stimulates antibody formation, its potential for repeated use is limited. Alteplase (recombinant tissue plasminogen activator, rtPA) is not antigenic but is very expensive. It is critically important to start thrombolysis within 12 h of myocardial infarction: additional benefit is obtained under 6 h.

Contraindications to thrombolysis are any recent bleeding, severe hypertension (blood pressure > 200/120 mmHg), active peptic ulceration, recent stroke (within last 2 months), proliferative diabetic retinopathy, severe liver or renal disease, pregnancy/lactation, bacterial endocarditis, acute pancreatitis.

β-Blockade
Intravenous β-blockade in the early stages of myocardial infarction may confer benefit (see ISIS-1, p. 261), but is contraindicated if there is bradycardia, hypotension, heart failure, asthma, sick-sinus syndrome or heart block (second-, third-degree or bifascicular). Long-term β-blockade beginning a few days postinfarction is routine in the absence of contraindications.

TRIALS BOX 16.3

Myocardial infarction
Gruppo Italiano per lo Studio della Sopravvivenza nell'Infarto Miocardio (GISSI-1) studied the use of conventional treatment (including heparin, nitrates, calcium antagonists, antiplatelet drugs, β-blockers) with or without streptokinase in 11 712 patients admitted within 12 h of chest pain suggestive of myocardial infarction. Streptokinase reduced both in-hospital and 1-year mortality, and was of most benefit if administered within 3 h. *Lancet* 1986; **i**: 397–401; *Lancet* 1987; **ii**: 871–874.

GISSI-2 compared streptokinase with alteplase, either with or without heparin, in up to 20 891 patients within 6 h of myocardial infarction. Concomitant aspirin and atenolol was recommended. Streptokinase and alteplase had similar beneficial effects, but the addition of heparin had no apparent benefit. *Lancet* 1990; **336**: 65–71; *Lancet* 1990; **336**: 71–75.

GISSI-3 studied the effects of lisinopril and/or transdermal glyceryl trinitrate on 19 394 patients admitted within 24 h of myocardial infarction. Lisinopril, but not nitrates, reduced early (6 weeks) development of heart failure and mortality. *Lancet* 1994; **343**: 1115–1122.

The **Global Utilization of Streptokinase and tPA for Occluded Coronary Arteries (GUSTO)** investigators compared alteplase with heparin and/or streptokinase with heparin in 41 021 patients within 6 h of myocardial infarction. Aspirin and atenolol were also given unless contraindicated. The results showed a small benefit in survival of alteplase over streptokinase. *N Engl J Med* 1993; **329**: 673–682.

The **GUSTO IIA** investigators evaluated cardiac troponin T levels for risk stratification in acute myocardial ischaemia, and reported that cardiac troponin T level is a powerful, independent risk marker in patients who present with acute myocardial ischaemia, allowing further stratification of risk when combined with standard measures such as electrocardiography and the CK-MB level. *N Engl J Med* 1996; **335**: 1333–1341.

The **GUSTO IIb** investigators compared recombinant hirudin with heparin in 12 142 patients with unstable angina or acute myocardial infarction. Recombinant hirudin provided a small advantage, as compared with heparin, principally related to a reduction in the risk of non-fatal myocardial infarction. The relative therapeutic effect was more pronounced early (at 24 h) but dissipated over time. The small benefit was consistent across the spectrum of acute coronary syndromes and was not associated with a greater risk of major bleeding complications. N Engl J Med 1996; **335**: 775–182.

The **GUSTO III** trial compared the effectiveness of early coronary angioplasty and abciximab for failed thrombolysis (reteplase or alteplase) during acute myocardial infarction. The use of abciximab for early angioplasty after clinically failed thrombolysis resulted in trends toward lower 30-day mortality and increased bleeding in 392 patients who underwent angioplasty a median of 3.5 h after thrombolysis. Am J Cardiol 1999; **84**: 779–784.

The **SPEED (GUSTO-4 Pilot)** trial examined the utility of early percutaneous coronary intervention (PCI) facilitated by a combination of abciximab and reduced-dose reteplase in 323 patients who underwent PCI with planned initial angiography, at a median 63 min after reperfusion therapy began. Early PCI was safe and effective in this setting, and was felt to have several advantages for acute myocardial infarction patients, warranting a dedicated, randomized trial. J Am Coll Cardiol 2000; **36**: 1489–1496.

The **GUSTO V** randomized trial compared reperfusion therapy for acute myocardial infarction with fibrinolytic therapy (reteplase) or combination reduced fibrinolytic therapy and platelet glycoprotein IIb/IIIa inhibition (abciximab). Combination therapy led to a consistent reduction in key secondary complications of myocardial infarction including reinfarction, which was partly counterbalanced by increased non-intracranial bleeding complications. Lancet 2001; **357**: 1905–1914.

The **First International Study of Infarct Survival (ISIS-1) Collaborative Group** studied the effect of atenolol (5–10 mg intravenously followed by 100 mg/day for 6 days) in 16 027

patients within 12 h of myocardial infarction. The results showed a short-term survival benefit of atenolol which was lost or reversed after the first year. Lancet 1986; **ii**: 57–66.

ISIS-2 compared the use of streptokinase, or aspirin, or aspirin and streptokinase, or placebo in 41 299 patients within 24 h of myocardial infarction. Mortality at 5 weeks was reduced by all treatments, although aspirin and streptokinase was the most effective procedure. Lancet 1988; **ii**: 349–360.

ISIS-3 studied the effects of streptokinase, or alteplase, or APSAC in 41 299 patients within 24 h of myocardial infarction. Patients also received aspirin, alone or in combination with heparin. There was no significant difference in survival up to 6 months between patients treated with streptokinase, alteplase or APSAC. Fewer reinfarctions and more strokes were observed following alteplase compared with streptokinase. Lancet 1992; **339**: 753–770.

ISIS-4 studied the effect of oral captopril for 1 month, oral mononitrate for 1 month, and intravenous magnesium sulphate for 24 h in 58 050 patients presenting within 24 h of suspected myocardial infarction in a randomized factorial trial. There was a significant 7% reduction in 5-week mortality in patients treated with captopril compared with placebo. Intravenous magnesium was ineffective, and although mononitrate was safe it conferred no clear survival benefit. Lancet 1995; **345**: 669–685.

Survival and Ventricular Enlargement (SAVE) Trial compared the effect of captopril or placebo in 2231 patients up to 16 days postmyocardial infarction with an asymptomatic ejection fraction $\leq 40\%$. Captopril was associated with a reduction of overall and cardiovascular mortality, and also reduced the risk of requiring treatment or hospitalization for heart failure. N Engl J Med 1992; **327**: 685–691.

In a **follow-up study of the SAVE trial patients** a substantial risk of stroke was observed during the 5 years after myocardial infarction (estimated 5-year rate of stroke 8.1%). Decreased ejection fraction and older age were independent risk factors. Anticoagulant therapy appeared to have a protective effect. N Engl J Med 1997; **336**: 251–257.

Angiotensin-converting enzyme inhibitors
Angiotensin-converting enzyme (ACE) inhibitors are beneficial in patients with established heart failure following anterior Q-wave myocardial infarction, with impaired left ventricular function on echocardiography (ejection fraction ≤ 40%), even if they are asymptomatic.

Anticoagulation
Anticoagulation should be considered to prevent deep venous thrombosis in patients slow to mobilize, or in the presence of atrial fibrillation or left ventricular aneurysm.

Primary angioplasty
Primary angioplasty (PTCA) is increasingly performed where facilities are available (see Trials).

Complications
Heart failure (p. 265)

Shock (10% of hospital admissions)
The patient is hypotensive, pale, cold, sweaty and cyanosed. A Swan–Ganz (left pulmonary artery flotation, p. 78) catheter will distinguish pump failure (pulmonary artery wedge pressure high) from hypovolaemia (wedge pressure low). Arrhythmias are common. Treatment is with:
• oxygen;
• diuretics if pulmonary oedema and high pulmonary artery wedge pressure;
• vasodilators—ACE inhibitors (arterial and venous) or nitrates (venous) if blood pressure allows; and
• inotropes—dopamine and dobutamine increase cardiac contractility by stimulating β_1-receptors in cardiac muscle. Low doses of dopamine (< 5 μg/kg/min) induce vasodilatation and increase renal perfusion, whereas higher doses cause vasoconstriction and may exacerbate heart failure.
   The overall mortality exceeds 70%. A pulmonary artery flotation catheter can also be used to monitor the response to treatment.

Arrhythmias
Sinus tachycardia. Usually requires no treatment. May be a sign of heart failure.

Supraventricular extrasystoles. Common, but rarely require treatment.

Supraventricular tachycardia. First try unilateral carotid sinus massage or Valsalva manoeuvre.
   Adenosine (3 mg by rapid injection into central or large peripheral vein) usually causes rapid reversion to sinus rhythm. Its short half-life (10 s) means that side-effects (facial flushing, bronchospasm, bradycardia) are usually short-lived.
   Verapamil may be preferable in asthmatics, but should be avoided if hypotension or heart failure are present. Verapamil is contraindicated in patients taking β-blockers.
   Disopyramide and amiodarone may be useful in resistant supraventricular tachycardia.
   Cardioversion under short-acting general anaesthesia is used when rapid results are required and other procedures have failed.

Atrial flutter and fibrillation. Oral digoxin usually slows the ventricular rate. Amiodarone can also be used. Consider direct current (DC) cardioversion.
NB Supraventricular arrhythmias may be caused by digoxin toxicity (serum levels helpful), particularly if there is hypokalaemia. In this situation, stop digoxin and consider β-blockade. Avoid DC shock, which may produce resistant ventricular fibrillation.

Sinus or nodal bradycardia. May be caused by sedation, particularly with opiates. If the rate is < 50 beats/min, and the patient is hypotensive, give atropine 0.6 mg intravenously and repeat twice if necessary. If unsuccessful, consider cardiac pacing.

Heart block. All degrees of heart block are more serious if they complicate anterior rather than inferior infarcts.
• First-degree: requires no therapy.
• Second-degree: monitor and consider atropine. Many physicians would consider cardiac pacing for Mobitz type II with anterior infarcts.
• Third-degree (complete heart block): atropine and isoprenaline may be helpful while awaiting cardiac pacing.
NB Complete heart block is more common

TRIALS BOX 16.4

The **Primary Angioplasty in Myocardial Infarction (PAMI) Study Group** compared immediate angioplasty with thrombolytic therapy for acute myocardial infarction in 395 patients who presented within 12 h of the onset of myocardial infarction. Compared with tissue plasminogen activator (tPA) therapy, immediate PTCA reduced the combined occurrence of non-fatal reinfarction or death, was associated with a lower rate of intracranial haemorrhage, and resulted in similar left ventricular systolic function. *N Engl J Med* 1993; **328**: 673–679.

Myocardial Infarction Triage and Intervention Investigators (MITI) found no benefit in terms of either mortality or the use of resources in a comparison of primary coronary angioplasty with thrombolytic therapy in patients with acute myocardial infarction. *N Engl J Med* 1996; **335**: 1253–1260.

Weaver *et al.* performed a quantitative review of 10 randomized trials performed between 1985 and 1996 comparing primary coronary angioplasty and intravenous thrombolytic therapy for acute myocardial infarction. Based on outcomes at hospital discharge or 30 days, primary angioplasty appeared to be superior to thrombolytic therapy, with the proviso that success rates for angioplasty are as good as those achieved in the trials. However, they concluded that data evaluating longer term outcomes, operator experience and time delay before treatment are needed before primary angioplasty can be universally recommended as the preferred treatment. *J Am Med Assoc* 1997; **278**: 2093–2098.

The **Stent Primary Angioplasty in Myocardial Infarction (Stent-PAMI) Study Group** compared coronary angioplasty with or without heparin-coated Palmaz–Schatz stent implantation in patients with acute myocardial infarction who underwent emergency catheterization and angioplasty. Those with vessels suitable for stenting were randomly assigned to undergo angioplasty with stenting (452 patients) or angioplasty alone (448 patients). Routine implantation of a stent had clinical benefits beyond those of primary coronary angioplasty alone. *N Engl J Med* 1999; **34**: 1949–1956.

The **Abciximab before Direct Angioplasty and Stenting in Myocardial Infarction Regarding Acute and Long-Term Follow-up (ADMIRAL)** investigators studied the use of abciximab, a platelet glycoprotein IIb/IIIa inhibitor with coronary stenting in acute myocardial infarction. Patients were randomly assigned in a double-blind fashion either to abciximab plus stenting (149 patients) or placebo plus stenting (151 patients) before they underwent coronary angiography. Abciximab improved coronary patency before stenting, the success rate of the stenting procedure, the rate of coronary patency at 6 months, left ventricular function and clinical outcomes. *N Engl J Med* 2001; **344**: 1895–1903.

In the **controlled adciximab and device investigation to lower rate of angioplasty complications (CADILLAC) trial**, primary PTCA with or without abciximab was compared with a Multi-Link stent with or without abciximab in acute myocardial infarction. At 6 months, major adverse cardiac events had occurred in about 11% of the stent group, whether or not they were administered abciximab, and about 20% of the PTCA group, whether receiving abciximab or not. At that time, 2.8% of those receiving only a stent had died compared with 4.3% of those only receiving PTCA. Reintervention was undertaken in 7% of the stent alone population compared with 14% in the PTCA alone group. *J Am Coll Cardiol* 2001; **37**: 342A.

in inferior myocardial infarctions because the atrioventricular nodal artery is a branch of the right coronary artery; complete heart block complicating anterior infarction is ominous because it implies a large muscle infarction.

Ventricular tachycardia. Try lidocaine (lignocaine) 100 mg intravenously as a bolus over a few minutes. If successful, continue as an infusion of 2–4 mg/min. If this fails, mexiletine (100–250 mg intravenously over 10 min), or amiodarone (5 mg/kg into central vein over at least 20 min) can be used, but proceed to DC cardioversion without delay if no success.

NB Lidocaine (lignocaine) does not reduce

mortality when used prophylactically following myocardial infarction.

Ventricular fibrillation. This is frequently within 6 h of myocardial infarction. A precordial thump should be followed by DC cardioversion (200 J, then further 200 J, followed by 360 J if unsuccessful). If ventricular fibrillation persists, perform external cardiac massage with artificial ventilation if not already started; give adrenaline (epinephrine) 1 mg intravenously and repeat DC cardioversion.

Electromechanical dissociation (complexes on ECG with no pulse). Consider and, if indicated, treat hypovolaemia, pneumothorax, cardiac tamponade, pulmonary embolism, electrolyte imbalance, hypothermia. External cardiac massage and artificial ventilation. Give adrenaline (epinephrine) 1 mg intravenously and consider calcium chloride (10 ml of 10% intravenously).

Late complications

Ventricular aneurysm occurs in 10–20%. Serious complications are heart failure, angina, arrhythmias, and emboli from thrombi within the aneurysm. There may be cardiac enlargement and abnormal cardiac pulsation (e.g. an impulse at the left sternal border). Its presence is suggested by ST segment elevation persisting in convalescence. The aneurysm may be demonstrated by echocardiography, radionuclide studies or left ventriculography. Surgical removal is indicated for heart failure or arrhythmias. Anticoagulants reduce the risk of emboli.

Papillary muscle dysfunction or rupture may cause heart failure. There is a pansystolic or late sysytolic mitral regurgitant murmur. Echocardiography confirms the diagnosis. Surgery may be indicated.

Ruptured ventricular septum is rare. Urgent surgical repair may be required for severe heart failure.

Myocardial rupture leads to death from tamponade (unless immediate surgery is available). Dressler (postmyocardial infarction) syndrome occurs weeks or months after myocardial infarction or cardiac surgery. It is characterized by fever, pleurisy and pericarditis, and the presence of antibodies to heart muscle.

Rehabilitation

Many patients find a formal coronary rehabilitation programme valuable. It may be preceded by an exercise stress test to assess suitability. Dietary and health education are given. An optimistic attitude to the future, together with an active involvement in self-rehabilitation, should be encouraged. The importance of stopping smoking must be stressed, and strategies to help smokers including repeated supportive advice and nicotine replacement therapy used if needed.

The uncomplicated case may be discharged without excess risk at 7–10 days. Patients should be encouraged to increase activity gradually over 1–2 months, when return to work can be considered. Patients should not drive for at least 1 month after the event.

Long-term pharmacological treatments

Unless contraindicated, discharge patients on aspirin, β-blockade and statins.

The benefits of aspirin persist for at least 4 years.

β-Blockers, if tolerated, reduce mortality (mostly sudden death) and morbidity (non-fatal infarction for at least 2–3 years).

Diet and lipid-lowering drugs reduce mortality in patients with high cholesterol (see Trials).

Cardiovascular disorders and driving

From the guide to UK medical standards of fitness to drive.

Group 1 entitlement

Angina. If angina occurs at wheel, driving must cease.

Myocardial infarction. At least 1 month off driving.

Successful coronary angioplasty. At least 1 week off driving.

Pacemaker insertion. One month off driving.

Arrhythmia. Off driving until satisfactory control of symptoms.

TRIALS BOX 16.5

Statins
Scandinavian Simvastatin Survival Study (S4) compared the effect of simvastatin or placebo in 4444 patients with established coronary heart disease (angina or postmyocardial infarction) and cholesterol 5.5–8.0 mmol/l. Simvastatin reduced mortality and morbidity. *Lancet* 1994; **344**: 1383–1389.

West of Scotland Coronary Prevention Group (WOSCOP) showed that treatment with pravastatin significantly reduced the risk of myocardial infarction and death from cardiovascular disease in middle-aged men with moderate hypercholesterolaemia and no history of myocardial infarction. *N Engl J Med* 1995; **333**: 1301–1307.

The **Cholesterol and Recurrent Events (CARE)** investigators showed that cholesterol-lowering therapy may be of benefit in patients with coronary heart disease and normal cholesterol levels. *N Engl J Med* 1996; **335**: 1001–1009.

The **MRC/BHF Heart Protection Study** studied over 20 500 subjects in a prospective, double blind, randomized, controlled trial with a 2×2 factorial design investigating prolonged use (> 5 years) of simvastatin 40 mg and a cocktail of antioxidant vitamins (vitamin E 650 mg, vitamin C 250 mg and ≥-carotene 20 mg). Men and women aged 40–80 years were eligible provided they were considered to be at elevated risk of coronary heart disease death because of past history of myocardial infarction or other coronary heart disease, occlusive disease of non-coronary arteries, diabetes mellitus or treated hypertension, and had baseline blood total cholesterol of 3.5 mmol/l. Simvastatin 40 mg treatment showed benefit across all patient groups regardless of age, gender or baseline cholesterol value and proved safe and well tolerated. Results show 12% reduction in total mortality, 17% reduction in vascular mortality, 24% reduction in CHD events, 27% reduction in all strokes and 16% reduction in non-coronary revascularizations. Preliminary results of the study are negative for the antioxidant vitamin cocktail but provided reassurance that vitamins do no harm. *Lancet* 2002; **360**: 7–22.

Heart failure

Heart failure has a prevalence in the UK, Scandinavia and the USA of about 1% overall, and 10% in the elderly. Annual mortality in severe cases exceeds 50%.

New York Heart Association classification
• Class I (asymptomatic): no limitation of normal physical activity
• Class II (mild): comfortable at rest but symptoms on mild exertion
• Class III (moderate): comfortable at rest but symptoms on moderate or severe exertion
• Class IV (severe): inability to perform any physical activity without discomfort, which may be present at rest.

Pathophysiology
Cardiac size increases as a result of dilatation or muscle fibre hypertrophy. In response to increased volume load, ventricular volume increases (the heart dilates). This is initially beneficial as the strength of contraction increases as the cardiac muscle is stretched (Starling's law). However, contraction declines as stretch becomes extreme.

Cardiac output is diminished by definition, resulting in reduced perfusion to vital organs.

Sympathetic nervous activity and plasma noradrenaline (norepinephrine) levels increase, leading to increased heart rate, myocardial contractility and arterial and venous tone.

Renal blood flow is reduced, leading to activation of the renin–angiotensin system (p. 269). *Angiotensin II* causes vasoconstriction and, by stimulating aldosterone, sodium and water retention. These mechanisms increase both pre- and afterload.

Preload is the extent to which cardiac muscle is stretched prior to contraction; it is reflected by the ventricular volume at the end of diastole—the *end-diastolic volume*.

Afterload is the load the ventricle contracts against during systole, which is produced by the aortic valve and the arterial tree.

Heart failure is therefore associated with vasoconstriction through angiotensin II and sympathetic nervous activity, and salt and water retention. These mechanisms initially increase cardiac output (Starling's law) and blood pressure, but do so at the expense of reduced peripheral blood flow and circulatory congestion.

Aetiology

It is important to identify the underlying cause:
• ischaemic heart disease with left ventricular dysfunction (the most common cause);
• hypertension;
• cardiomyopathy;
• valvular heart disease;
• congenital heart disease (atrial septal defect (ASD), VSD);
• pericardial disease; and
• in high-output heart failure excessive cardiac workload may result from anaemia, Paget's disease and thyrotoxicosis.

There may also be precipitating factors:
• anaemia;
• fluid retention (non-steroidal drugs, renal disease);
• infection (especially of the lungs with reduced Po_2; endocarditis);
• pulmonary emboli; and
• drugs with negative inotropism (β-blockers, most anti-arrhythmic drugs except digoxin).

Clinical features

In *left heart failure* left ventricular end-diastolic pressure (LVEDP) is increased. Pulmonary congestion causes dyspnoea, orthopnoea and paroxysmal nocturnal dyspnoea, and leads to acute pulmonary oedema. Fatigue results from reduced muscle blood flow. Signs are tachycardia, third heart sound, crackles at the lung bases and pulmonary effusions.

Right heart failure is usually caused by pulmonary congestion of left heart failure. It also complicates lung disease (cor pulmonale), pulmonary hypertension, right ventricular infarction, or pulmonary or tricuspid valve disease.

Signs are raised JVP, hepatomegaly (cardiac cirrhosis may occur if chronic), oedema and ascites.

Investigation

All patients with newly diagnosed heart failure require the following.
• Full blood count to exclude anaemia.
• Urea and electrolytes to look for evidence of impaired renal function as a cause of fluid retention or a consequence of reduced renal perfusion.
• Chest X-ray for evidence of cardiomegaly, venous hypertension or pulmonary oedema.
• ECG for evidence of myocardial ischaemia or infarction, left ventricular hypertrophy, arrhythmia.
• Echocardiography to exclude valvular or pericardial disease and assess left ventricular function.

Further investigations, including cardiac radio-nuclide studies, exercise testing and coronary angiography, may be indicated.

Echocardiography (p. 78)
Thickening of stenotic valves, often with calcification, gives rise to intense echoes with limited movement of the valve leaflets. Doppler can be used to assess pressure gradients across stenosed valves, and is extremely sensitive in detecting valve regurgitation.

In dilated cardiomyopathy both end-diastolic and end-systolic dimensions are increased, and shortening fraction reduced.

Hypertrophic cardiomyopathy is suggested by thickening of the left and/or right ventricle or interventricular septum in the absence of aortic stenosis or hypertension. There is typically anterior motion of the mitral valve during systole, and mid-systolic closure of the aortic valve. Doppler can be used to detect a pressure gradient across the left ventricular outflow tract.

Pericardial effusion appears as an echo-free space around the heart. If tamponade develops ventricular wall movement is reduced.

Radionuclide studies (p. 78)
Ejection fraction is reduced and there may be

dilatation of the heart. A fall in ejection fraction on exercise is a poor prognostic sign.

Regional abnormalities of the ventricular muscle usually indicate myocardial ischaemia or infarction. Regional paradoxical movement suggests an aneurysm.

Treatment

• *Diuretics* are used to control sodium and water retention. Furosemide (frusemide) 40 mg/day or bumetanide 1 mg/day are usually effective. Higher doses may be required and synergism between thiazide and loop diuretics can be exploited. Careful monitoring of fluid status and renal function is required.

• *ACE inhibitors* have beneficial effects on all classes of heart failure (see Trials above). They should be considered in all patients, even if asymptomatic, because they reduce afterload and may enable remodelling of the left ventricle muscle. Use may be limited by side-effects which include hypotension, renal impairment, hyperkalaemia and cough (when angiotensin II antagonists can be substituted).

• *β-Blockade* with carvedilol or bisoprolol, titrated from very small doses under cardiological hospital care, may be added to reduce excess sympathetic activity and to encourage cardiac muscle remodelling.

• *Spironolactone* 25 mg/day carries the risk of hyperkalaemia and renal dysfunction.

• *Digoxin* is indicated for control of concomitant atrial fibrillation. Recent studies have also shown a benefit in patients with heart failure in sinus rhythm (see Trials Box 16.6).

TRIALS BOX 16.6

ACE inhibitors

The **Cooperative North Scandinavian Enalapril Survival Study (CONSENSUS)** compared the effect of enalapril (2.5–20 mg b.d.) or placebo (in addition to conventional treatment including digoxin, diuretics, vasodilators), on mortality, morbidity (New York Heart Association class) and heart size in 253 patients with NYHA class IV heart failure. Enalapril reduced mortality, improved NYHA class and decreased heart size. N Engl J Med 1987; **316**: 1429–1435.

The **Studies of Left Ventricular Dysfunction (SOLVD)** trials studied the effects of enalapril in patients with symptomatic or asymptomatic left ventricular failure. SOLVD treatment compared enalapril (2.5 or 5 mg b.d. titrating up 10 mg b.d.) with placebo in the treatment of 2569 patients with symptomatic heart failure (ejection fraction ≤ 35%). Mortality and hospitalization rate were both reduced by enalapril. N Engl J Med 1991; **325**: 293–302.

SOLVD Prevention compared enalapril (2.5–10 mg b.d.) with placebo in 4228 patients with asymptomatic heart failure (ejection fraction ≤ 35%). Enalapril reduced the incidence of heart failure and related hospitalization and mortality, but did not affect overall mortality. N Engl J Med 1992; **327**: 685–691.

The **Acute Infarction Ramipril Efficacy (AIRE) and AIRE Extension (AIREX)** studies assessed the long-term (mean follow-up 59 months) effect of ramipril compared with placebo in 603 patients with heart failure after myocardial infarction. Treatment with ramipril resulted in a large and sustained reduction in mortality (relative risk reduction 36%). Lancet 1997; **349**: 1493–1497.

The **ATLAS (Assessment of Treatment with Lisinopril and Survival) Study Group** compared the effects of low and high doses of the angiotensin-converting enzyme inhibitor, lisinopril, on morbidity and mortality in 3164 patients with New York Heart Association class II–IV heart failure. The results indicated that patients with heart failure should not generally be maintained on very low doses of an ACE inhibitor (unless these are the only doses that can be tolerated) and suggested that the difference in efficacy between intermediate and high doses of an ACE inhibitor (if any) is likely to be very small. Circulation 1999; **100**: 2312–2318.

Other vasodilators

The **Vasodilator–Heart Failure Trial (V-HeFT II)** compared enalapril (5 mg b.d. increasing to 10 mg b.d.) with hydralazine and isosorbide dinitrate in 804 men. Enalapril improved prognosis, despite evidence that hydralazine and isosorbide had superior haemodynamic effects. *N Engl J Med* 1991; **325**: 303–310.

The **Vasodilator–Heart Failure Trial (V-HeFT III) Study Group** studied the effect of the calcium antagonist felodipine as a supplementary vasodilator therapy in 450 male patients with chronic heart failure treated with enalapril. Felodipine exerted a well-tolerated additional sustained vasodilator effect in patients with heart failure treated with enalapril, but the only possible long-term benefit was a trend for better exercise tolerance and less depression of quality of life in the second year of treatment. *Circulation* 1997; **96**: 856–863.

β-Blockers

The **US Carvedilol Heart Failure Study Group** enrolled 1094 patients with chronic heart failure in a trial in which patients with mild, moderate or severe heart failure with left ventricular ejection fractions ≤ 0.35 were randomly assigned to receive either placebo (n = 398) or the β-blocker carvedilol (n = 696); background therapy with digoxin, diuretics and an angiotensin-converting enzyme inhibitor remained constant. Carvedilol reduced the risk or death as well as the risk of hospitalization for cardiovascular causes. *N Engl J Med* 1996; **334**: 1349–1355.

The **Carvedilol Prospective Randomized Cumulative Survival Study Group** evaluated 2289 patients who had symptoms of heart failure at rest or on minimal exertion, who were clinically euvolaemic, and who had an ejection fraction of less than 25%. Patients were randomly assigned to treatment with carvedilol for a mean period of 10.4 months, during which standard therapy for heart failure was continued. The study showed that the previously reported benefits of carvedilol with regard to morbidity and mortality in patients with mild to moderate heart failure were also apparent in the patients with severe heart failure. *N Engl J Med* 2001; **344**: 1651–1658.

The **Cardiac Insufficiency Bisoprolol Study II (CIBIS-II)** studied patients with New York Heart Association class III or IV heart failure, with left ventricular ejection fraction of 35% or less receiving standard therapy with diuretics and inhibitors of angiotensin-converting enzyme. Patients were randomly assigned to bisoprolol 1.25 mg/day (n = 1327) or placebo (n = 1320), the drug being progressively increased to a maximum of 10 mg/day and followed up for a mean of 1.3 years. β-Blocker therapy had benefits for survival in stable heart-failure patients. *Lancet* 1999; **353**: 9–13.

The **Metoprolol CR/XL Randomized Intervention Trial in congestive heart failure (MERIT-HF)** studied the effects of controlled-release metoprolol on total mortality, hospitalizations and well-being in 3991 patients with New York Heart Association (NYHA) functional class II–IV heart failure in a randomized, double blind, placebo controlled trial. Metoprolol CR/XL improved survival, reduced the need for hospitalizations caused by worsening heart failure, improved NYHA functional class, and had beneficial effects on patient well-being. *J Am Med Assoc* 2000; **283**: 1295–1302.

Digoxin

The **Randomized Assessment of the Effect of Digoxin on Inhibitors of the Angiotensin Converting Enzyme (RADIANCE)** studied 178 patients with stable NYHA class II or III heart failure who were in sinus rhythm while taking digoxin, diuretics and an ACE inhibitor. Patients were randomized to continue digoxin or switch to placebo for 12 weeks. Patients withdrawn from digoxin suffered a significant reduction in functional capacity and quality of life. *N Engl J Med* 1993; **329**: 1–7.

Spironolactone

The **Randomized Aldactone Evaluation Study Investigators** studied patients who had severe heart failure and a left ventricular ejection fraction of no more than 35% and who were being treated with an angiotensin-converting enzyme inhibitor, a loop diuretic and, in most cases, digoxin. 822 patients were randomly assigned to receive spironolactone 25 mg/day, and 841 to receive placebo. The trial was discontinued early, after a mean follow-up period of 24 months, because an interim analysis determined that spironolactone, in addition to standard therapy, substantially reduces the risk of both morbidity and death among patients with severe heart failure. *N Engl J Med* 1999; **341**: 709–717.

Hypertension

Aetiology

In over 90% of cases no specific cause is found and the hypertension is known as essential. The aetiology is probably multifactorial. Predisposing factors include:

- increasing age;
- obesity; and
- excessive alcohol intake.

Hypertension may be secondary to:

- renal disease;
- endocrine disease—Cushing syndrome, Conn syndrome, phaeochromocytoma, acromegaly;
- oral contraceptive pill;
- eclampsia; and
- coarctation of the aorta.

Genetic factors

Blood pressure levels show a strong familial aggregation that cannot be accounted for by shared environment alone. However, the genetic and environmental factors contributing to hypertension are likely to be extremely diverse, confounding the search for responsible genes. Attention has principally been directed towards the identification of candidate genes. These include genes involved in the reninangiotensin system, together with a number of important vasoconstrictor and vasodilator substances which have recently been identified.

Renin–angiotensin–aldosterone system

A number of factors, including hypotension, hypovolaemia and hyponatraemia, stimulate renin release from the juxtaglomerular apparatus. Renin converts angiotensinogen to angiotensin I, which is then converted by ACE to angiotensin II. Angiotensin II causes arteriolar vasoconstriction, activation of the sympathetic nervous system, and antidiuretic hormone (ADH) and aldosterone secretion. In the kidney angiotensin II causes a relatively greater increase in efferent (postglomerular) compared to afferent (preglomerular) arteriolar constriction, thereby maintaining glomerular filtration in the face of reduced renal perfusion.

Endothelins, prostacyclins and nitric oxide. These are derived from the vascular endothelium. They regulate vascular contraction and relaxation, particularly in the coronary circulation.

Endothelins are a family of structurally related 21-amino-acid peptides and the most potent vasoconstrictors. At least three different isoforms exist. Endothelin-1 (ET-1) is the predominant peptide generated by vascular endothelial cells. It is generated from proendothelin-1 by the action of endothelin-converting enzyme, a metalloprotease. Two distinct endothelin receptors have been identified. ETA receptors are highly expressed in smooth-muscle cells where they preferentially bind ET-1 and mediate vasoconstriction. ETB receptors have equal affinity for all three endothelins. They are present on the luminal surface of vascular endothelial cells, where they promote release of endothelium-derived vasodilators, and to a lesser extent smooth-muscle cells, where they mediate vasoconstriction.

ET-1 has been implicated in the pathophysiology of a number of conditions involving vasoconstriction, including heart failure, pulmonary hypertension, subarachnoid haemorrhage, Raynaud disease and Prinzmetal angina.

Prostacyclin is produced by endothelial cells, platelets and monocytes via a phospholipase A_2 (PLA_2)-dependent pathway, and causes smooth-muscle cell relaxation, and also inhibition of platelet aggregation, via intracellular increases in cyclic $3',5'$-adenosine monophosphate (cAMP). Prostacyclin is synthesized in response to the same inflammatory mediators that raise cytoplasmic free calcium as nitric oxide. Interleukin 1 (IL-1) and tumour necrosis factor increase the activity of the enzymes mediating prostacyclin generation.

Nitric oxide (NO, originally named endothelial-derived relaxing factor) is produced by oxidation of the guanidine-nitrogen terminal of L-arginine, forming NO and citrulline. Production of NO is regulated via activity of NO synthase, a predominantly cytosolic calcium-calmodulin-requiring enzyme which is similar in structure to cytochrome P450 enzymes. Two distinct types of the enzyme have been identified: designated constitutive and inducible.

Constitutive NO synthase is a calcium-calmodulin-requiring enzyme that is responsible for the transient release of small (picomolar) quantities of NO from vascular endothelium, platelets, mast cells, adrenal medulla and some neurons.

Enzyme activity is increased by:
• inflammatory mediators, such as thrombin, histamine, bradykinin, serotonin and leuko-triene C_4, which raise intracellular calcium;
• mechanical forces, such as shear stress; and
• acetylcholine.

Inducible NO synthase is not dependent on calcium-calmodulin and causes a sustained release of larger (nanomolar) amounts of NO from activated macrophages, neutrophils, vascular endothelium and microglial cells. It is induced by bacterial endotoxin, IL-1, tumour necrosis factor and interferon-γ.

Pharmacology of nitric oxide

Nitric oxide mediates the action of some commonly used vasodilators. Glyceryl trinitrate and organic nitrate esters react with thiols such as cysteine and glutathione to yield unstable intermediates which release NO. Sodium nitroprusside spontaneously releases NO.

Analogues of L-arginine such as L-NG-monomethyl arginine (L-NMMA) and L-nitroarginine methyl ester (L-NAME) act as inhibitors of NO production. Although yet to enter clinical practice, such agents offer the possibility of novel therapies for conditions such as septic shock.

Pathophysiology

In its early stages hypertension is thought to be characterized by increased cardiac output with normal peripheral resistance. As hypertension progresses peripheral resistance increases and cardiac output returns to normal.

Left ventricular hypertrophy (LVH) may be present even in mild hypertension, and is associated with increased risk of cardiac dysfunction, atherosclerosis, arrhythmias and sudden death.

Diagnosis
• ECG: S wave in V1 and R wave in V5 or V6

≥ 35 mm. May be associated with ST segment depression or T-wave inversion ('strain pattern').
• Echo: much more sensitive than ECG. The left ventricular mass index (LVMI) is calculated from left ventricular wall thickness and left ventricular internal diameters in systole and diastole.
• LVH present if LVMI $> 110 \, g/m^2$ in women or $> 131 \, g/m^2$ in men.

There is good evidence that treatment of hypertension results in regression of LVH.

Symptoms

There are usually no symptoms of hypertension.

Headaches or visual disturbance occur in severe or accelerated hypertension.

Examination

The blood pressure is measured at rest. If high (systolic > 140 mmHg, diastolic > 90 mmHg), check in both arms, and unless very severe recheck on at least three separate occasions before considering treatment. A large cuff should be used in the 10% of the population with arm circumference over 33 cm. Phase V diastolic (disappearance) should be recorded together with the patient's posture and the arm used.

Mild or moderate hypertension usually gives no other abnormalities on examination. In long-standing or severe hypertension look for evidence of LVH with an aortic ejection murmur and loud aortic second sound. The optic fundi may show evidence of retinopathy with arterial narrowing and arteriovenous narrowing (indicating atherosclerosis), haemorrhages and exudates. Papilloedema indicates the presence of malignant hypertension.

Ten per cent have an underlying definable cause: it is essential to think of these less common causes.
• Observe the face for evidence of Cushing syndrome—usually caused by steroid administration.
• Examine for aortic coarctation—feel both radials and measure blood pressure in both arms. Look for radial–femoral delay, weak femoral pulses, bruits of the coarctation and scapular anastomoses which may produce visible pulsations.

- Listen for an epigastric or paraumbilical bruit of renal artery stenosis.
- Feel for polycystic kidneys.
- Think of chronic renal disease, phaeochromocytoma (rare) and primary hyperaldosteronism (very rare).

Investigation

Routine investigation of hypertension is aimed at detecting treatable disease (usually renal), and assessing cardiac and renal function.

All patients require:
- ECG to assess left ventricular size, and if abnormal a chest X-ray;
- urinalysis for blood and protein—if abnormal a midstream specimen of urine for cells, casts, proteinuria and evidence of infection, and 24-h urine collection to measure creatinine clearance and protein loss;
- blood, urea and electrolytes to assess renal function and look for hypokalaemic alkalosis of Conn or Cushing syndromes (or diuretic therapy);
- 24-h urine collection to measure vanillymandelic acid (VMA) or 4-hydroxy-3-methoxymandelic acid (HMMA) output (phaeochromocytoma).

Investigate renovascular disease (p. 275), Cushing syndrome (pp. 148–149), Conn syndrome (pp. 149–150), phaeochromocytoma (pp. 151–152) or aortic coarctation.

Treatment

Patients should attempt to achieve an ideal weight, avoid excessive alcohol or salt and take regular exercise. Aim at a blood pressure of 140/85 mmHg (140/80 mmHg in diabetes). Systolic blood pressure is at least as important as diastolic as a predictor of cardiovascular disease.

The British Hypertension Society guidelines for management of hypertension recommend antihypertensive drug therapy in people with sustained systolic BP $\geq$ 160 mmHg or sustained diastolic BP $\geq$ 100 mmHg. In people with diabetes mellitus, antihypertensive drug therapy should be initiated if systolic BP is sustained $\geq$ 140 mmHg or diastolic BP is sustained $\geq$ 90 mmHg. In non-diabetic hypertensive people, optimal BP treatment targets are: systolic BP < 140 mmHg and diastolic BP < 85 mmHg. In diabetic hypertensive people, optimal BP targets are: systolic BP < 140 mmHg and diastolic BP < 80 mmHg. Low-dose thiazide diuretics or β-blockers are preferred as first-line therapy for the majority of hypertensive people (*J Hum Hypertens* 1999; **13**: 569–592).

In the absence of contraindications or compelling indications for other antihypertensive agents, low-dose thiazide diuretics or β-blockers are preferred as first-line therapy for the majority of hypertensive people. In the absence of compelling indications for β-blockade, diuretics or long-acting dihydropyridine calcium antagonists are preferred to β-blockers in older subjects. Compelling indications and contraindications for all antihypertensive drug classes are specified. For most hypertensives, a combination of antihypertensive drugs will be required to achieve the recommended targets for blood pressure control. Other drugs that reduce cardiovascular risk must also be considered. These include aspirin for secondary prevention of cardiovascular disease, and primary prevention in treated hypertensive subjects over the age of 50 years who have a 10-year CHD risk $\geq$ 15% and in whom blood pressure is controlled to the audit standard. In accordance with existing British recommendations, statin therapy is recommended for hypertensive people with a total cholesterol $\geq$ 5 mmol/l and established vascular disease, or 10-year CHD risk $\geq$ 30% estimated from the Joint British Societies CHD risk chart. Glycaemic control should also be optimized in diabetic subjects. Specific advice is given on the management of hypertension in specific patient groups, i.e. the elderly, ethnic subgroups, diabetes mellitus, chronic renal disease and in women (pregnancy, oral contraceptive use and hormone replacement therapy). Suggestions for the implementation and audit of these guidelines in primary care are provided.

Successful treatment reduces the incidence of stroke by 37% and of myocardial infarction by 25%. There is an overall reduction of 32% in all cardiovascular events.

Thiazide diuretics inhibit distal tubular sodium reabsorption. Low doses (e.g. bendrofluazide 2.5 mg/day) have maximal antihypertensive effect. Higher doses confer little additional antihypertensive effect, but cause more marked adverse metabolic effects, including hypokalaemia, hyponatraemia, hypochloraemic alkalosis, hyperuricaemia, hyperglycaemia and hyperlipidaemia.

β-Blockers reduce blood pressure and cardiac output, block peripheral adrenoceptors and alter baroreceptor reflex sensitivity. β-Blockers with intrinsic sympathomimetic activity (e.g. acebutalol, pindolol) stimulate as well as block adrenergic receptors, and may cause less bradycardia and coldness of the extremities. Water-soluble β-blockers (e.g. atenolol, nadolol) are less likely to cross the blood–brain barrier and cause sleep disturbance. Some β-blockers have less effect on $β_2$-(bronchial) receptors (e.g. atenolol, bisoprolol, metoprolol). They are therefore relatively cardioselective, and less likely to provoke bronchospasm. However, all β-blockers should be avoided in patients with asthma or chronic obstructive airways disease.

Calcium-channel blockers inhibit inward movement of calcium ions through slow channels in cell membranes. They influence the function of cardiac myocytes, the specialized conducting cells of the heart, and vascular smooth-muscle cells. Three classes, which differ in their relative effects on the heart and blood vessels, are available.

• The phenylalkylamine, verapamil, slows conduction in the sinoatrial and atrioventricular nodes and depresses myocardial contraction, but is less potent as a vasodilator.

• The benzothiazepine, diltiazem, slows conduction in the sinoatrial and atrioventricular nodes, but causes less myocardial depression and vasodilatation.

• The dihydropyridines (nifedipine, nicardipine, amlodipine, felodipine, isradipine, lacidipine) have little effect on cardiac contraction or conduction, but are more potent arterial vasodilators. Dihydropyridines vary in their effects on different vascular beds. Nimodipine acts preferentially on cerebral arteries and

is used to prevent vascular spasm following subarachnoid haemorrhage.

ACE inhibitors (e.g. captopril, lisinopril) inhibit conversion of angiotensin I to II, which is a vasoconstrictor and stimulates aldosterone production. They should be considered for treatment of hypertension when β-blockers or thiazides are contraindicated or ineffective. They may cause excessive hypotension, particularly in the presence of sodium depletion. In heart failure, first doses are usually given at bedtime, and where possible diuretic therapy should be stopped for a few days before initiating treatment. Side-effects include hyperkalaemia (particularly in the presence of renal disease), persistent dry cough, blood dyscrasias, rashes and angioedema. ACE inhibitors should be used with caution in renal disease (see below).

Angiotensin-II receptor antagonists (e.g. losartan, valsartan) are similar in effect to the ACE inhibitors but, because they do not inhibit the breakdown of bradykinin and other kinins, avoid the dry cough that can prohibit the use of an ACE inhibitor.

Moxonidine, methyldopa and clonidine are centrally acting anti-hypertensive drugs.

Severe hypertension

Very severe hypertension (diastolic > 140 mmHg) or malignant hypertension (with papilloedema) should be treated in hospital. BP should be reduced gradually with an oral β-blocker (with α-blockade if phaeochromocytoma is suspected) or calcium-channel blocker. Rapid falls in BP can precipitate myocardial ischaemia, and reduce cerebral and renal perfusion, leading to stroke and deteriorating renal function. Intravenous vasodilators, e.g. hydrallazine and sodium nitroprusside, are rarely required.

Hypertension in relation to other conditions

DIABETES

Hypertension is more common in diabetics than non-diabetics. Possible reasons include:

• obesity;

• increased sympathetic nervous stimulation and catecholamine production;

TRIALS BOX 16.7

The earliest studies showing beneficial effects of antihypertensives used diuretics or β-blockers, but more recent trials have shown benefits from calcium-channel blockers and ACE inhibitors. Recent trials studying the effect of antihypertensives on blood pressure (BP) control, morbidity and mortality are summarized below.

The **Metoprolol Atherosclerosis Prevention in Hypertension (MAPHY)** study compared propranolol and thiazide diuretics (hydrochlorothiazide or bendroflumethiazide (bendrofluazide)) in 3234 men aged 40–64 with diastolic BP 100–130 mmHg. Additional hypertensives were allowed if BP did not respond. The findings suggest that metoprolol produces greater 5-year survival benefits than thiazide diuretics, being associated with significant reductions in total mortality, cardiovascular mortality, cardiovascular events, coronary mortality and stroke mortality. *Hypertension* 1991; **17**: 579–588; *Am J Hypertens* 1991; **4**: 151–158.

The **International Prospective Primary Prevention Study in Hypertension (IPPPSH)** compared oxprenolol with placebo in 6357 patients with diastolic BP 100–125 mmHg. Additional hypertensives were allowed if BP did not respond. BP was reduced more effectively in the group receiving oxprenolol, but there was no difference in the incidence of sudden death, cerebrovascular accidents or myocardial infarction between the two groups. *J Hypertens* 1985; **3**: 379–392.

The **Heart Attack Primary Prevention in Hypertension (HAPPHY)** trial compared β-blockers and diuretics in 6569 men aged 40–64 years with diastolic BP 100–130 mmHg. If monotherapy failed, additional drugs were used. After a mean follow-up of 45.1 months there were no significant differences in BP control, cardiovascular events or the severity of the adverse effects of the drugs between the two groups. *J Hypertens* 1987; **5**: 561–572.

The **MRC (Medical Research Council) young hypertensives trial** compared bendrofluazide, propranolol and placebo in the treatment of 17 354 patients aged 35–64 with diastolic BP 90–109 mmHg. Additional hypertensives were allowed if BP did not respond. Bendrofluazide and propranolol were equally effective at lowering BP. Active treatment did not significantly influence overall mortality, nor overall coronary events at 5 years. However, the incidence of cardiovascular events and the incidence of stroke were both reduced by active treatment. *Br Med J* 1985; **291**: 97–104.

The **MRC elderly hypertensives trial** compared atenolol, amiloride plus hydrochlorothiazide and placebo in the treatment of 4396 patients aged 65–75 years with systolic BP 160–209 mmHg. After a mean follow-up of 5.8 years both active treatments were effective in reducing BP compared to placebo. Active treatment reduced stroke, coronary artery events and all cardiovascular events compared to placebo. These benefits were entirely attributable to the diuretic treatment group. *Br Med J* 1992; **304**: 405–412.

The **European Working Party on Hypertension in the Elderly (EWPHE)** compared active therapy (first-line, hydrochlorothiazide and triamterine; second-line, methyldopa) with placebo in the treatment of 840 patients aged over 60 years with diastolic BP 90–119 mmHg. Active treatment was associated with a reduction in cardiovascular mortality, deaths from myocardial infarction and non-fatal strokes, but total mortality was not reduced. *Am J Med* 1991; **90** (suppl 3A): 1S–64S.

Systolic Hypertension in the Elderly Program (SHEP) compared chlorthalidone (switching to atenolol or reserpine if necessary) with placebo in 4736 patients aged over 60 with systolic BP 160–219 mmHg and diastolic BP < 90 mmHg. Treatment lowered both BP and the risk of stroke and myocardial infarction. *J Am Med Assoc* 1991; **265**: 3255–3264.

Swedish Trial in Old Patients with Hypertension (STOP–Hypertension) used atenolol, or hydrochlorothiazide plus amiloride, or metoprolol, or pindolol, or placebo in 1627 patients aged 70–84 with systolic BP 180–230 mmHg and diastolic BP 90 mmHg or above. Active treatment reduced BP and the incidence of fatal and non-fatal strokes. *Lancet* 1991; **338**: 1281–1285.

Shanghai Trial of Nifedipine in the Elderly (STONE) compared nifedipine with placebo in 1632 elderly hypertensives (aged 60–79 years). Nifedipine reduced the risk of stroke and severe arrhythmia. *J Hypertens* 1996; **14**: 1237–1245.

The **Intervention as a Goal in Hypertension Treatment (INSIGHT)** study compared the effects of the calcium-channel blocker nifedipine once daily with the diuretic combination co-amilozide on cardiovascular mortality and morbidity 6321 high-risk patients aged 55–80 years with hypertension (BP ≥ 150/95 mmHg or ≥ 160 mmHg systolic). Nifedipine once daily and co-amilozide were equally effective in preventing overall cardiovascular or cerebrovascular complications. The investigators concluded that the choice of drug can be decided by tolerability and blood-pressure response rather than long-term safety or efficacy. *Lancet* 2000; **356**: 366–372.

The **Swedish Trial in Old Patients with Hypertension-2 study (STOP-2)** compared the effects of conventional and newer antihypertensive drugs on cardiovascular mortality and morbidity in elderly patients. 6614 patients aged 70–84 years with hypertension (BP ≥ 180 mmHg systolic, ≥ 105 mmHg diastolic or both) were randomly assigned conventional antihypertensive drugs (atenolol 50 mg, metoprolol 100 mg, pindolol 5 mg, or hydrochlorothiazide 25 mg plus amiloride 2.5 mg/day) or newer drugs (enalapril 10 mg or lisinopril 10 mg, or felodipine 2.5 mg or isradipine 2–5 mg/day). Old and new antihypertensive drugs were similar in prevention of cardiovascular mortality or major events. Decrease in blood pressure was of major importance for the prevention of cardiovascular events. *Lancet* 1999; **354**: 1751–1756.

The **antihypertensive and lipid-lowering treatment to prevent heart attack trial (ALLHAT)** compared the effect of doxazosin, an α-blocker, with chlorthalidone, a diuretic, on incidence of cardiovascular disease in patients with hypertension as part of a study of four types of antihypertensive drugs:

chlorthalidone, doxazosin, amlodipine and lisinopril. In January 2000, after an interim analysis, an independent data review committee recommended discontinuing the doxazosin treatment arm based on comparisons with chlorthalidone. Compared with doxazosin, chlorthalidone yielded essentially equal risk of coronary death/non-fatal myocardial infarction but significantly reduced the risk of combined cardiovascular disease events, particularly congestive heart failure, in high-risk hypertensive patients. *J Am Med Assoc* 2000; **283**: 1967–1975.

The **Nordic Diltiazem (NORDIL)** study compared the effects of diltiazem with that of diuretics, β-blockers, or both on cardiovascular morbidity and mortality in 10 881 patients, aged 50–74 years, who had diastolic blood pressure of 100 mmHg or more. Diltiazem was as effective as treatment based on diuretics, β-blockers, or both in preventing the combined primary endpoint of all stroke, myocardial infarction and other cardiovascular death. *Lancet* 2000; **356**: 359–365.

The **Captopril Prevention Project (CAPPP)** randomized trial compared the effects of ACE inhibition and conventional therapy on cardiovascular morbidity and mortality in 10 985 patients aged 25–66 years with a measured diastolic blood pressure of 100 mmHg or more on two occasions. Patients were randomly assigned captopril or conventional antihypertensive treatment (diuretics, β-blockers). Cardiovascular mortality was lower with captopril than with conventional treatment, the rate of fatal and non-fatal myocardial infarction was similar, but fatal and non-fatal stroke was more common with captopril. The difference in stroke risk was thought to be caused by the lower levels of blood pressure obtained initially in previously treated patients randomized to conventional therapy. *Lancet* 1999; **353** (9153): 611–616.

• diabetic nephropathy; and
• insulin resistance and the associated hyper-insulinaemia.

Treatment (see Trials Box 11.1, p. 155)
Thiazide diuretics (which may provoke hyperglycaemia) and β-blockers (which reduce

awareness of hypoglycaemia) have potential disadvantages in diabetics. ACE inhibitors are preferred. In patients with nephropathy, BP control slows the decline in renal function. ACE inhibitors appear to have a specific renal protective effect that is independent of their antihypertensive action.

RENAL DISEASE

Hypertension is an important cause and consequence of renal disease.

Hypertension as a cause of renal disease

Estimates of the prevalence of chronic renal failure because of hypertension vary widely from 0.002% to 20%. Renal failure caused by hypertension is more common in black than white people, and there appears to be familial clustering of hypertensive renal disease within the black population, raising the possibility of a genetic susceptibility to hypertensive renal damage.

Renal failure is an invariable feature of *accelerated hypertension* in which acute, severe hypertension is associated with gross intimal hyperplasia leading to occlusion of the lumen of small arteries and arterioles within the kidney. Renal failure is a rapid consequence if the BP is not controlled.

Renal disease as a cause of hypertension

Hypertension may occur in renal disease as a result of:

- activation of the renin–angiotensin–aldosterone system;
- retention of salt and water;
- altered production or excretion of vasoactive substances (e.g. endothelin); and
- alterations in the structure and function of resistance vessels.

Renovascular hypertension

Ischaemia of the kidney caused by renal artery disease is an important treatable cause of hypertension, although renovascular hypertension occurs in < 1% of the total hypertensive population. The diagnosis should be considered when the onset of hypertension is abrupt, or occurs before age 30 or after age 50. The presence of an abdominal bruit, atherosclerosis elsewhere, hypokalaemia, or deteriorating renal function following treatment with ACE inhibitors are also suggestive.

Atherosclerotic renal disease accounts for approximately 70% of cases, is bilateral in 25% of cases, is most common in elderly men and usually results from a plaque in the first part of the renal artery. Fibrous renal artery disease occurs predominantly in young women, is frequently bilateral and often involves the distal portion of the artery, giving rise to a beaded appearance on arteriography.

Diagnosis

Renal arteriography remains the principal method, although duplex ultrasonography, magnetic resonance imaging scanning and differential isotope renography before and after captopril may also provide useful information.

Treatment

ACE inhibitors provide an attractive means of reducing BP, but should be used with caution as renal perfusion in the presence of renal artery stenosis is dependent on angiotensin II. Rarely, ACE inhibitors cause membranous glomerulonephritis. Angioplasty is the treatment of first choice in many centres. The procedure can be repeated if restenosis occurs, and does not preclude surgical revascularization, which may have a better success rate in atherosclerotic lesions.

PREGNANCY

Stroke volume and heart rate increase during pregnancy, leading to increased cardiac output. BP usually falls during early pregnancy as a result of reduced peripheral resistance, but rises towards non-pregnant values by term.

Pregnancy-induced hypertension has been defined as diastolic BP 110 mmHg or above, or two readings of 90 mmHg or above after 20 weeks in previously normotensive women (International Society for the Study of Hypertension in Pregnancy). Diastolic BP above 90 mmHg before 20 weeks suggests chronic hypertension, which is confirmed if hypertension persists after delivery.

Pre-eclampsia is defined by pregnancy-induced hypertension and proteinuria greater than 300 mg/24 h. Serum uric acid is usually raised. It may lead, often rapidly, to haemolysis, epileptic seizures, abnormal liver function tests and low platelet count (HELP syndrome). Pre-eclampsia affects about 5% of primiparae, but is less common in subsequent pregnancies by the same father.

Treatment

β-Blockers are used in the third trimester, but may cause intrauterine growth retardation if started earlier. Methyldopa is also used. ACE inhibitors may adversely affect the fetal kidney. Diuretics interfere with physiological plasma volume expansion and should be avoided. Pre-eclampsia warrants admission to hospital. Parenteral hydralazine or α-blockers can be used for control of severe hypertension. Seizures (eclampsia) are managed with intravenous magnesium sulfate, 4 g bolus followed by 1 g/h. Delivery cures both eclampsia and pre-eclampsia.

Valvular heart disease (see Fig. 7.2)

Aortic stenosis

Aetiology

Valvular stenosis

Valvular stenosis is caused by calcification of a congenital bicuspid valve or rheumatic valve disease. Over the age of 60 years, degenerative calcification of an otherwise normal valve is more common.

Congenital aortic stenosis (very rare)

Subvalvar stenosis (with fibromuscular hypertrophy, or hypertrophic obstructive cardiomyopathy), and supravalvar stenosis (with 'fish face' and infantile hypercalcaemia).

Symptoms

There may be no symptoms initially. Later angina, dyspnoea and syncope (which may be a result of the low cardiac output) occur. Left ventricular failure and sudden death are relatively common, and probably caused by ventricular arrhythmia.

Signs

• Regular slow-rising, slow-falling (plateau) pulse.
• Small pulse pressure (e.g. BP 105/90 mmHg).
• Left ventricular hypertrophy (sustained and heaving apex).
• There may be an aortic thrill in systole.

Auscultation. An aortic systolic ejection mur-mur occurs, maximal in the right second intercostal space radiating to the neck, with a quiet delayed or absent second sound. An ejection click indicates valvar stenosis. The murmur becomes less marked when the stenosis is very tight because the flow falls as the heart pump fails.

NB Neither supravalvar nor subvalvar stenosis has an ejection click. Poststenotic dilatation is uncommon in subvalvar stenosis (see below).

Investigations

• ECG shows LVH and usually left atrial hypertrophy. Severe stenosis in adults is unlikely if LVH is not present.
• Chest X-ray. Left ventricular enlargement may not be present, even in the presence of a prominent apex beat. The aorta is small and may be dilated distal to the valve (poststenotic dilatation). The aortic valve may be calcified (best seen on lateral chest X-ray).
• Echocardiography defines the size of the orifice and degree of thickening and calcification of the valve, which may be bicuspid. Doppler can be used to assess the gradient across the valve.
• LVH and function can also be assessed.
• Cardiac catheterization. The pressure gradient across the valve can be measured during angiography by withdrawing the catheter across the valve. In addition, coronary arteriography should be performed, because 25% of patients over 50 will also have significant coronary artery disease.

Complications

• Left ventricular failure.
• Infective endocarditis.
• Syncope.
• Sudden death.

Management

Valve replacement is indicated for asymptomatic severe stenosis (gradient > 50 mmHg), or for symptomatic deterioration including syncope. Catheter studies are performed to confirm the site of the obstruction and gradient, and assess the state of the coronary arteries (*Antibiotic prophylaxis*, p. 285).

Aortic regurgitation

Aetiology

Congenital bicuspid valve and infective endocarditis are the most common identifiable causes. Rheumatic valve disease is now a rare cause. Less common associations include seronegative arthritis (ankylosing spondylitis, Reiter syndrome, colitic and psoriatic arthropathy), congenital lesions (coarctation of the aorta, Marfan syndrome), traumatic rupture and syphilis.

Atherosclerosis and hypertension are of disputed importance.

Symptoms

There are usually none until dyspnoea from pulmonary oedema occurs. Angina is not common.

Signs

The pulse has a sharp rise and fall ('waterhammer' or 'collapsing') and there is a wide pulse pressure. There may be marked carotid pulsation in the neck (Corrigan's sign). The left ventricle is enlarged and the apex displaced laterally.

There is an early blowing diastolic murmur at the left sternal edge maximal in the left third and fourth intercostal spaces, heard best with the patient leaning forward and with the breath held in expiration. The second sound is quiet. There is usually a systolic flow murmur, which does not necessarily indicate aortic stenosis. There may be a diastolic murmur at the apex, which sounds like mitral stenosis, as the regurgitant aortic jet strikes the mitral valve (Austin Flint murmur).

Investigations

• ECG shows left ventricular hypertrophy.
• Chest X-ray shows cardiac enlargement.
• Echocardiography: will demonstrate dilatation of the aortic root and the separation of the cusps. Left ventricular function and dimension can be assessed. The mitral valve can be affected with fluttering of the anterior leaflet, and premature closure if the regurgitation is severe.

Management

• *Medical.* Identify any underlying cause. Give antibiotic prophylaxis, and treat endocarditis if present. Treat any heart failure.
• *Surgical.* Valve replacement should be considered for symptomatic deterioration if the heart size increases rapidly or if the left ventricular internal diameter is > 55 mm on echocardiography in a young patient, even if asymptomatic.

Dominance of the lesion in combined rheumatic aortic stenosis/aortic regurgitation

Aortic regurgitation is dominant if the pulse volume is high, the pulse pressure collapsing and the left ventricle enlarged and displaced. Aortic stenosis is dominant if the pulse is of small volume ('plateau pulse') and the pulse pressure low. The ventricular apex of a hypertrophied ventricle is not necessarily displaced.

Mitral stenosis

Aetiology

This is almost invariably a late consequence of rheumatic fever. Mitral stenosis is the most common rheumatic valve lesion and is four times more common in women than in men. It develops 2–20 years after the acute episode of rheumatic fever. Thirty per cent of patients give no history of the illness because it was either very mild or has been forgotten.

Symptoms

• Dyspnoea occurs at night and on exertion and is caused by pulmonary oedema.
• Palpitation is caused by atrial fibrillation. There is a risk of embolism.
• Haemoptysis is caused by pulmonary hypertension, pulmonary oedema or pulmonary embolism.
• Fatigue and cold extremities are caused by a low cardiac output. Angina may rarely occur.

Signs

• Mitral facies. This is a dusky purple flush of the cheeks with dilated capillaries—malar flush.
• Arterial pulse is of small volume caused by obstruction to flow at the mitral valve. It may be irregular because of atrial fibrillation.

• The apex beat is tapping. This represents a palpable first sound.
• If pulmonary hypertension has developed, there is a left parasternal heave of right ventricular hypertrophy. A diastolic thrill can be present in severe disease.

Auscultation

The mitral first sound is loud because the mitral valve is held wide open by high atrial pressure until ventricular systole slams it shut.

The length of the murmur is proportional to the degree of stenosis. The murmur starts when blood starts to flow through the mitral valve, i.e. when atrial pressure exceeds ventricular pressure. The tighter the stenosis, the higher atrial pressure and therefore the longer the murmur. The murmur can be difficult to hear in mild cases, but it can be made easier to hear by exercise tachycardia and with the patient lying on the left side. The presence of an opening snap and a loud first sound suggest a pliable valve. If the valve is rigid these cannot occur. Presystolic accentuation is caused by the increased flow through the valve produced by atrial systole and it is therefore absent in atrial fibrillation.

NB Some of the signs of mitral stenosis can be given by the Austin Flint murmur of aortic regurgitation (the regurgitant aortic jet strikes the normal mitral valve), and very rarely by a left atrial myxoma.

Assessment

The *degree of stenosis* can be assessed from the severity of dyspnoea, the duration of the murmur, and evidence of the degree of left atrial enlargement on ECG and chest X-ray. The tighter the stenosis, the longer the murmur and the closer the opening snap to the second sound.

The *mobility of the valve* is denoted by the presence of an opening snap and a loud mitral first sound (and absence of valve calcification on the chest X-ray).

Pulmonary hypertension. Fatigue, symptoms of right heart failure and a reduction in dyspnoea indicate raised pulmonary vascular resistance.

The development of pulmonary hypertension is indicated by a dominant 'a' wave in the jugular venous pulse (unless in atrial fibrillation), a loud pulmonary second sound, right ventricular hypertrophy, rarely pulmonary incompetence and low-volume peripheral arterial pulse (mnemonic: April).

Presence of other lesions. Mitral regurgitation and other valve lesions must be noted and assessed, particularly if symptoms indicate surgical intervention. Atrial fibrillation may suggest a greater degree of myocardial disease, which is always present to some extent.

ECG. In early disease, the P mitrale of left atrial hypertrophy develops. This disappears with the later onset of atrial fibrillation. Right ventricular hypertrophy may be present.

Chest X-ray. Characteristically, there is left atrial enlargement plus upper lobe venous congestion with septal lines (Kerley B) just above the costophrenic angles and enlargement of the pulmonary arteries. The mitral valve may be calcified. Haemosiderosis in the lung fields is rare.

Echocardiogram allows measurement of the reduced diastolic closure rate of the mitral valve. It also demonstrates valve thickening and calcification (a mitral valve area of < 1.5 cm^2 indicates critical stenosis), and gives an assessment of ventricular function.

Complications
• Pulmonary oedema.
• Right heart failure.
• Atrial fibrillation.
• Systemic embolization.
• Infective endocarditis.

Management

Use prophylactic antibiotics for dental extraction, surgery or invasive investigations (p. 285).

Anticoagulation is indicated when atrial fibrillation develops or there is left atrial enlargement. Some physicians prophylactically anticoagulate all patients with mitral stenosis.

The fast ventricular rate of untreated atrial fibrillation is controlled by digoxin.

Valvotomy (trans-septal balloon or open valvotomy) is indicated if persistent pulmonary oedema or pulmonary hypertension is present.

Mitral stenosis in pregnancy. Fluid retention in normal pregnancy produces a 30% increase in blood volume during the last trimester and can precipitate heart failure in the presence of mitral stenosis. Valvotomy can be performed at any time during pregnancy if indicated by the above criteria. The cardiac output falls in the last 2 months of pregnancy and most patients who can manage at that time go to term. If there are obstetric complications, antibiotics to cover the organisms of the genital tract should be given throughout labour.

Mitral regurgitation
Aetiology
• Floppy (prolapsing) mitral valve leaflets.
• Ischaemic papillary muscle dysfunction, particularly after inferior myocardial infarction.
• Severe left ventricular failure with dilatation of the mitral ring.
• Rheumatic fever.
• Rarely, cardiomyopathy, congenital malformation (Marfan syndrome), infective endocarditis and rupture of the chordae tendinae.

Symptoms
Progressive dyspnoea develops as a result of pulmonary congestion and this is followed by right heart failure. Angina and haemoptysis are more common than in mitral stenosis. Fatigue and palpitation are common.

Signs
Palpation. LVH and a systolic thrill are characteristic. A left parasternal heave may be present, and is caused by systolic expansion of the left atrium rather than by right ventricular hypertrophy.

Auscultation. There is an apical pansystolic murmur radiating to the left axilla. The mitral sound is soft. There may be a third sound caused by rapid ventricular filling. A short mid-diastolic murmur in severe mitral regurgitation does not necessarily indicate valve stenosis.

Mitral valve prolapse produces a late systolic click and murmur. It is late because the posterior leaflet of the valve only starts to leak when the ventricular pressure is at its highest. It occurs in two clinical situations. In the middle-aged and elderly it is associated with a wear and tear disorder of the leaflet, chordae or papillary muscles (particularly after myocardial infarction). A floppy valve can be detected in up to 5% of young people by echocardiography. The prognosis is usually excellent, although it has been associated with arrhythmias, syncope, atypical chest pain and bacterial endocarditis. Prophylactic antibiotics should be used (p. 285).

Investigations
• *ECG* may show LVH, and the P mitrale of left atrial hypertrophy. Atrial fibrillation is less common than in mitral stenosis.
• *Chest X-ray.* The left atrium and ventricle are enlarged, the former sometimes being enormous.
• *Echocardiography* helps to distinguish between the various causes, and to assess left ventricular function.
• *Assessment* of the dominance of the lesions in combined mitral stenosis/mitral regurgitation. Mitral stenosis is more likely to be the dominant lesion if the pulse volume is small (in the absence of failure) and if there is no LVH.

Complications
These are similar to those in mitral stenosis except that infective endocarditis is more common and embolism less common.

Management
Give prophylactic antibiotics. Valve replacement is indicated if the symptoms are severe and uncontrolled by medical therapy, or if pulmonary hypertension develops.

Indications for anticoagulation are atrial fibrillation, systemic embolism and prosthetic valves.

Other valve disease

Tricuspid regurgitation

Tricuspid regurgitation may be caused by *dilatation of the tricuspid valve ring* in right ventricular failure from any cause, *rheumatic fever* (where it is invariably associated with disease of mitral and/or aortic valves), or *endocarditis* in drug addicts.

The signs include:
• giant 'v' waves in the jugular venous pulse and systolic pulsation of an enlarged liver (both caused by the transmission of ventricular filling through the open tricuspid valve); and
• right ventricular enlargement causing marked pulsation at the lower left sternal edge and a pansystolic murmur, loudest in inspiration, heard at the lower end of the sternum.

There is often ankle and sacral oedema, ascites and jaundice from hepatic congestion.

Pulmonary stenosis

Pulmonary stenosis is usually congenital but may follow maternal rubella. Rarely, it is associated with Noonan syndrome (Turner's phenotype with normal chromosomes). Rheumatic fever and carcinoid are extremely rare causes. Fatigue and syncope occur if the stenosis is severe. Patients may show peripheral cyanosis, a low-volume pulse and a large 'a' wave in the jugular venous pulse wave. Right ventricular hypertrophy causes a parasternal heave. There is a systolic thrill and murmur in the pulmonary area (second left intercostal space) and an ejection click. The pulmonary component of the second sound is quiet and late.

Atrial myxoma

Atrial myxoma may mimic valve disease. It is very rare. It usually occurs in the left atrium and presents with features of mitral stenosis, systemic emboli and constitutional upset with fever. It can mimic bacterial endocarditis. It is best diagnosed by echocardiography where the tumour produces characteristic echoes as it moves between the mitral valve leaflets in ventricular diastole and in the atrium in systole. It is fatal unless removed surgically.

Congenital heart disease

Congenital heart disease may present as an isolated cardiac abnormality or as part of a systemic syndrome.

Maternal rubella

It is dangerous in the first 3 months of pregnancy (particularly the first month when 50% of fetuses are affected). The cardiac lesions are in three groups:
• patent ductus arteriosus;
• septal defects: atrial septal defect, ventricular septal defect, Fallot's tetralogy; and
• right-sided outflow obstruction: pulmonary valve, artery or branch stenoses.

The systemic syndrome includes cataract, nerve deafness and mental retardation.

All children are offered rubella vaccine at the age of 12 years. Boys are included to reduce transmission. Fertile women given vaccine must not become pregnant in the immediate future.

If a pregnant woman is in contact with rubella, serum should be taken for antibody levels to rubella if these are not known. If raised, this is evidence of previous infection and there is little or no risk to the fetus. If the titre is not raised, a repeat sample is measured 3–4 weeks later (or if symptoms appear in the mother) and if the titre has risen significantly, this is evidence of recent infection. The earlier that this occurs in the pregnancy, the greater the risk to the fetus. Some parents elect for termination of pregnancy.

Down syndrome (usually 21-trisomy)

Associated with septal defects, particularly ventricular.

Turner syndrome (XO)

Associated with coarctation of the aorta. Affected females are short and the neck may appear webbed. Ovaries fail to develop properly leading to primary amenorrhoea.

Marfan syndrome (arachnodactyly)

An autosomal dominant connective tissue

disorder which affects the aortic media, eyes and limb skeleton.

Incidence: 5000 in UK (5% of cases are a new mutation). Ten per cent are seriously affected.

It is characterized by disproportionate length of the long bones, which results in span exceeding height and long fingers and toes. Joints tend to be hyperextensible. There is frequently a high arched palate, pectus excavatum, scoliosis, little subcutaneous fat and lens dislocation with myopia. The aortic media is weak with a tendency to dilatation of the ascending aorta and aortic valve ring, resulting in aortic valve regurgitation and dissection of the aorta. Mitral regurgitation may develop.

Working classification

An asterisk denotes the most frequent.

Stenosis
• Semilunar valves: aortic stenosis (supra- and subvalvar and valve stenoses), pulmonary stenosis.
• Atrioventricular valves: mitral stenosis, tricuspid stenosis.
• Major arteries: coarctation of aorta,* pulmonary artery stenosis.

Regurgitation
• Semilunar valves: aortic regurgitation, pulmonary regurgitation (very rare).
• Atrioventricular valves: mitral regurgitation, tricuspid regurgitation, Ebstein's anomaly.

Shunts
• *Left-to-right*: ASD,* VSD,* patent ductus arteriosus (PDA),* aortopulmonary window.
• *Right-to-left* (cyanotic: transposition of the great vessels (frequent but die at birth), Fallot's tetralogy,* Eisenmenger syndrome.

Atrial septal defect

This accounts for 10% of all congenital heart disease. It occasionally occurs in Marfan syndrome.

Ostium secundum (70% of ASDs) is usually uncomplicated. Compared with other congenital heart defects, there is a high (and late)

incidence of atrial fibrillation (20%) and an extremely low incidence of endocarditis.

Ostium primum (30% of ASDs) is often complicated because it tends to involve the atrioventricular valves to produce mitral and tricuspid regurgitation and may even have an associated VSD. In most respects (embryology, cardiodynamics, complications and prognosis) it is quite different from ostium secundum ASD.

Symptoms

In simple lesions there are usually no symptoms, although dyspnoea occurs in 10% of cases. Symptoms usually occur for the first time in middle age. It is usually detected at routine chest X-ray.

Signs

Characteristically, there is fixed, wide splitting of the second sound. Flow through the defect does not itself produce a murmur but increased right heart output gives a pulmonary flow murmur and large shunts may produce a tricuspid diastolic flow murmur. In ostium primum there may be signs of the associated lesions, and mitral (plus occasional tricuspid) regurgitation. The precordium may be deformed and the pulse volume small. A left parasternal lift of right ventricular hypertrophy may be present.

Assessment

ECG
• *Ostium secundum*. There is partial right bundle branch block with right axis deviation and right ventricular hypertrophy. Atrial fibrillation may occur.
• *Ostium primum*. Usually, there is left axis deviation with evidence of right ventricular hypertrophy. Conduction defects and junctional dysrhythmias occur.

Chest X-ray
This shows enlargement of the right atrium and ventricle with enlarged pulmonary arteries and plethoric lung fields (evidence of increased right-sided flow). The aorta appears small (evidence of decreased left-sided blood flow).

Cardiac catheterization reveals a step up in oxygen saturation in the right atrium.

Complications
• Eisenmenger syndrome. If the left-to-right shunt through the defect results in a pulmonary hypertension with pressure above systemic level, a reversed shunt develops.
• Atrial fibrillation.
• Tricuspid regurgitation (from right ventricular enlargement).
• Infective endocarditis occurs in ostium primum, but rarely in ostium secundum defects.

Management
• *Ostium secundum*. Operate if the pulmonary : systemic flow ratio is more than 2 : 1.
• *Ostium primum*. Operate for symptoms, or for cardiac enlargement with mitral regurgitation. NB Eisenmenger syndrome precludes surgery.

Patent ductus arteriosus
This represents 15% of all congenital heart disease. It is associated with the rubella syndrome. It is more common in females.

Symptoms
Usually there are none. Bronchitis and dyspnoea on exertion occur later and with with severe lesions.

Signs
The pulse may be collapsing (water hammer) and the left ventricle hypertrophied. There is a continuous (machinery) murmur with systolic accentuation, maximal in the second left intercostal space and posteriorly. This continuous murmur must be distinguished from the other causes, i.e. jugular venous hum, mitral regurgitation plus aortic regurgitation, VSD plus aortic regurgitation, pulmonary arteriovenous fistulae.

Assessment
The *ECG* is normal or there may be left ventricular hypertrophy.

Chest X-ray. The aorta and left ventricle may be enlarged. The pulmonary artery is enlarged and there is pulmonary plethora.

Echocardiography shows a dilated left atrium and left ventricle.

Complications
• Endarteritis (of the ductus)
• Heart failure (Eisenmenger syndrome, p. 285, as a result of pulmonary hypertension and shunt reversal).

Management
Indometacin, is given within 1–3 weeks of birth to close the duct, possibly by blocking prostaglandin E production in the duct muscle. If this is unsuccessful, surgical ligation (1–5 years) is required or possibly an umbrella occlusion device. Cyanosis contraindicates surgery. Antibiotic prophylaxis is given (p. 285).

Ventricular septal defect
This accounts for 25% of congenital heart disease.

Small defect. This is also called *maladie de Roger*. There is a loud murmur with a normal-sized heart, chest X-ray and ECG.

Large defect. The clinical importance of this depends on the pulmonary vascular resistance, which determines how much shunting is present and its direction of flow.

Symptoms
There are none unless the VSD is large, when there may be dyspnoea and bronchitis.

Signs
There may be a small-volume pulse and LVH may be present (and right ventricular hypertrophy too, if there is pulmonary hypertension). A pansystolic murmur (and thrill) is present in the fourth left intercostal space. A mitral diastolic flow murmur implies a large shunt.

Assessment
ECG shows LVH.

Chest X-ray. Enlargement of the left atrium and ventricle may be present. The pulmonary arteries are enlarged if there is pulmonary hypertension.

Complications
• Endocarditis occurs in 20–30% with emboli into the pulmonary circulation.
• Eisenmenger syndrome.

Management
• Chemoprophylaxis to prevent endocarditis (p. 285).
• A small VSD may close spontaneously. Surgery is not indicated for the endocarditis risk alone.
• A large VSD needs surgery in most cases to prevent the development of irreversible pulmonary vascular damage. Surgery is contraindicated once Eisenmenger syndrome has developed.

Fallot's tetralogy
This accounts for 10% of congenital heart disease, and 50% of cyanotic congenital heart disease.

The four features (tetralogy) are:
1 VSD in which the shunt is from right to left because of;
2 pulmonary stenosis, infundibular or valvar;
3 right ventricular hypertrophy caused by the consequent load on the right ventricle; and
4 associated dextroposition of the aorta so that it sits over the defect in the septum.

Symptoms
• Syncope in 20%.
• Squatting (this may help decrease the right-to-left shunt by increasing systemic resistance and reducing venous return).
• Dyspnoea.
• Retardation of growth.

Signs
Cyanosis and finger clubbing.

The typical murmur is of pulmonary stenosis with a quiet or inaudible pulmonary second sound. There is no VSD murmur.

Assessment
The *ECG* usually shows moderate right atrial and ventricular hypertrophy.

Chest X-ray shows a normal-sized but boot-shaped heart and a large aorta with a small pulmonary artery and pulmonary oligaemia. It is boot-shaped because of the small left pulmonary artery.

Polycythaemia is common.

Complications
• Cyanotic and syncopal attacks (sometimes fatal).
• Cerebral abscesses (10%).
• Endocarditis (10%).
• Paradoxical emboli.
• Strokes (thrombotic–polycythaemia).
• Epilepsy is more common than in the general population.
NB Only 1 in 10 people survive to 21 years of age if they are untreated.

Management
Total correction on cardiopulmonary bypass.

Coarctation of the aorta
These represent 5% of congenital heart disease. It is associated with berry aneurysms, Marfan and Turner syndromes. Ninety-eight per cent are distal to the origin of the left subclavian artery.

Symptoms
Sixty per cent have none. Forty per cent have symptoms including stroke, endocarditis, occasionally intermittent claudication and those secondary to hypertension.

Signs
• Classically, there is radial–femoral arterial pulse delay, with a smaller volume femoral pulse than radial. The blood pressure may be raised in the arms (especially on exercise), different between the two sides and low in the legs. Asymmetry of radial pulses may be present.
• Visible and/or palpable scapular collateral arteries.
• Left ventricular hypertrophy
• The murmurs are:
  (a) a systolic murmur at front and back of the left upper thorax;
  (b) collateral murmurs over the scapulae; and

(c) an aortic systolic murmur (of an associated bicuspid valve in 70% of cases) that is usually obscured by the coarctation murmur.

Assessment

ECG. Fifty per cent have LVH.

Chest X-ray. There is a double aortic knuckle as a result of stenosis and poststenotic dilatation, rib notching (and notching at the scapular margin) and normal or large cardiac shadow.

Associations

Bicuspid aortic valve, cerebral artery aneurysms (berry aneurysms) and patent ductus arteriosus.

Prognosis

Ninety per cent die by the age of 40 years from endocarditis, heart failure or cerebrovascular haemorrhage.

Management

Surgical resection with an operative mortality of 5%. Use antibiotic prophylaxis (p. 285).

Eisenmenger syndrome

This refers to the situation in which there is a reversal of a left-to-right shunt (e.g. VSD, ASD, PDA) because of pulmonary hypertension. With left-to-right shunts there is a pulmonary circulatory overload, and an increase in pulmonary vascular resistance follows with the development of pulmonary hypertension. When the pressure on the right side of the shunt exceeds that on the left side, the shunt flow reverses. The patient becomes cyanosed and deteriorates rapidly with symptoms of dyspnoea, syncope and angina. The lesion must be surgically corrected before this stage is reached. If not, heart–lung transplantation should be considered.

Infective endocarditis

Acute

This is a rare disease in which the heart valves are infected as part of an acute septicaemia, of which the features are swinging fever, rigors, delirium and shock. Healthy valves are affected in 50% of cases. It follows infection with staphylococcus, usually from primary infection of the lungs or skin. *Streptococcus pneumoniae*, *Haemophilus influenzae*, gonococcus and meningococcus may also be responsible.

The prognosis is that of the generalized septicaemia unless valve destruction leads in addition to acute, intractable cardiac failure.

Subacute

This is usually bacterial and subacute in onset (subacute bacterial endocarditis, SBE).

Predisposing abnormalities
• *Congenital*: VSD, PDA, coarctation of the aorta and bicuspid aortic valves.
NB ASD of the secundum (common) variety does not develop endocarditis, but the rare primum lesion, where the mitral valve is also involved, do.
• *Acquired*: any rheumatic valve may be affected, the mitral more than the aortic, and mitral regurgitation more frequently than mitral stenosis. Chronic rheumatic heart disease now accounts for less than one-quarter of all UK cases. Mitral valve prolapse is present in 5–15% of young adults, particularly females. Calcified aortic stenosis and syphilitic aortitis (rare) predispose to endocarditis. It occurs postoperatively following cardiac catheterization or surgery and often on prosthetic valves, which are at risk. The normal tricuspid valve is at special risk in drug addicts.

Organisms
• *Streptococcus viridans* (non-haemolytic) is the most common (45%), and the usual source is teeth.
• *Staphylococcus aureus* and *S. albus* (25%).
• *Streptococcus faecalis* (7%) especially in young women (abortion) and old men (genitourinary catheterization). Other bacteria include gonococcus, *Brucella* and *Proteus*.
• *Coxiella burnetii* (Q fever).
• Fungi (*Candida*, *Aspergillus*, *Histoplasma*).
The origin of infection varies with the infecting organisms and includes teeth and tonsils (*Streptococcus viridans*), urinary tract (*S. faecalis*), central venous catheterization (*Staphylococcus*) and the skin (*Staphylococcus*).

Diagnosis

The diagnosis should be considered in any patient with a predisposing cardiac lesion who develops any illness. It is made on the basis of the clinical picture alone, even if unconfirmed by the isolation of the organism from blood culture. The most efficient way to establish the diagnosis is:

• repeated examination, particularly for changing murmurs;
• blood cultures (at least three sets);
• midstream urine examination for microscopic haematuria;
• immune complexes and low complement in serum;
• echocardiogram for vegetations on the damaged valves; and
• positive rheumatoid factor.

NB Endocarditis sometimes presents with atrial fibrillation in the elderly.

Clinical features

Classically, the disease affects young adults (20–30 years) with rheumatic valve or congenital heart disease, although it is now more commonly recognized in the over-60s (30%). The symptoms and signs may be considered in three groups.

1 *Signs of general infection.* Lethargy, malaise, anaemia and low-grade fever are frequent but not invariable (fever exists at presentation in 70%). Clubbing of the fingers (20%) and splenomegaly (40%) are fairly late signs (6–8 weeks). There may be transient myalgia or arthralgia (25%). The white cell count may be low, normal or high. *Café-au-lait* complexion is now exceedingly rare as it occurs only in the latest stages.

2 *Signs of underlying cardiac lesions* must be sought, although they are not present in 50% of patients. New lesions and changing murmurs are highly suggestive and the patient must be examined for these daily.

3 *Embolic phenomena.* Large emboli (30%) may travel to the brain (15%) and viscera or cause occlusion of peripheral arteries. Emboli from left-to-right shunts (VSD and PDA) and on right-sided heart valves go to the lungs, giving pleurisy and lung abscesses. Paradoxical emboli, which pass through a septal defect.

Vasculitic phenomena occur in up to 50% and cause splinter haemorrhages in the nail bed, and microscopic haematuria. Osler's nodes in the finger pulp are pathognomonic but rare. Roth spots in the eye also occur rarely.

The renal lesions in SBE are of two kinds:
• a diffuse, proliferative glomerulonephritis (not specifically diagnostic of SBE); and
• a focal, embolic glomerulonephritis. The tissue is sterile on culture.

Immune complexes are present in serum and complement levels reduced.

Prognosis

The mortality is 95% in untreated cases. It is still over 30%, even with modern therapy. Adverse features include the presence of congestive heart failure, advanced age or of peripheral emboli. Death is often from heart failure of valve destruction or from major (e.g. cerebral) emboli.

Management

Prophylaxis

When valves are abnormal antibiotics must be given during intercurrent infections and before any surgical procedures in the mouth, genitourinary tract or gastrointestinal tract.

Dentistry. Under local or no anaesthesia oral amoxicillin 3 g l h before the procedure. For those who are penicillin-allergic, or have received penicillin in the previous month, give clindamycin 600 mg l h before. Under general anaesthesia give amoxicillin l g intravenously or intramuscularly at induction, then 500 mg 6 h later. Intravenous vancomycin and gentamicin can be used in those who have received penicillin recently or are allergic. Good dental hygiene is essential.

Genitourinary, gastrointestinal or obstetric procedures. Amoxicillin l g and gentamicin at time of induction, followed by amoxicillin 500 mg 6 h later. (Vancomycin and gentamicin if penicillin allergy or recent exposure.)

Chemotherapy

It is essential to obtain blood culture before starting chemotherapy, but it should not be delayed in the presence of good clinical evidence even if cultures are negative. Penicillin G, 7.2 g/day intravenously in six divided doses is given with an aminoglycoside (e.g. gentamicin). Vancomycin can be used in place of penicillin if allergic. When the results of bacterial sensitivities are available, therapy is guided by this, an attempt being made to achieve serum levels of the antibiotic at least three times the minimal inhibitory concentration (MIC) of the organism. Therapy should be continued for at least 4 weeks (intravenously for the first 2 weeks), if effective blood concentrations can be achieved. The patient should be carefully followed for recurrence. Emboli may occur for up to 1–2 months after cure.

Indications for surgery
Surgery must be considered early for valve rupture, intractable heart failure, resistant infection particularly of a valve prosthesis, and if the organisms are drug-resistant.

Culture-negative endocarditis
This diagnosis is considered after six successive negative cultures when culture technique is known to be good. The following should be considered.
• Unsuspected organisms—e.g. *Coxiella burnetii* (Q fever), especially if the aortic valve is diseased. The diagnosis depends on finding a rise in antibody titre. *Bacteroides*—anaerobic culture is required (and kept for up to 3 weeks). Fungi—*Candida, Aspergillus, Histoplasma*.
• Partly treated bacterial causes.
• Right-sided endocarditis.
• Systemic vasculitis, systemic lupus erythematosus (SLE), atrial myxoma, or the antiphospholipid syndrome (p. 124).
• Non-bacterial thrombotic endocarditis associated with carcinoma.

Constrictive pericarditis

Aetiology
This is now rare. It may be caused by tuberculosis following spread from the pleura or mediastinal lymph glands. It may follow acute viral or pyogenic pericarditis, but the cause is often unclear. Haemopericardium, irradiation and carcinoma account for a few. It never follows acute rheumatic fever. It may be stimulated by restrictive cardiomyopathy (p. 289).

Clinical features
Symptoms result from cardiac constriction with decreased filling and low cardiac output. Right heart failure predominates over left. Fatigue and ascites with little or no ankle swelling are characteristic, but dyspnoea and ankle swelling may occur later. Pulmonary oedema and paroxysmal nocturnal dyspnoea are rare.

Examination
The pulse is rapid and volume small and there may be arterial paradox (pulsus paradoxus), as with acute pericarditis. Atrial fibrillation is present in 30% of cases. Ascites may be the presenting feature and the elevated JVP may be missed because it is so high. The classical JVP signs of diastolic collapse (steep 'y' descent), and a further rise on inspiration (Kussmaul's sign) are often not observed. The liver, and sometimes the spleen, is enlarged. Ventricular contraction may cause localized indrawing of the chest wall at the apex. The heart sounds may be normal, although quiet. A third sound, brought about by an abrupt end to ventricular filling, may be present. There is no rub.

Investigation
• ECG: there may be widespread ST changes with low-voltage complexes, and atrial fibrillation.
• Chest X-ray: there may be calcification of the pericardium (often seen only in the lateral film). Cardiomegaly, if present, is less than one would expect from the degree of right (and possibly left) heart failure.
• Echocardiography shows the rigid, thickened pericardium, particularly if calcified, large atria with normal (or small) ventricles, and ventricular filling predominantly in early diastole.
• CT scan demonstrates the thickened pericardium in almost all cases.

Management

No action is needed if the patient is symptom-free and the assessment confirms mild disease. Close follow-up is essential. Pericardiectomy is performed if severe constriction is present.

Acute pericarditis

Aetiology

Pericarditis is common within the first week of acute myocardial infarction. Dressler syndrome is uncommon and occurs 2 weeks–2 months after myocardial infarction or cardiac surgery. It is characterized by fever, pleurisy, pericarditis and the presence of antibodies to heart muscle.

Infective pericarditis is usually a complication of chest infection. Acute benign pericarditis affects young men, often follows a respiratory infection and is probably viral. A rising antibody titre to Coxsackie B virus is sometimes found. Suppurative pericarditis is rare. It results from infection with staphylococcus or, occasionally, haemolytic streptococcus. Tuberculous pericarditis is very rare and non-suppurative.

Pericarditis occurs as part of systemic syndromes: rheumatic fever, SLE, severe uraemia, local extension of carcinoma of the bronchus and following trauma.

Clinical features

There is central, poorly localized tightness in the chest that varies with movement, posture and respiration. There may be pain referred to the left shoulder if the diaphragm is affected. The pericardial rub varies with time, position and respiration.

The signs of pericardial effusion without tamponade are an absent apex beat, a silent heart and disappearance of the rub.

Tamponade, which is rare, produces the following.

• Pulsus paradoxus. The pulse volume decreases in the normal person on inspiration. This is more marked with tamponade and is then known as pulsus paradoxus. The paradox that Kussmaul noted was that the heart continued to beat strongly while the peripheral arterial pulse virtually disappeared during inspiration.

• A rise in the JVP on inspiration (Kussmaul's sign).

Both pulsus paradoxus and Kussmaul's sign result from decreased cardiac filling on inspiration because of the descending diaphragm stretching the pericardium and increasing the intrapericardial pressure.

Assessment

ECG: there is raised concave elevation of the ST segment in most leads (especially II and V3–4) and T-wave inversion. The voltage is low in the presence of effusion.

Chest X-ray: it is unchanged in the absence of effusion. Effusion classically produces an enlarged pear-shaped cardiac shadow with loss of normal contours.

Echocardiography is the most sensitive way of detecting pericardial fluid with free space between the heart and percardium.

Management

Aspirate for tamponade (if the systolic arterial blood pressure falls below 90–100 mmHg). Treat the underlying condition. Steroids are used for SLE and in acute benign pericarditis if it is severe or prolonged. Recurrent effusion with tamponade is treated by insertion of a drain or creation of a pericardial window.

Syphilitic aortitis and carditis

Late syphilis is now very rare in the UK. Acquired syphilis affects the aorta, the aortic ring to produce dilatation or aneurysm, and aortic regurgitation and the coronary artery orifices to cause angina.

NB Congenital syphilis does not produce aortitis.

Pathology

Endarteritis, and occlusion of the vasa vasorum affects the aortic muscle wall, which becomes degenerate and fibrotic. Atheromatous plaques form over the damaged areas.

Clinical features
• Aortic regurgitation.
• Syphilitic angina. The angina is severe, attacks are long, often nocturnal, and respond poorly to glyceryl trinitrate.
• Syphilitic aneurysms of the ascending aorta, the arch of the aorta or in the abdomen.

Cardiomyopathy

This word means disorder of heart muscle. It is usually restricted to cardiomyopathies of unknown cause or association. They are classified into three major groups depending upon the clinical effects of the abnormality of the function of the left ventricle, which may be: hypertrophied, dilated or restricted.

Hypertrophic cardiomyopathy
Also known as HCM, it is usually familial. It results in asymmetrical LVH associated with:
• loss of left ventricular distensibility which leads to symptoms of dyspnoea, pulmonary oedema and syncope—some patients develop angina;
• hypertrophy, particularly of the left ventricle and septum with mitral regurgitation—in some patients this disappears with progression of the disease as the heart muscle fails.

Signs
There is a steep-rising, jerky pulse (unlike the slow-rising, plateau pulse of aortic valve stenosis), cardiac hypertrophy, a palpable atrial beat followed by a late systolic aortic ejection murmur, usually heard best in the left third and fourth intercostal spaces. There may be associated signs of mitral regurgitation. Complications include atrial fibrillation (10%), systemic embolism, congestive heart failure and sudden death.

Investigation
Echocardiography shows asymmetrical septal hypertrophy, systolic anterior movement of the mitral valve and a narrow left ventricular cavity with hypertrophied trabeculae and papillary muscles. A 24-h ECG record may identify those most at risk from sudden death from dysrhythmias.

Management
β-Adrenergic blockade is given to increase left ventricular compliance and reduce the incidence of dysrhythmias and angina. The response is variable. If the patient develops atrial fibrillation, anticoagulants and digoxin or verapamil are added. Serious arrhythmias may need amiodarone. Patients are at risk from endocarditis. Treat for cardiac failure and if medical therapy fails, consider transplantation.

Dilated (congestive) cardiomyopathy
This is very rarely familial.

The label 'congestive cardiomyopathy' covers a large group of aetiologically unrelated disorders which tend to present as low-output congestive heart failure. By convention, the more common and more easily diagnosed myocardial disorders are excluded, i.e. ischaemic, hypertensive and rheumatic heart diseases.

Angina (10%), systemic and pulmonary infarcts, conduction defects and arrhythmias occur.

Aetiology
• Alcoholism and thiamine deficiency (beriberi).
• Infections: viruses, e.g. influenza A_2, Coxsackie B, *Toxoplasma*, diphtheria.
• Infiltrations: sarcoidosis, amyloidosis (primary and secondary to myeloma), haemochromatosis.
• Collagen disease: SLE, polyartertis nodosa, diffuse systemic sclerosis.
• Muscular dystrophies and Friedreich's ataxia (p. 106).
• Endocrine: hyper- and hypothyroidism.
• Postpartum.

Management
Bed rest, diuretics and ACE inhibitors form the basis of treatment of the cardiac failure. Anticoagulants are given because of the risks of embolism. Any underlying pathology (e.g. thyroid disease, collagen disease) should be treated appropriately.

Restrictive cardiomyopathy

The efficiency of the ventricles as pumps is restricted by endocardial fibrosis or by granulation tissue—respectively endomyocardial fibrosis (EMF) of equatorial Africa or Löffler eosinophilic endomyocardial disease. In the UK, amyloidosis is the most common cause of this rare condition, and is best diagnosed by endomyocardial biopsy.

Peripheral arterial disease

There are four common clinical syndromes: intermittent claudication, acute obstruction, ischaemic foot and Raynaud's phenomenon.

Intermittent claudication

Ninety per cent are males over 50 years of age. The disorder is associated with smoking and diabetes mellitus, occasionally with hyperlipidaemia and occasionally precipitated by anaemia. Obstruction may be femoropopliteal (80%), aortoiliac (15%) or distal (5%).

Diagnosis

The history is of pain in the calf on effort with rapid relief by rest. The Leriche syndrome is buttock claudication with impotence. The major peripheral arterial pulses are reduced or absent. There may be arterial bruits over the aorta, iliac or femoral arteries. The tissues of the leg atrophy with reduced muscle bulk and hair loss is common. There may be cyanosis, pallor or redness, oedema, ulcers or gangrene.

Doppler ultrasound is useful to exclude obstruction in doubtful cases. Arteriography is required if surgery is contemplated.

Prognosis

The symptom indicates generalized vascular disease and 80% die from cardiovascular or cerebrovascular disease. Life expectancy is similar to a healthy population 10 years older. Diabetes mellitus and persistent smoking are associated with a worse prognosis. Age, cerebrovascular disease and ischaemic heart disease are poor prognostic features. Leg gangrene is uncommon.

Management

• Stop smoking.
• Manage hyperlipidaemia and take prophylactic aspirin.
• Exercise within the effort tolerance to help develop collateral vessels. Treat obesity, hypertension and hyperuricaemia, despite the lack of firm evidence that this affects the prognosis: a positive attitude to therapy is itself reassuring.
• Check for diabetes, polycythaemia and anaemia and treat if necessary.
• Keep the body and arms warm, and the legs cool.
• Attend carefully to foot hygiene.
• Surgery. Endarterectomy is indicated if there is a high block with good distal blood flow on angiography. Bypass (prosthetic or vein graft) surgery may be indicated if angiography shows the vessels to be satisfactory distal to the block.
• Dilatation of narrowed arteries using balloon catheter angioplasty may be successful. Sympathectomy is rarely successful in relieving symptoms of muscle ischaemia.

Acute obstruction

This may be caused by thrombosis or to embolism (usually blood clot in atrial fibrillation). Ninety per cent are in the legs.

Diagnosis

Pain (usually severe) is associated with numbness, paraesthesiae and paresis. There is pallor and coldness of the limb below the obstruction followed by cyanosis. The limb becomes anaesthetic and the arterial pulses weak or absent.

Management

Maintain the limb at room temperature or below to decrease local cell metabolism and therefore its oxygen demand.

Assess early for disobliteration, which is the treatment of choice, even if shocked. The embolus is sent to the laboratory for histology and culture. The muscles are probably viable if firm and tender and resist movement. The skin is probably not viable if it is densely cyanosed and anaesthetic.

Hyperbaric oxygen, if available, may be helpful. Heparin and low-molecular-weight dextrans are used while awaiting surgery and, in addition, thrombolytic agents and vasodilators may be tried if surgery is contraindicated or delayed.

Ischaemic foot

This is caused by chronic arterial obstruction distal to the knees. It is most commonly seen in diabetes, and is associated with neuropathy and local infection.

Symptoms
- Areas of necrosis and ulceration.
- Pain in the foot (often not present in diabetics because of associated peripheral neuropathy).
- Intermittent claudication.

Signs
If the large arteries are narrowed there is pallor and/or cyanosis, empty veins in the feet with trophic changes in nails and absence of hair. The feet are cold and pulses diminished or absent.

In diabetes, it is often chiefly the small vessels that are affected. The foot pulses are often present despite severe ischaemia of the toes.

Management
Foot hygiene is important, especially in diabetes. Pain may be severe and require morphine. Sympathectomy may improve skin blood supply and reduce pain. Endarterectomy or vascular grafting are seldom technically feasible and angiography therefore seldom indicated. If amputation is required it is frequently above-knee. Conservative management includes stopping smoking and various drugs which are not fully evaluated. These include agents to reduce platelet stickiness and blood viscosity, e.g. aspirin.

Raynaud's phenomenon
Definition
Intermittent, cold-precipitated, symmetrical attacks of pallor and/or cyanosis of the digits without evidence of arterial obstructive disease. The digits become white (arterial spasm), then blue (cyanosis) and finally red (reactive arterial dilatation).

Aetiology
- Idiopathic and familial, usually in young women (Raynaud's disease).
- Collagen disease, especially SLE and scleroderma.
- Arterial obstruction, e.g. cervical rib.
- Trauma, usually in occupations involving vibrating tools (vibration white finger).
- Drugs, including β-blockers, the contraceptive pill and ergot derivatives.

Management
Treatment is disappointing. The hands and feet should be kept warm and free from infection. The patient is reassured about the long-term prognosis (usually good) and advised to stop smoking. Electrically heated gloves can be very helpful. Calcium antagonists (e.g. nifedipine) or patches of glyceryl trinitrate can be tried. Sympathectomy is sometimes successful as a last resort, particularly in the presence of recurring skin sepsis. Intravenous prostacyclin (epoprostenol) has been used in severe cases.

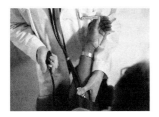

Dermatology

The most common dermatological diseases are dermatitis, psoriasis, acne vulgaris, drug eruptions, athlete's foot, warts and basal cell carcinoma.

Psoriasis

This affects about 1–2% of the population and may be almost inapparent, or cosmetically debilitating or chronic. Rarely, it may be acute and life-threatening. Partial remissions are characteristic.

Psoriasis may present acutely with multiple, small, round, silver-scaly lesions on an erythematous base on the body, limbs and scalp (guttate psoriasis). Removal of the scales leaves small bleeding points. This tends to remit spontaneously over 2–4 months, but some patients subsequently develop chronic psoriasis.

Similar chronic skin lesions occur mainly on the extensor surfaces (back, elbows, knees) and scalp, but any area of skin may be affected and symmetry is a feature. Thimble-pitting of the nail plate is common. In flexures it looks different with smooth, confluent red areas and pruritus is then fairly common, although not necessarily in the flexural parts.

Psoriatic arthropathy occurs in 5–10% and resembles seronegative rheumatoid arthritis and is associated with thimble-pitting in the nail plate (p. 135).

Treatment
Topical treatments
Salicylic acid (2–6% ointment or lotion) reduces hyperkeratotic, scaling lesions. It is often used in combination with coal tar or dithranol.

Coal tar paste is effective but is unpleasant to use. Coal tar shampoo can be used for scalp lesions, and coal tar baths if lesions are extensive.

Dithranol is applied to lesions, covered with a dressing, and left for an hour or more. Skin irritation can occur (start with 0.1% and gradually build up to 5%). It stains skin, hair and clothes brown.

Calcipotriol and *tacalcitol* are vitamin D derivatives that can be used topically for mild to moderate psoriasis.

Systemic treatments
Psoralens and ultraviolet A phototherapy (PUVA) is successful in clearing and delaying recurrence in chronic psoriasis. There is a very slightly increased risk of skin cancer.

Retinoids (vitamin A derivatives) are used for severe, resistant psoriasis. Side-effects include dryness and cracking of skin and lips, transient hair loss, myalgia, hepatotoxicity and a rise in plasma lipids. They are teratogenic and must be avoided in pregnancy.

Methotrexate and cyclosporin A are used for severe resistant psoriasis but only under expert supervision.

Lichen planus

Lichen planus is an uncommon disorder, usually of the middle-aged, who present with an irritating rash affecting the flexures of the wrist and forearms, the trunk and the ankles. About 10% have nail involvement. The rash consists of discrete, purple, shiny, polygonal papules with fine white lines passing through them (Wickham's striae), often occurring in scratch marks and other sites of injury (Köbner's phenomenon). The lesions may be widespread or confined to one or two papules. Lesions may occur on the buccal mucosa with a white, lacy network or in the nails without other lesions on the skin.

The disorder usually resolves within 6 months but recurrences may occur. The cause is unknown but many drugs may produce an identical eruption, e.g. gold, antimalarials and antituberculous drugs. The dermis is infiltrated with T cells. Only 50% resolve in 9 months (85% in 18 months).

Treatment
Topical steroids may be sufficient to suppress symptoms until resolution has occurred. Systemic steroids may be required to suppress the pruritus of widespread lichen planus, especially plantar and palmar lesions.

Pityriasis rosea

The rash is preceded by a *herald patch*—a solitary, red, scaly, oval lesion on the abdomen or over the scapular area. This is followed after 1–2 weeks by a mildly itching macular rash which may cover the entire trunk, the upper thighs and upper arms. The macules tend to be oval and aligned along the natural skin creases with peripheral scales. The disorder occurs in small outbreaks in schools and families and may be caused by a virus.

The disorder is self-limiting, usually within 6 weeks.

Treatment
Mild sedation can help. Mild to moderate topical steroids may be needed.

Dermatitis and eczema

Dermatitis is often used to refer only to skin inflammation caused by an exogenous agent. The term is, however, synonymous with eczema, a term used colloquially for endogenous dermatitis, i.e. atopic dermatitis. It affects 10% of the population.

Clinical features
Clinically, the term describes a patchy, diffuse, irritating and sometimes painful lesion, often with vesicles that rupture to leave a raw weeping surface. Itching may be the dominant symptom. Secondary infection is common. In chronic lesions scaling may be present and the skin may become thickened (lichenification). Healed lesions do not scar but may pigment.

Histologically, the initial abnormality is oedema of the epidermis and this finally results in vesicle formation. Vesicles or oedema dominate, depending upon the thickness of the horny layer. In eczema of the face and genitalia oedema is marked, but on the palms and soles vesicles are more prominent.

Contact dermatitis
There are two groups, *irritant* and *allergic*.
1 *Irritant* contact dermatitis follows prolonged or repeated exposure to physical or chemical trauma (e.g. industrial solvents) and may occur in anyone exposed. It is a common problem in certain occupations such as hairdressers and engineers.
2 *Allergic* contact dermatitis requires previous sensitization and may subsequently be provoked by very small quantities of the allergen. The rash is usually confined to the sites of exposure. A careful history is often necessary to discover possible sensitizers. Patch tests should be performed on all suspected cases. Epoxy resins, parabens (preservatives in cosmetics and creams), chromates, nickel, rubber, dyes, perfumes, antibiotics (topical), some plants and antiseptics are frequent sensitizers.

Seborrhoeic dermatitis
A red, itchy, inflamed and scaly remittent dermatitis which appears on oily areas of the skin, especially around the head, including the scalp, eyebrows and creases of the nose and ears. It also occurs in flexures (axillae, inframammary and perineal) as intertrigo and, with ammonia from urine, as nappy rash.

Atopic dermatitis
Atopy refers to a hereditary tendency to develop allergic responses to various allergens

and is usually shown by asthma, rhinitis and conjunctivitis and well as dermatitis. About one-quarter of the UK population is atopic. Atopic dermatitis usually presents in infancy in an individual (and from a family) with other atopic manifestations. Prick tests to common allergens are usually positive and serum immunoglobulin E (IgE) levels often raised, although this does not help management. There is itching and inflammation, usually flexural, and lichenification is common.

Treatment
The local irritant or sensitizer must be removed if possible and practicable. Dietary manipulation and hyposensitization have only a minor role in routine management. Many commercial soaps contain such irritants and it is best, therefore, to wash with water only or to use soap substitutes. If the lesion is weeping, local soaks (e.g. 1 : 8000 potassium permanganate) will aid healing, and then apply topical mild to moderate steroids. If dry, an emollient such as aqueous cream may be sufficient, but topical steroids may also be required. Sedative antihistamines by mouth may relieve pruritus and allow sleep. Systemic antibiotics are given if secondary infection occurs in the skin.

Acne vulgaris

A disease chiefly of puberty (but onset can be up to 40 years) in which androgens cause increased sebaceous gland activity. Plugging of hair follicles by keratin causes retention of sebum producing the characteristic comedo (blackhead). These may become secondarily infected with skin bacteria. The comedos are distributed on the face, the shoulders and upper thorax. The skin is usually greasy. It usually disappears in early adult life, often with residual scarring. Acne is seen in Cushing syndrome (p. 149).

Treatment
Frequent washing with soap and water or local detergents (e.g. cetrimide) to degrease the skin.

Topical benzoyl peroxide cream or lotion (2.5–10%) or antibiotics (clindamycin or erythromycin) usually helps, often with oral antibiotics.

Oral antibiotics such as oxytetracyline (or erythromycin) 1 g/day are given for 6 months or longer and are usually effective for mild to moderate disease, although results may take 3 months to appear.

Isotretinoin (Roaccutane) is a vitamin A derivative taken orally for severe disease when topical therapy and oral antibiotics have failed. Side-effects are common, including facial erythema, dry skin, myalgia and a rise in plasma lipids and abnormal liver function tests. It is teratogenic.

Rosacea

This is a disorder, more common in women, beginning usually after 30 years of age, with erythema, papules, pustules and telangiectasia over the cheeks, nose, chin and forehead.

Treatment
Avoid precipitating factors (e.g. hot drinks, sunlight, alcohol and topical steroid preparations).

Oxytetracycline (500 mg b.d.) may be effective when given in the long-term intermittently, 2 months at a time with or without topical metronidazole.

Fungus infections

Candidiasis (*Monilia*, thrush)
This yeast infection, although common in fit people, should raise the suspicion of underlying diabetes mellitus (and the rare hypoparathyroidism), or other factors which suppress normal immune mechanisms, e.g. leukaemia, Hodgkin disease, steroid therapy, and acquired immunodeficiency syndrome (AIDS) when overwhelming systemic infection may occur.

The nail folds are commonly involved, sometimes producing obvious paronychia. Thrush occurs frequently in the vagina, on the penis, and on the oral mucosa, especially in users of inhaled steroids. It may spread to affect the entire gastrointestinal tract, especially after antibiotics.

NB Oesophageal moniliasis has a characteristic radiological appearance with barium adhering to the patches of *Monilia*.

Treatment

Nystatin orally (500 000 units 6-hourly) and imidazole creams (e.g. clotrimazole) are the drugs of choice but may be ineffective if the underlying disorder does not respond to specific therapy. Itraconazole is used orally.

Pityriasis versicolor

This is a yeast infection with *Pityrosporum orbiculare* (*Malassezia furfur*) usually of the trunk which causes brownish, scaly lesions of varying size which may coalesce. Depigmentation, which may last many months after effective treatment, may resemble vitiligo because only the unaffected skin pigments in sunbathers. Diagnosis is made by skin scrapings. An application of 2.5% selenium sulphide repeated after a week may be sufficient. Topical imidazole for several weeks may be used.

Ringworm (tinea)

The ringworm fungi are a group of related organisms (*Trichophyton*, *Microsporum*, *Epidermophyton*) which live in the keratin layer of the skin. The disorders produced are described after their site on the body—tinea pedis, tinea cruris and tinea capitis. Diagnosis is confirmed either by observing fungal hyphae in skin scrapings treated with potassium hydroxide or by culture.

Tinea pedis (athlete's foot)

The most common of the group affecting the interdigital skin, usually between the fourth and fifth toes. The nails may be involved. The lesion is irritating and the skin appears white and macerated. It may provide an entry for bacterial infection (streptococcal cellulitis). The infection tends to be recurrent or chronic. The disorder must be distinguished from simple skin maceration, atopic dermatitis, psoriasis and footwear (contact) dermatitis.

Tinea cruris

This may result from spread of infection from the feet. The lesion affects the upper inner thighs and has a slightly raised, well-defined, spreading scaly margin. In contrast, *Monilia* is symmetrical, with ill-defined edges and small satellite lesions. Tinea gives pruritus.

Tinea capitis

A disease of prepubertal children who present with an area of baldness with scaly skin and stumps of broken hair. Some infections show characteristic fluorescence when viewed under Wood's light. The underlying scalp is scaly and may become secondarily infected.

Treatment of dermatophytes in general

Topical imidazole (e.g. clotrimazole, miconazole) or terbinafine treatment is usually effective for localized areas, but if the infection is severe, widespread or if there is nail and hair involvement, systemic therapy may be needed. For nail infections, oral terbinafine (6 weeks for fingers, 12 weeks for toes) is usually effective but has the risk of serious adverse effects such as Stevens–Johnson syndrome and hepatitis. It should only be started after laboratory confirmation of the diagnosis.

Drug eruptions

Many drugs can produce eruptions which may be erythematous, maculopapular, urticarial or purpuric. The pattern for any one drug may not always be the same and most drugs may at times produce one or other type of reaction, i.e. virtually any drug can produce any eruption—an overstatement but necessary to consider in any patient with a rash. The most common now are the thiazides, allopurinol, captopril and penicillamine. Topical antibiotics, particularly the penicillins and the neomycin group, frequently produce skin eruptions. The common drug rash of ampicillin is maculopapular and may be specific to it and not to all penicillins. (It is almost universal in patients with infectious mononucleosis.)

Urticarial reactions

The penicillins are probably the most common group of drugs which produce urticaria. Of all patients receiving a penicillin, 1–2% have adverse reactions, and many of them (if asked) give a history of previous sensitivity. Reactions are more frequent in adults and are probably a measure of previous exposure. Sensitivity to one penicillin may mean sensitivity to all, and cephalosporin sensitivity occurs in about 1 in 10 patients. The urticarial eruption usually occurs 3–7 days after therapy is started. Rarely, an acute hypersensitivity reaction occurs within minutes and is associated with serum sickness-like features of fever, wheezing, arthralgia and hypotension. If chronic, patients should avoid dairy produce as antibiotics are generously used in farming.

Other drugs that produce urticarial reactions include barbiturates, salicylates, streptomycin, sulphonamides, tetracyclines, phenothiazines and chloramphenicol.

Purpura

This may be a feature of any severe drug reaction and results from capillary damage. Bone marrow suppression by gold, carbimazole or phenylbutazone may cause thrombocytopenic purpura (p. 310).

Other disorders

• Light sensitivity (amiodarone, sulphonamides, tetracyclines, thiazides, chlorpropamide, tolbutamide, griseofulvin, chlorpromazine).
• Fixed drug eruption. This describes an eruption that has the same character and occurs in the same site when the causative drug is taken. Phenolphthalein, used in some laxatives, is frequently incriminated. Other drugs include penicillin, phenylbutazone, aspirin and sulphonamides.
• Lichen planus (gold, phenylbutazone, quinidine, p. 291).
• Exfoliative dermatitis (gold, barbiturates, phenytoin, chlorpropamide).

• Erythema multiforme (p. 298).
• Systemic lupus erythematosus (p. 122).

Management
• Stop all drugs.
• Oral antihistamines for urticaria.
• Mild topical steroids may help itching.
• Adrenaline (epinephrine) may be life-saving in acute hypersensitivity reactions including shock and angioedema (p. 239), and systemic steroids may be required in severe but less acute cases.

Skin manifestations of systemic disease

Erythema nodosum
Clinical presentation
Tender, red, raised lesions usually on the shins and less frequently the thighs and upper limbs. The lesions pass through the colour changes of a bruise. It is five times more common in females and occurs usually between 20 and 50 years of age. Arthropathy, especially in the legs, occurs in 50% and bilateral hilar lymph gland enlargement is usually seen on chest X-ray in sarcoidosis.

Aetiology
• Sarcoidosis is probably the most common cause in the UK (35%).
• Streptococcal infection and hence rheumatic fever.
• Tuberculosis.
• Drugs, particularly sulphonamides and including penicillin and salicylates.
• Other causes include ulcerative colitis, Crohn disease, Behçet disease and fungal infections (e.g. *Histoplasma*). Erythema nodosum occasionally occurs as an isolated, sometimes recurrent, disorder.

Lyme disease (erythema chronicum migrans, ECM)
Borrelia burgdorferi is a spirochaete spread by ixodid ticks from deer and rodents to humans. The infection may produce clinical features in the skin (ECM), joints, central nervous system and heart.

ECM begins as an indistinct red macule, from around the tick bite, which enlarges progressively.

There may be other features of infection with fever, malaise, myalgia and lymphadenopathy plus:
- migratory arthralgia, usually of large joints;
- neurological features including aseptic meningitis and cranial nerve lesions (especially seventh nerve); or
- cardiac disease with atrioventricular block and myocarditis.

The diagnosis is confirmed serologically by the presence of a high titre of antibodies to *B. burgdorferi*, and treatment is with tetracycline, penicillin or a third-generaton cephalosporin (e.g. cefotaxime).

Haemolytic streptococcal infection

Skin lesions frequently occur as a sign of streptococcal sensitivity and present as erythema nodosum, erythema marginatum (very rare but virtually diagnostic of rheumatic fever) and erythema multiforme (also occurs in rheumatic fever). Skin infections produce cellulitis or erysipelas (slightly raised, well-circumscribed, acutely painful, bright red lesions of half to one hand's-breadth in diameter). The elderly are more commonly affected and the legs and face the most common sites. There may be generalized symptoms of headache, fever and vomiting. Response to parenteral penicillin is usually rapid. Transient skin rashes are common with streptococcal infection but the classical endotoxic rash of scarlet fever is now rarely seen.

Herpes zoster (shingles)

Although it usually occurs in isolation, herpes zoster may occur in any debilitating disease and particularly with Hodgkin disease, the leukaemias and patients on steroids. The lesion consists of groups of vesicles on an inflamed base. Pain precedes the lesions in nerve root distributions. Postherpetic neuralgia may be severe and intractable. The virus (varicella-zoster) is identical with the virus of chickenpox and denotes earlier clinical or subclinical infection in childhood. The virus remains latent within dorsal root ganglia until diminished resistance allows reactivation. Patients should be isolated from the non-immune and immuno-compromised population until the lesions are crusted to prevent spread. Oral acyclovir can speed healing and parenteral acyclovir is usually required in the immunosuppressed (p. 331).

Malignancy

Generalized pruritus is associated with tumours of the reticuloendothelial system such as Hodgkin disease (also renal and hepatic failure, and old age).

Dermatomyositis (see p. 128)

Twenty per cent of adult cases occur in association with carcinoma, leukaemia or lymphoma.

Acanthosis nigricans

Brown pigmented warts or plaques most marked in the axilla are associated with underlying carcinoma, particularly of the bronchus, gastrointestinal tract, prostate, breast and uterus. It is very rare. Benign forms occur, especially in the obese.

Other manifestations

These include acquired ichthyosis (Hodgkin disease), chronic myeloid leukaemia, skin infiltration, secondary skin metastases, migratory thrombophlebitis and exfoliative dermatitis.

Xanthomatosis

Tendon xanthomas, usually most easily felt in the Achilles tendon and in the finger extensors on the dorsum of the hand, are characteristic of familial hypercholesterolaemia and associated with premature cardiac death. Xanthelasmas are dull yellow plaques commonly in the inner angles of the eyelids. They may, although not always, indicate hyperlipidaemia with raised serum cholesterol and are associated with myxoedema, diabetes and primary biliary cirrhosis. Eruptive xanthomas may occur with greatly elevated serum lipid levels.

Other rare manifestations

The following conditions are well recognized:

- necrobiosis lipoidica in diabetes mellitus (p. 158);
- pretibial myxoedema in thyrotoxicosis (p. 142);
- lupus pernio (a purple eruption) in sarcoid (p. 246);
- lupus vulgaris and erythema induratum (Bazin disease) in tuberculosis (p. 247);
- *café-au-lait* spots and multiple neurofibromas of neurofibromatosis (von Recklinghausen's disease, p. 104);
- light sensitivity and blistering in porphyria (p. 165); and
- ECM in Lyme disease (p. 295).

Mucosal ulceration

This is usually localized to the buccal mucosa but may be associated with generalized disease. Causes include aphthous ulcers, herpes simplex ulceration, herpangina (Coxsackievirus type A), agranulocytic ulcers in aplastic anaemia usually drug-induced or leukaemic, erythema multiforme and Stevens–Johnson syndrome, Behçet disease (p. 126) and under dental plates (often *Candida*).

Bullous lesions

Drugs may produce bullous eruptions. There are four other primary bullous skin disorders that are well recognized. All are rare.

Dermatitis herpetiformis
All patients have a gluten-sensitive enteropathy, although in 50% it is subclinical. The skin of the limbs and trunk is affected. In 80% histocompatibility locus antigen (HLA) B8 is present. Subepidermal IgA is usually present.

Clinical presentation
Symmetrical clusters of urticarial lesions on the occiput, interscapular and gluteal regions and extensor aspects of the elbows and knees. Vesicles follow and only rarely become bullous as skin trauma is provoked by the intolerable itching. There are seldom lesions in the mouth and there is no fever.

Prognosis and management
The disease starts acutely and may remit spontaneously, but tends to become chronic. Secondary bacterial infection is common. Oral dapsone or sulphonamides are the drugs of choice for the skin lesion. All patients require a gluten-free diet.

Pemphigus vulgaris
Clinical presentation
A rare disease of middle age, some of the characteristics of which are explained by the very superficial site of the lesion: there is splitting in the epidermis above the basal layer. Degeneration of the cells of the epidermis (acantholysis) is seen on skin biopsy. IgG is present on the intercellular substance and patients have antibodies against desmoglein. Clinically, it presents with widespread erosions and relatively few bullae (because they rupture so easily) spread over the limbs and trunk. Most (90%) patients have lesions in the mouth and these may be the only lesions at first. The surrounding skin is normal. The superficial skin layer can be moved over the deeper layers (Nikolsky's sign) and tends to disintegrate, allowing secondary infection. Lesions appear at sites of pressure and trauma and are then extremely painful. There is fever and severe constitutional disturbance. It may be precipitated by drugs, e.g. penicillamine.

Complications and management
Secondary bacterial infection is common and septicaemia may result. Protein loss from weeping skin may occur in widespread disease. Very high doses of prednisolone (initially 60–100 mg, later reduced) is given to control the eruptions. Immunosuppression with azathioprine, and intravenous immunoglobulin may be required.

Pemphigoid
Pemphigoid is a disease of the elderly in which the lesion is at the basement membrane between the dermis and epidermis—deeper in the

skin than in pemphigus. IgG is deposited in the basement membrane zone and patients have antibodies against bullous pemphigoid antigens (BPAG1 and BPAG2). Acantholysis is not seen on histology. Clinically, it presents after prodromal itch for a few weeks, with the sudden onset of bullae on the limbs and, to a lesser extent, on the trunk. The large, tense, subepidermal bullae have less tendency to break than in pemphigus but can be provoked by trauma. Nikolsky's sign is negative. The surrounding skin shows erythematous patches. Mucosal ulceration is rare (10%). Secondary infection is common, and the patients are not usually ill.

Management

Steroids (prednisolone 40–60 mg/day) are required to control the eruption and may be required in low dosage for years.

Pemphigoid gestationis (herpes gestationis) presents with vesicular and urticarial lesions during the second or third trimesters of pregnancy. It resolves after delivery and is associated with an IgG antibody against bullous pemphigoid antigens.

Erythema multiforme

Clinical presentation

Erythema multiforme is a generalized disease that may present as an isolated skin disorder or with prodromal symptoms of fever, sore throat, headache, arthralgia and gastroenteritis. These are followed by a pleomorphic erythematous eruption that may become bullous. The forearms and legs are commonly affected first and the rash may spread centripetally to involve the entire body. The buccal mucosa may be involved. Target lesions—concentric rings of differing shades of erythema—are

characteristic but late. The disease remits spontaneously in 5–6 weeks but may recur.

Stevens–Johnson syndrome is a severe form of erythema multiforme characterized by systemic illness with lesions in the mouth, conjunctiva, anal and genital regions.

Aetiology

The disease sometimes follows drug therapy (sulphonamides, penicillin, salicylates and barbiturates) and herpes simplex infection. The aetiology often remains unknown.

Management

• Withdraw drugs.
• Local treatment with mild potency steroids for pruritus.
• Stevens–Johnson syndrome may require steroids to suppress the eruption but infection must be identified and specifically treated.

Skin pigmentation

This is usually racial or caused by sun tanning. Other causes include pregnancy and the oral contraceptive (chloasma), Addison disease, Nelson syndrome (postadrenalectomy), haemochromatosis, cirrhosis, uraemia, heavy-metal and chronic arsenic poisoning. In neurofibromatosis the patches are of varying size, discrete and associated with subcutaneous neurofibromas. In Peutz–Jeghers syndrome there are small, discrete patches around the mouth and multiple small intestinal polyps. Other dermatological causes include the post-inflammatory changes that follow a number of dermatoses. Remember cosmetic preparations intended to simulate suntan. The *café-au-lait* pigmentation of bacterial endocarditis is now rarely seen because patients are treated early.

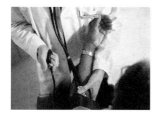

Haematology

Diagnosis of haematological disorders is made or confirmed on the basis of laboratory findings.

Peripheral blood film features
- Reticulocytes, (active marrow)—haemolysis or chronic blood loss.
- Anisocytes (variation in red cell size) or poikilocytes (variation in red cell shape)—iron deficiency.
- Target cells ('Mexican hat' cells)—thalassaemia.
- Rouleau formation (clumping together of red cells)—raised ESR (check for myeloma).
- Burr cells (irregular 'crinkled' red cell membrane)—renal failure, carcinoma.
- Hypersegmented polymorphs—B_{12} or folic acid deficiency.
- Howell–Jolly bodies (remnants of nuclear material)—splenectomy (or non-functioning spleen).
- Blast cells (immature cells)—acute leukaemia.
- Eosinophilia—parasitic infection, allergy, occasionally systemic vasculitis or Hodgkin's disease.

Reticulocytes. Normal range $10–100 \times 10^9/l$. Reticulocytes are premature red cells in which traces of nucleoprotein remain as fine, reticular strands. They are larger than mature red cells and, if increased, may cause macrocytosis.

An increase (reticulocytosis) suggests marrow hyperactivity because of:
- loss or destruction of red cells, e.g. bleeding;
- a response to treatment of anaemia e.g. of pernicious anaemia with vitamin B_{12}; or
- haemolysis.

Normocytic anaemia. MCV in the normal range. Usually anaemia secondary to chronic disease. It is usually insidious, not progressive and fairly mild ($> 9\,g/dl$) except in chronic renal failure. It may become slightly hypochromic and/or microcytic. The white cell count and platelets are normal. The serum transferrin is normal or low but, unlike iron deficiency, the serum ferritin is normal or high (with increased iron stores in the bone marrow). A marrow examination may show malignant disease (leukaemia, mycloma, metastasis) or myelofibrosis.

Anaemia of chronic diseases occurs in:
- chronic renal failure—check serum urea, creatinine, creatinine clearance;
- chronic liver failure—check liver function tests, γ-glutamyl transferase, prothrombin time;
- connective tissue disease (e.g. rheumatoid arthritis, SLE)—check ESR, C-reactive protein and autoantibodies: rheumatoid factor, anti-deoxyribonucleic acid (DNA) antibodies (SLE), anti-neutrophil cytoplasm antibodies (ANCA; present in systemic vasculitis);
- chronic infection—abscesses, tuberculosis, bacterial endocarditis; and
- malignant neoplasms.

NB The anaemia of chronic renal failure can be effectively reversed by treatment with recombinant human erythropoietin.

Microcytic anaemia. MCV is low, e.g. $< 80\,fl$. The serum iron is either low (iron deficiency or anaemia secondary to chronic disease) or normal (haemoglobinopathies, usually thalassaemia minor, p. 306). The spread of red cell size (red cell distribution width, RDW) tends to be increased in most conditions

REFERENCE VALUES

Hb (male)	$12.5–16.5 \times 10^9/l$
Hb (female)	$11.5–15.5 \times 10^9/l$

An automated cell counter (e.g. Coulter counter) gives the following readings:

Haematocrit (PCV; male)	0.42–0.53
Haematocrit (PCV; female)	0.39–0.45
Red cell count (male)	$4.5–6.5 \times 10^{12}/l$
Red cell count (female)	$3.9–5.6 \times 101^{12}/l$
MCV	80–96 fl*
RDW	11.1–13.7†
MCH	27–31 pg‡
MCHC	32–36 g/dl§
Transferrin (iron-binding plasma protein)	2–3g/l
	Raised in iron deficiency (and pregnancy)
	Reduced in anaemia of chronic disease, acute inflammation and protein loss
Ferritin	Correlates with tissue iron stores (iron is stored in the tissues in two forms, ferritin and haemosiderin). Only low in iron-deficiency states

*MCV is haematocrit/red cell count.
†This is an automated measure of anisocytosis: the variability of red cell size.
‡MCH is Hb/red cell count.
§MCHC is Hb/haematocrit. MCH and MCHC are of limited use in the differential diagnosis of anaemia.
Hb, haemoglobin; MCH, mean corpuscular haemoglobin; MCHC, mean corpuscular haemoglobin concentration; MCV, mean corpuscular volume; PCV, packed cell volume; RDW, red cell distribution width.

Table 18.1 Haematological values in anaemia. A significant difference between one Hb reading and the next is 1 g/dl. If you are attempting to analyse anaemia and are looking at a Coulter-style full blood count, first check the MCV. See if the cells are normal (normocytic), small (microcytic) or large (macrocytic).

causing microcytic anaemia, but normal when the microcytosis is caused by chronic disease and thalassaemia minor. The MCH is usually low (hypochromic), i.e. < 25 pg.

Iron deficiency is caused by poor intake, poor absorption, poor iron use by the marrow or increased blood loss (menstrually or from the gut). Check with serum iron (very low) and transferrin, which tends to be high. If in doubt check the serum ferritin (low) and demonstrate low iron stores in the marrow.

Macrocytic anaemia. MCV > 96, and often > 100 fl. NB Only perform check tests after full clinical review:
• vitamin B_{12} deficiency (usually pernicious anaemia)—check serum B_{12};
• folic acid deficiency—check red cell folate;
• hypothyroidism—check thyroid function tests;
• liver disease (usually excess alcohol)—check liver function, including γ-glutamyl transferase. Check the haemoglobin, and reticulocyte response to therapy. If in doubt, marrow examination may provide a definitive diagnosis (megaloblastic). If necessary, when pernicious anaemia has already been treated with vitamin B_{12}, it may still be diagnosed with a Schilling test (B_{12} absorption before and after intrinsic factor).

Anaemia secondary to chronic disease
Anaemia about 10 g/dl, usually normocytic (or slightly microcytic), associated with chronic

infection, malignant disease, chronic renal failure and the collagen diseases. The serum iron is characteristically reduced, and so is the transferrin (iron-binding capacity), unlike the findings in iron-deficiency anaemia. The marrow iron stores are increased, but the iron is not incorporated fully into red cell precursors.

Pancytopenia. This is a rare combination of anaemia, leucopenia and thrombocytopenia. It is caused by either:

1 reduced production of cells, caused by:
(a) bone marrow infiltration (leukaemia, myeloma, carcinoma, myelofibrosis)
(b) bone marrow aplasia: (idiopathic or drug-induced (e.g. NSAIDs, chloramphenicol, chemotherapy for malignancy); severe vitamin B_{12} or folate deficiency); or

2 increased destruction of cells, caused by hypersplenism; or autoimmune disease (e.g. SLE).

Bone marrow examination is the most important investigation in distinguishing these causes.

Marrow suppression

Secondary bone marrow failure may affect one or all of the formed elements of the blood; red cells, white cells or platelets. It may be idiopathic or secondary to infiltration, drugs, (gold, penicillamine, chloramphenicol, carbimazole), radiation, leukaemias, infections or other disorders such as uraemia, hypothyroidism and chronic disease.

Erythrocyte sedimentation rate measures the rate of sedimentation (in mm/h) of red cells in a column of anticoagulated blood. Rapid sedimentation (increased ESR) suggests increased levels of immunoglobulins or acute phase proteins, which cause the red cells to stick together. A raised ESR is therefore a non-specific indicator of inflammation or infection. The ESR is usually very high in myeloma.

A very high ESR (> 100 mm/h), suggests:

1 multiple myeloma;
2 systemic lupus erythematosus (SLE);
3 temporal arteritis;

4 polymyalgia rheumatica; or
5 rarely, carcinoma or chronic infection, including tuberculosis.

Anaemia

There are three major types of anaemia, classified by cause: deficiency, haemolysis and marrow disorders.

The symptoms are tiredness, physical fatigue and dyspnoea, with angina, heart failure and confusion in older people.

Deficiency

• Iron (including sideroblastic anaemia).
• Vitamin B_{12}.
• Folic acid.

Iron-deficiency anaemia

Diagnosis

The cause of the iron deficiency must be identified and corrected. In premenopausal women, excess menstrual loss is often the cause, although this should not be accepted uncritically because other important causes may be present as well. Slow gastrointestinal loss is a common cause, with peptic ulceration, gastric carcinoma and carcinoma of the descending colon most common. Carcinoma of the ascending colon or caecum frequently produces no symptoms and its presence must be considered in all cases of iron-deficiency anaemia. In the elderly, dietary deficiencies remain an important cause, and remember that hypothyroidism can present as iron-deficient anaemia.

Examination includes assessment of pallor (very imprecise), glossitis, angular stomatitis, koilonychia and rectal examination. Investigate the gastrointestinal tract if no other cause is identified. Early colonoscopy, especially in the asymptomatic patient, can detect carcinoma of the large bowel at a curable stage.

Laboratory investigation (Table 18.1). The peripheral blood count shows hypochromia (mean corpuscular haemoglobin (MCH) < 27 pg) and microcytosis (mean corpuscular volume (MCV) < 80 fl), possibly with poikilocytosis (variation in shape) and anisocytosis (variation in size). The serum iron is low and the transferrin raised, with a low saturation. The serum iron is also low in anaemia secondary to chronic disease, but normal in haemoglobinopathies and, usually, thalassaemia minor (p. 306). Serum ferritin reflects the state of the iron stores and is therefore low. There is a reduction in stainable iron in the marrow. The bone marrow shows adequate iron in macrophages but reduced amounts in developing erythroblasts. Other causes of hypochromic, microcytic anaemia include thalassaemia, and anaemia secondary to chronic disease where the erythrocyte sedimentation rate (ESR) is usually raised, and the serum iron and total iron-binding capacity (TIBC) are usually reduced and ferritin normal or even raised; it is an acute-phase protein.

Management

In the absence of active bleeding, ferrous sulphate 200 mg b.d. before food is usually all that is required. The reticulocyte count rises first and then the haemoglobin (at about 1 g/week), but iron should be continued for another 3 months to replenish the stores.
NB *Hypochromic anaemia*, unresponsive to oral iron therapy, occurs in:
• incorrect diagnosis or mixed deficiency;
• continued bleeding (reticulocytosis persists), e.g. microscopic from tumour of the bowel;
• patients who do not take their tablets;
• rheumatoid arthritis, SLE infections (and other chronic illness);
• malabsorption;
• thalassaemia; and
• myelodysplastic syndrome—refractory anaemia (if ringed sideroblasts present in marrow, sideroblastic anaemia).

Hazards of blood transfusion

Transfusion reaction (minimize risk by cross-matching patient's serum with donor blood). If clinical manifestations of a transfusion reaction occur (fever, backache, hypotension and haemoglobinuria), stop the transfusion immediately and initiate supportive treatment to alleviate shock.

Transmission of infection (blood is screened for hepatitis B and C and human immunodeficiency virus (HIV)).
Circulatory overload (give furosemide (frusemide) with transfusion in patients at risk of heart failure).
Coagulation defects and electrolyte abnormalities (particularly hyperkalaemia—red cell breakdown releases potassium) where large volumes are transfused.

Vitamin B_{12} deficiency
(usually pernicious anaemia)
Vitamin B_{12} is present in liver, and small amounts also in milk and dairy products, and requires intrinsic factor for absorption.

The most common cause of vitamin B_{12} deficiency in the UK is lack of intrinsic factor as a result of parietal cell and intrinsic factor antibodies. It is associated with other organ-specific autoimmune disorders. Achlorhydria is invariably present. Rare causes of B_{12} deficiency include gastrectomy, intestinal blind loops (in which bacteria multiply using up B_{12}), a vegan diet, Crohn disease involving the absorbing surface in the terminal ileum, other causes of malabsorption and *Diphyllobothrium latum*—a Finnish tapeworm that consumes B_{12}. Stores of B_{12} last 3–4 years.

Clinical features

Pernicious anaemia occurs in the middle-aged and elderly and is more common in women. Exhaustion and lethargy are the most common presenting complaints, although pallor may be noticed incidentally, or the blood picture noticed in the laboratory.

In chronic, severe B_{12} deficiency, which is uncommon, the skin has a pale lemon tint, the hair is snow white and the sclera may be slightly jaundiced as a result of mild haemolysis. The tongue may be tender, smooth and red because of atrophy of the mucosa. Peripheral neuropathy may be the presenting feature with pain, soreness or numbness of the feet on walking. Later, features of subacute combined degeneration of the cord may develop. Cardiac failure is common if the anaemia is marked. The spleen is sometimes palpable.

Neutrophils (Normal range: 2.0–7.5 × 10⁹/l (40–75% of total white cells)
Causes of neutrophilia (raised neutrophil count)
Acute bacterial infections
Inflammation, e.g. arteritis
Acute tissue necrosis, e.g. myocardial infarction, large pressure sores, burns
Acute haemorrhages
Leukaemias

Causes of neutropenia (low neutrophil count)
Viral infections, e.g. glandular fever, measles, acquired immunodeficiency syndrome (AIDS)
Drug reactions, e.g. carbimazole, chemotherapy
Blood diseases, e.g. leukaemias, pernicious anaemia, aplastic anaemia

Lymphocytes (Normal adult range: 1.5–4.0 × 10⁹/l (20–45% of total))
There are two main subpopulations of T lymphocytes, which bear different surface markers, or cluster of differentiation (CD) antigens. CD8 cells are 'cytotoxic'—their main function is to recognize and kill cells expressing foreign (usually viral) proteins. CD4 cells are 'helper' cells—they help B lymphocytes to differentiate into plasma cells and produce antibodies. The normal ratio of CD4 : CD8 cells is 2 : 1

Causes of lymphocytosis (raised lymphocyte count)
Acute viral infections, e.g. glandular fever, chickenpox, rubella, mumps
Lymphatic leukaemia
Vasculitis and drug hypersensitivity

Causes of lymphopenia (low lymphocyte count)
AIDS—a severely depressed CD4 count predicts the onset of opportunistic infections
Ionizing radiation (treatment for malignancy or accidental)
Chemotherapy for malignancy
Steroid therapy or Cushing syndrome

Eosinophils (Normal range: 0.04–0.4 × 10⁹/l)
Causes of eosinophilia (raised eosinophil count)
Allergies, e.g. bronchial asthma, urticaria, hay fever, drug reaction
Parasitic infestation of gut or other tissues (muscles, subcutaneous tissues, liver, urinary tract)
Connective tissue diseases, especially systemic vasculitis (see polyarteritis nodosa, p. 125; Churg–Strauss syndrome, p. 126; Hodgkin's disease, p. 311)

Table 18.2 White cells. Normal white cell count: 4–10 × 10⁹/l.

There is an increased incidence of gastric carcinoma.

Diagnosis
The haemoglobin may be very low, i.e. 3–4 g or less. The blood film shows macrocytes usually with anisocytosis and poikilocytosis, and the MCV is usually > 100 fl. The total white blood cell (WBC) count may fall because of reduced numbers of both lymphocytes and neutrophils (Table 18.2). Some neutrophils may show hypersegmentation of the nuclei (> 5 lobes). There may also be a moderate fall in the platelet count. Reticulocytes are generally not increased until treatment is started.

The marrow is hypercellular, with giant metamyelocytes and megaloblasts present—evidence that anaemia is in part caused by suppression of cell release. *Megaloblasts* are found only rarely in the peripheral blood. They are characterized by a large and inactive nucleus (maturation arrest) in a relatively hypermature, and even haemoglobinized, cytoplasm. They are not present in normal marrow and their presence denotes vitamin B₁₂ or folate deficiency, which may be secondary to antifolate or phenytoin therapy. If sufficiently severe, vitamin B_{12} and folate deficiencies produce depression of all the marrow elements, including neutrophils and platelets. There is usually some haemolysis with a raised unconjugated serum bilirubin. The haptoglobins are reduced. Urobilinogen is present in the urine as a result of reduced red cell survival and ineffective erythropoiesis. Antibodies to parietal cells are present in > 90% of patients and to intrinsic factor in approximately 55%. Not all individuals who have parietal cell antibodies have pernicious anemia.

Patients with pernicious anaemia treated with vitamin B_{12} usually have normal peripheral blood and a normal marrow within 24 h. The serum folates and B_{12} are normal. Parietal cell and intrinsic factor antibodies are still present.

Treatment

Vitamin B_{12} as hydroxocobalamin 1 mg (1000 μg) is given five times at 2-day intervals and then every 3 months for life.

The response of the marrow to therapy is very rapid with an early reticulocyte response maximal on the fourth to sixth day. The haemoglobin follows this and rises about 1 g/dl every 1–2 weeks. The WBC and platelets are normal in about 7 days.

The rapid production of cells with therapy may reveal an associated deficiency of, and demand for, iron, potassium or folic acid and supplements should be given where necessary.

Neurological features of B_{12} deficiency usually improve to some degree; sensory abnormalities more completely than motor, and peripheral neuropathy more than myelopathy. However, neurological features may remain static and occasionally even deteriorate.

NB If folic acid alone is given to patients with pernicious anaemia the neurological features may become worse.

Blood transfusion contains enough B_{12} to correct the marrow and to make interpretation of serum B_{12} levels difficult. It may precipitate heart failure and death—some authorities believe that transfusion must *never* be given to patients with pernicious anaemia. A poor response to B_{12} therapy suggests that the diagnosis is wrong.

Folic acid deficiency

Folic acid is found in green vegetables and liver.

• *Dietary deficiency*. In the UK this is most commonly seen in chronic alcoholics, the poor and the elderly who eat no green vegetables. In the tropics it is often seen in association with multiple deficiencies and with gut infection and infestation.

• *Malabsorption* (p. 225).

• *Increased requirement*. Pregnancy and infancy. Haemolysis results in increased red cell formation, which requires folate more than B_{12}.

• *Folate metabolism*. Phenytoin therapy interferes with folate metabolism.

Haemolytic anaemia (Table 18.3)

Haemolytic anaemias are rare in the UK. Haemolysisis is characterized by jaundice with a raised unconjugated serum bilirubin, increased urobilinogen in urine and stools, increased haptoglobins and reticulocytosis. The degree of reticulocytosis is an indirect measure of the rate of haemolysis. There is no bile pigment in the urine (the jaundice is acholuric). The rate of disappearance of chromium-tagged red cells gives a more accurate measure of the rate of haemolysis. Splenomegaly and pigment stones may occur. The blood film may show polychromasia, spherocytes, crenated and fragmented red cells. There may be features of:

• rapid red cell destruction—increased plasma haemoglobin, methaemalbuminaemia, decreased haptoglobins, haemoglobinuria and haemosiderinuria; and

• excess red cell formation—reticulocytosis, erythroid hyperplasia and increased folate requirements.

Hereditary haemolytic anaemias

These are caused by defects in the red cell membrane or specific red cell enzyme deficiencies.

Hereditary spherocytosis

An autosomal dominant disorder that causes increased osmotic fragility and produces spherocytes in the peripheral blood. Patients present with an intermittent jaundice which

HAEMOLYTIC ANAEMIAS

Intrinsic red cell disorders (abnormal RBCs) (all Coombs-negative)	Extrinsic disorders (normal RBCs)

Membrane disorder
Hereditary spherocytosis*; hereditary elliptocytosis
	Immune
	Autoimmune (Coombs-positive)
	Warm antibodies
	  Idiopathic
	  Secondary (SLE, CLL, lymphoma, Hodgkin's, carcinoma, drugs: methyldopa, mefenamic acid)
	Cold—agglutinins
	  Idiopathic

Enzyme deficiency G6PD*; pyruvate kinase	Secondary (*Mycoplasma*, glandular fever, lymphoma) Lysis
Haemoglobinopathy Sickle-cell anaemia; thalassaemia	*Isoimmune* (Coombs-negative) Mismatched transfusion Haemolytic disease of the newborn
	Non-immune (Coombs-negative) *Mechanical haemolytic anaemias*: disseminated intravascular coagulation, microangiopathic haemolytic anaemia (thrombotic thrombocytopenic purpura), haemolytic–uraemic syndrome, postcardiotomy—prosthetic heart valves (red-cell fragmentation), march haemoglobinuria, hypersplenism and burns *Infections*: malaria, *Clostridium perfringens*, viral infections *Paroxysmal nocturnal haemoglobinuria* (p. 306) *Drugs*: e.g. oxidative damage, dapsone, salazopyrine Secondary to renal or liver disease

*Most frequent.
CLL, chronic lymphoid leukaemia; G6PD, glucose-6-phosphate dehydrogenase; RBC, red blood cell; SLE, systemic lupus erythematosus.

Table 18.3 Classification of haemolytic anaemias.

may be confused with Gilbert syndrome or with recurrent hepatitis. Gallstones, leg ulcers, splenomegaly and haemolytic or aplastic crises during intercurrent infections may occur.

Splenectomy relieves the symptoms but does not cure the underlying defect.

Hereditary elliptocytosis

This is also inherited as an autosomal dominant trait and produces elliptical red blood cells, variable degrees of haemolysis and, rarely, splenomegaly.

Glucose-6-phosphate dehydrogenase deficiency

A disease found in Africa, the Mediterranean, the Middle and Far East. Inheritance is sex-linked on the X chromosome (affected males always show clinical manifestations but females will have variable degrees of haemolysis). Because of the phenomenon of random inactivation of the X chromosome, females will have two populations of red blood cells (RBCs), one normal and one glucose-6-phosphate dehydrogenase (G6PD) deficient: the susceptibility to haemolysis will be greater, the greater the size of the deficient population. In the UK, acute haemolytic episodes are usually drug-induced (sulphonamides, primaquine) or occur during acute infections. Other features are neonatal jaundice and favism.

The diagnosis is confirmed by reduced or absent enzyme activity in the red cells.

Paroxysmal nocturnal haemoglobinuria

This is an acquired clonal disorder of haematopoiesis in which cells have deficient production of the phospholipid glycosylphosphatidylinositol that anchors certain proteins to the cell surface. These include CD59, which protects cells from complement-mediated lysis. This accounts for the increased sensitivity of red cells to complement, which forms the basis of Ham's acid lysis test.

The clinical features occur usually in the over-30s, who develop paroxysmal haemolysis (with anaemia, macrocytosis, reticulocytosis, haemoglobinuria and haemosiderinuria) and life-threatening venous thromboses. Patients may develop aplastic anaemia. Spontaneous remission occurs in about 15% of cases. Long-term anticoagulation should be considered.

Haemoglobinopathies

Clinical features

Normal adult haemoglobin is made up of two polypeptide chains, the α- and β-chains, which are folded such that each chain can hold an oxygen-binding haem molecule. The haemoglobinopathies are a diverse group of autosomal recessive disorders of haemoglobin synthesis which include sickle-cell anaemia (abnormal β-chain synthesis) and the thalassaemias (deficient or absent α- or β-chain synthesis). Together they form the most common group of single-gene disorders worldwide.

Genetic basis of haemoglobinopathies

Genes encoding five different β-globin chains and three different α-globin chains are expressed in a precisely regulated manner during different stages of development. During fetal life the two β-globin variants called γ-globin combine with two α-globin chains to give rise to fetal haemoglobin (HbF). During adult life the β-globin variants themselves combine with α-globin chains to form adult haemoglobin (HbA). HbA_2 is < 3% of haemoglobin in adults and possesses two α- and two δ-chains.

The five β-globin chain genes are clustered on chromosome 11, whereas the α-globin chain genes occur together on chromosome 16.

Numerous different mutations in the α-globin and β-globin genes have been described, which give rise to α- or β-thalassaemia respectively. Sickle-cell anaemia is caused by a point mutation, which involves substitution of T for A in the second nucleotide of the sixth codon, changing the sixth amino acid from glutamine to valine.

NB HbA is 95% of haemoglobin in adults and possesses two α- and two β-chains $(\alpha_2\beta_2)$.

HbF is < 0.5% of haemoglobin in adults and possesses two α- and two γ- chains $(\alpha_2\gamma_2)$.

Sickle-cell haemoglobin (HbS) possesses two α- and two abnormal β-chains.

Haemoglobin A_2 (HbA_2) is < 3% of haemoglobin in adults and possesses two α- and two δ-chains $(\alpha_2\delta_2)$.

Sickle-cell disease

A disease found in Africa, the Middle East, the Mediterranean and India, transmitted as an autosomal dominant trait. Sickle-cell trait occurs in heterozygotes (HbA–HbS) whose haemoglobin contains characteristically 60% HbA and 40% HbS. Patients with the trait are usually symptom-free except when the oxygen tension is very low, e.g. through altitude and anoxic anaesthesia. The outlook is excellent. The prevalence of the gene is probably because the HbS protects against the serious and occasionally lethal effects of falciparum malaria.

Sickle-cell anaemia occurs in homozygotes (HbS–HbS). The abnormal haemoglobin renders the RBCs susceptible to very small reductions in oxygen tension. This leads to the sickling phenomenon and to abnormal sequestration with thrombosis in small arterioles. The subsequent infarction may affect any part of the body.

Clinical features

Anaemia occurs within the first months of life as levels of HbF fall. Acute haemolytic crises begin after 6 months, causing bone infarcts, which are common, and children may present with pain and swelling in the fingers and toes (dactylitis). Infarcts may cause abdominal pain, haematuria or cerebrovascular accidents. Splenic infarction is common and by the age of

I year most children are functionally asplenic. Repeated renal infarction causes tubular damage and failure to concentrate urine, compounding sickle-cell crises.

Prognosis

The disease carries a high infant and child mortality from thrombosis to a vital organ or infection, with pneumococcus the most common as a result of hyposplenism. Children who survive beyond 4–5 years continue to have chronic ill health with anaemia, haemolytic and thrombotic crises, leg ulcers and infections (which may precipitate crises), and rarely survive beyond 35–40 years. Folate supplements are required throughout life. Pneumococcal vaccine should be given and penicillin prescribed to reduce mortality from pneumococcus.

Thalassaemia

Thalassaemia is found in the Middle and Far East and the Mediterranean, and is caused by deficient α- or β-chain synthesis. The deficiency is genetically determined and results in α- or β-thalassaemia. In the latter, γ-chains continue to be produced in excess into adult life and excess HbF is present.

β-Thalassaemia minor trait (heterozygote)

This usually presents as a symptom-free, mild, microcytic, hypochromic anaemia that may be confused with iron deficiency. It is diagnosed by finding a raised HbA_2 level generally (4–7%). HbF levels may also be slightly raised (1–3%).

β-Thalassaemia major (homozygote)

Both parents possess the trait. Patients are relatively normal at birth (little β-chain anyway) but develop severe anaemia later with failure to thrive and are prone to infection. The anaemia is hypochromic and the film contains target cells ('Mexican hat' cells) and stippling. Erythroid hyperplasia occurs in the marrow and chain precipitation appears as inclusion bodies on supravital staining.

Infants who survive develop hepatosplenomegaly, bossing of the skull, brittle and overgrown long bones, gallstones and leg ulcers.

Treatment consists of transfusion to main-

POLYCYTHAEMIA VERA

Haemoglobin	> 18 g/dl*
Red cell count	7–12 × 10¹²/l*
Haematocrit	> 0.55*
Platelets	> 650 000 × 10⁹/l
White cell count	> 12 × 10⁹/l with basophilia
Arterial oxygen saturation usually normal	92%
Leucocyte alkaline phosphatase score	> 100
Serum B_{12}	Increased

*Also present in secondary polycythaemia.

Table 18.4 Haemological values in polycythaemia vera. Increased red blood cell mass (> 36 ml/kg in men; > 32 ml/kg in women). NB Splenomegaly occurs in 75%.

tain the haemoglobin at 10 g/dl but this, combined with increased iron absorption, results in iron overload. Desferrioxamine is given to reduce haemosiderosis with folic acid replacement, and splenectomy may be indicated if hypersplenism supervenes. Bone marrow transplantation has been used successfully.

Marrow disorders

Myeloproliferative disorders

This term includes polycythaemia vera, primary thrombocythamia, myelofibrosis and chronic myeloid leukaemia (p. 311). They are interlinked clonal diseases all derived from haemopoietic stem cells in the marrow, each one of which can transform into another.

Polycythaemia (increased haemoglobin) may be:

• primary (polycythaemia vera, leucocytes and platelets usually increased as well); or

• secondary (e.g. caused by increased erythropoietin production in hypoxia or renal disease).

Polycythaemia vera (Table 18.4)

Polycythaemia vera presents in late middle age (50–60 years), most commonly as a chance haematological finding. If symptomatic, it presents usually with vascular occlusion, arterial or venous or, much less often, with gout, pru-

PLATELET DISORDERS

Thrombocytosis (increased platelets)
After haemorrhage, surgery or trauma
Splenectomy or splenic atrophy
Inflammation (as part of an inflammatory response)
Malignancy
Myeloproliferative disorders, e.g. megakaryocytic leukaemia
    (rare)

Thrombocytopenia (decreased platelets)
Adverse drug reactions (e.g. non-steroidal anti-inflammatory
    drugs, phenothiazines, gold, thiazides)
Autoimmune thrombocytopenic purpura, in which circulating
    anti-platelet antibodies lead to premature platelet
    destruction
Marrow aplasia

NB If also anaemic, exclude disseminated intravascular
coagulation (p. 310) and prosthetic valve dysfunction.

Table 18.5 Causes of platelet disorders. (Normal range $150–400 \times 10^9$/l.)

ritus or a finding of splenomegaly. Diagnosis is established by the presence of:

1 a raised red cell mass (RCM); and
2 the absence of any cause for a secondary polycythaemia, plus one of the two other major diagnostic criteria:
3 a palpable spleen; or
4 an abnormal acquired marrow karyotype.

The presence of two of the minor criteria (thrombocytosis, neutrophil leucocytosis, ultrasound splenomegaly) can suffice in the absence of either of the two latter major criteria. A raised RCM is defined as one 25% greater than that predicted from the patient's height and weight. Secondary causes to be excluded include hypoxaemia ($Sao_2 < 92\%$ at rest in sleep studies) and renal disease (ultrasound for polycystic disease and hypernephroma). Cerebellar haemangioblastoma and hepatoma are associated but very rare. Treatment is with repeated venesection, hydroxyurea and low-dose aspirin to reduce the incidence of intravascular coagulation.

NB In polycythaemia vera, all cellular elements are raised (RBCs, WBCs and platelets). In secondary polycythaemia, only the red cell count is raised.

• Primary thrombocythaemia, if not found incidentally, presents with small vessel vascular occlusion. There is a high platelet count of over 600×10^9/l.

• Myelofibrosis presents with the finding of huge and increasing splenomegaly, and evidence of bone marrow failure: anaemia, infection, bleeding. There is marrow fibrosis and a leucoerythroblastic peripheral blood picture: myelocytes, nucleated red cells.

Myelodysplastic syndrome

This refers to peripheral cytopenia with a cellular marrow. It is usually discovered on a routine peripheral blood film, usually as macrocytosis (with normal B_{12}, folates, liver and thyroid function tests, and γ-glutamyl transferase). Less commonly, patients may present with a refractory anaemia, pancytopenia, neutropenia or thrombocytopenia (Table 18.5). Marrow examination shows a dysmyelopoietic picture with excess blasts, with normal or increased cellularity.

There are six major subgroups with decreasingly satisfactory prognoses:

1 refractory anaemia with sideroblasts, with > 15% ringed sideroblasts, but none in the periphery;
2 refractory anaemia with < 5% blasts in a dyserythropoietic marrow, but no blasts in the peripheral blood;

3 refractory anaemia with excess blasts, amounting to 5–20% nucleated marrow cells;

4 refractory anaemia in transformation, with 20–30% sideroblasts or > 5% in the periphery or of Auer's rods in the blast cells, regardless of the marrow blast count;

5 chronic myelomonocytic leukaemia, with a peripheral monocyte count $> 1 \times 10^9$ and monocytic precursors in the marrow. Philadelphia chromosome-negative; and

6 acute myeloblastic leukaemia.

Treatment
Haematinics (iron, folate, B_{12}) are ineffective. Blood transfusion is necessary and has to be repeated regularly.

Prognosis depends on the occasional transformation to blasts and is then that of the leukaemia, with bone marrow failure.

Complications
Anaemia (requiring the transfusion of about 1 unit blood/week), infection, haemorrhage and blast transformation.

Marrow failure
Marrow aplasia
Primary aplastic anaemia gives a pancytopenia with reduction in all the formed elements. It is rare. Patients present with:
• anaemia; and/or
• spontaneous bleeding because of lack of platelets; and/or
• infection caused by lack of polymorphonuclear leucocytes.

A peripheral blood film reveals a pancytopenia, although one cell line may be affected more than the others. A bone marrow aspiration is performed. If it is difficult to aspirate (possible myelofibrosis or malignancy), a trephine biopsy may be necessary to obtain a diagnostic specimen of marrow. The drugs that most commonly cause marrow suppression include phenylbutazone (now only on hospital prescription), gold, indometacin, chloramphenicol and cytotoxic drugs. Remember ionizing radiation.

Some marrow suppression is associated with uraemia, rheumatoid arthritis and hypothyroidism.

Bleeding disorders

Haemophilias
Haemophilia A (classical haemophilia) or haemophilia B (Christmas disease) results from defects in the clotting factor VIII (on chromosome Xq28) or factor IX (on chromosome Xq27), respectively. They are sex-linked recessive clotting disorders of men, carried by women in which patients suffer mainly from spontaneous bleeding into joints and soft tissues, and excessive bleeding in response to trauma or surgery. All carriers who wish to have children should receive genetic counselling. The diseases can be detected *in utero*.

Therapy
Treatment is by replacement of the deficient clotting factor. As soon as possible after bleeding has started, purified factor VIII or IX is given as required. Purified factor VIII is also used to raise factor VIII levels in von Willebrand disease. Fresh frozen plasma contains both factors but is best reserved for when the single factors are not available. Aspirin-containing preparations should be avoided because they impair platelet function and may cause gastric erosion. Desmopressin can be used to increase factor VIII levels in mild to moderate haemophilia.

von Willebrand disease
This is an autosomal dominant disease of both sexes that causes abnormal bleeding, particularly from mucous membranes. There is a prolonged bleeding time, low factor VIII clotting activity and poor platelet adhesion. (von Willebrand factor is a cofactor for this adhesion.)

Skin haemorrhage
• Purpura refers to small areas of cutaneous bleeding. The purplish red spots do not fade on pressure. Ecchymosis refers to larger lesions (bruises). Purpura is rare, but bruising is very common.

• The most common causes of skin haemorrhage are senile purpura, therapy with steroids or anticoagulants and, less commonly, thrombocytopenia caused by leukaemia and marrow aplasia.

Thrombocytopenia

May result from decreased production (marrow aplasia, leukaemia or infiltration) or increased destruction (idiopathic thrombocytopenic purpura, hypersplenism and consumption coagulopathy).

Idiopathic thrombocytopenic purpura

Idiopathic thrombocytopenic purpura (ITP) is rare and not to be confused with thrombotic thrombocytopenic purpura (TTP), which is very rare. ITP occurs chiefly in children following a respiratory or gastrointestinal viral infection. Patients present with purpura and a low platelet count. If the platelet count is very low, major bleeding may occur from the nose, gut or into the brain. The bleeding time is prolonged but coagulation times are normal. Spontaneous recovery is the rule. Platelet counts above 80 000 mm³ do not need treatment. Steroids or intravenous immunoglobulin may be of benefit in the more severe cases, occasionally with lasting remission. Splenectomy should be avoided if possible, especially in children, in view of the risk of pneumococcal septicaemia in asplenic patients, but may be curative when medical management is unsuccessful.

Thrombotic thrombocytopenic purpura

Thrombotic thrombocytopenic purpura is a very rare disease of young adults who present with fever, abdominal pain, purpura and focal neurological signs. Initial haematuria may progress to renal failure. The mechanism is unknown but it may be a disorder of vascular endothelium that is unable to produce a prostacycline platelet inhibitor: hence the widespread intravascular thrombosis. The mortality is high. Treatment consists of plasma exchange and renal dialysis, if indicated, with or without heparin and steroids.

Henoch–Schönlein purpura (see p. 126)

Osler disease (Osler–Weber–Rendu)

• Hereditary haemorrhagic telangiectasia: autosomal dominant.
• May present as intermittent bleeding, usually gastrointestinal.

• There are small capillary angiectases throughout the gastrointestinal tract, including the buccal mucosa and tongue.

Disseminated intravascular coagulation (DIC)

Synonym: consumption coagulopathy. This occurs in obstetric practice, thoracic surgery, pulmonary embolism, in shock (especially when associated with infection or bleeding) and following mismatched blood transfusion.

The syndrome may present less acutely with intravascular coagulation rather than excessive bleeding, e.g. the thrombophlebitis migrans of malignancy.

Platelets and factor V and VIII are consumed in the pathological coagulation as well as fibrinogen. Fibrinolysis takes place simultaneously with coagulation and produces fibrin degeneration products which can be measured in the serum and urine.

Treatment is of the underlying disease, usually septicaemia. Replace the platelets and the deficient factors by fresh (12 h) whole blood or fresh frozen plasma and fibrinogen concentrates. Heparin is given, progress being monitored by changes in the fibrinogen level.

Leukaemia

This refers to malignant proliferation of blood-forming cells, and is broadly classified according to:
1 whether the disease, if untreated, is likely to follow an acute, rapidly fatal, or more prolonged chronic course, and
2 whether lymphocytic or myeloid (marrow-related) cell lines are primarily involved.

Acute lymphatic leukaemia

This, the most common form of childhood leukaemia, accounts for 75–80% of all childhood leukaemias. Infiltration of bone marrow with lymphoblastic cells causes anaemia, bruising (thrombocytopenia) and infections (neutropenia). Lymphoblasts are usually present in the peripheral blood and always in the marrow. Lymphadenopathy, splenomegaly and hepatomegaly occur. Seventy per cent of children with acute lymphatic leukaemia can now be 'cured'.

Chronic lymphatic leukaemia

This occurs in the elderly with a generalized lymphadenopathy and a raised white cell count with lymphocytosis. It usually follows a benign course and treatment is only indicated if symptoms develop.

Acute myeloid leukaemia

This occurs at all ages but less commonly in childhood. Myeloblasts infiltrate the marrow and are found in the blood. Anaemia, bleeding or infections are common. Involvement of other organs is unusual.

Chronic myeloid leukaemia

This usually presents in middle age, often insidiously with anaemia, weight loss and fever. White cell count is markedly raised with myeloid precursors in the marrow and peripheral blood. The spleen, and in later stages the liver, are markedly enlarged. In over 90% of patients leucocytes contain the Philadelphia chromosome, a translocation of the breakpoint cluster region (*bcr*) gene on the long arm of chromosome 22 to a position adjacent to the *c-abl* gene on chromosome 9. This results in formation of a *bcr-abl* fusion gene, and the subsequent expression of the BCR-ABL fusion protein is involved in the malignant transformation of myeloid cells.

Lymphoma

These are solid tumours of the lymphoreticular system that are divided histologically into two main types: Hodgkin's disease, characterized by the presence of multinucleated giant cells (Reed–Sternberg cells); and non-Hodgkin's lymphoma.

Clinical features

Patients may present with painless lymphadenopathy. Symptoms, if present, include lethargy, anorexia, weight loss, fever, night sweats and pruritus. Hepatomegaly and splenomegaly may occur.

Lymphomas are staged according to the extent of disease:

• Stage I: involvement of a single lymph node region;
• Stage II: two regions involved on the same side of the diaphragm;
• Stage III: disease on both sides of the diaphragm, but limited to nodes, spleen or a single extralymphatic organ or site;
• Stage IV: diffuse involvement of one or more extralymphatic sites, with or without lymph node involvement.

In Hodgkin's disease the suffix A (e.g. stage IIA) denotes the absence of symptoms, whereas the suffix B denotes the presence of weight loss (> 10%), fever or night sweats.

The diagnosis is usually made on lymph node biopsy. Staging requires careful examination for superficial nodes and chest X-ray for mediastinal involvement. Computed tomographic (CT) scanning above and below the diaphragm can avoid the need for laparotomy.

Treatment is with combination chemotherapy, radiotherapy or a combination of the two depending on clinical, radiological and histological staging.

Myeloma

There is malignant proliferation of a specific clone of plasma cells resulting in the production of a monoclonal immunoglobulin known as a paraprotein.

Clinical features

Eighty per cent of cases occur after the age of 50. Non-specific symptoms include malaise, lethargy and weight loss. Bone destruction from the expanding plasma cell clone causes pain, fractures and hypercalcaemia. Normochromic anaemia, thrombocytopenia and leukopenia (infections are common) occur as the normal bone marrow is replaced. Renal failure may result from hypercalcaemia or the presence of light chains, which may be nephrotoxic or become precipitated in tubules.

TRIAL BOX 18.1

The **International Lymphoma Study Group** (Revised European–American Classification of Lymphoid Neoplasms (REAL), *Blood* 1994; **84**: 1361–1392) has agreed a classification for non-Hodgkin's lymphoma and lymphoid neoplasms. They have been broadly classified into the following.

B-cell neoplasms
• Precursor B-cell neoplasm (most present as acute leukaemia but a few present as solid tumours).
• Peripheral B-cell neoplasms (includes B-cell chronic lymphocytic leukaemia, mantle cell lymphoma, follicular lymphoma, mucosa-associated lymphoid tissue (MALT) lymphoma,

hairy-cell leukaemia, plasmacytoma, Burkitt's lymphoma).

T-cell and putative natural killer-cell neoplasms
• Precursor T-cell neoplasm (precursor T-lymphoblastic lymphoma).
• Peripheral T-cell and natural killer-cell neoplasms (includes T-cell chronic lymphocytic leukaemia, large granular lymphocyte leukaemia (LGL), mycosis fungoides/Sézary syndrome.

Hodgkin's disease
• Stage I: lymphocyte predominance
• Stage II: nodular sclerosis
• Stage III: mixed cellularity
• Stage IV: lymphocyte depletion.

Investigation

There is usually anaemia with a markedly raised ESR. The monoclonal antibody is detected as a discrete M band on plasma protein electrophoresis. Free immunoglobulin light chains may be detectable in the urine as Bence Jones protein (precipitate on heating to $56°C$, redissolve on boiling). There may be hypercalcaemia and renal failure. Osteolytic lesions are seen on X-ray. Alkaline phosphatase is usually normal (lesions are destructive without osteoclastic activity).

Diagnosis

Diagnosis depends on the presence of one major and one minor criterion, or three minor criteria, one of which must be increased plasma cells in bone marrow.

Major criteria

• Tissue plasmacytoma.
• Excess ($> 30\%$ plasma cells in bone marrow).
• Monoclonal M band on plasma protein electrophoresis (> 3.5 g/dl immunoglobulin G (IgG) or > 2 g/dl IgA); or > 1 g/24 h of κ or λ light chains in urine.

Minor criteria

• 10–30% plasma cells in bone marrow.
• Presence of M band or urinary light chains at lower levels.

• Osteolytic lesions on X-ray.
• Evidence of immunosuppression with reduced normal (polyclonal) immunoglobulins.

In *Waldenström's macroglobulinaemia* a monoclonal IgM paraprotein is produced. Radiological involvement of bone is rare, but anaemia and a bleeding tendency occur. Plasmapheresis is indicated if symptoms related to hyperviscosity are present.

Management of haematological malignancies

Management of haematological malignancies is under continuous review, and many patients are entered into multicentre trials. Patients should be treated in units with specialist experience of the drug regimens, and supportive treatment, including transfusions and antibiotics.

Cytotoxics (to destroy rapidly dividing cells) are used alone or in combination with radiotherapy. In some cases induction of remission by intensive chemotherapy is followed by bone marrow transplantation. The following drugs are commonly used.

Alkylating agents

Alkylating agents transfer alkyl groups to DNA, interfering with its replication. They reduce fertility in males (consider sperm storage) and may be associated with premature menopause in females. They are teratogenic, but there does not appear to be an increase in fetal abnormalities in patients who are fertile after treatment. Bone marrow depression is common and prolonged use is associated with an increased incidence of acute non-lymphocytic leukaemia.

- *Cyclophosphamide* for chronic lymphocytic leukaemia and lymphoma.
- *Chlorambucil* for chronic lymphatic leukaemia and lymphoma.
- *Melphalan* for myeloma.
- *Busulfan* for chronic myeloid leukaemia.
- *Lomustine (CCNU)* is a nitrosourea used for Hodgkin's disease.

Antimetabolites

Antimetabolites are usually competitive analogues of normal metabolites. They cause gastrointestinal upsets and bone marrow depression.

- *Mercaptopurine* is a purine analogue used as maintenance therapy in acute leukaemias.
- *Cytarabine*, *fludarabine* and *fluorouracil* interfere with pyrimidine synthesis.
- *Methotrexate* inhibits dihydrofolate reductase, preventing synthesis of tetrahydrofolic acid that is needed as a coenzyme for synthesis of nucleic acids.

Vinca alkaloids

The *vinca alkaloids* arrest the cell cycle in mitosis. They cause peripheral and autonomic neuropathy and alopecia. *Vincristine*, *vinblastine* and *vindesine* are used for lymphomas and acute leukaemias.

Cytotoxic antibiotics

Cytotoxic antibiotics interfere with DNA or RNA synthesis through various mechanisms.

Doxorubicin is used to treat lymphomas and acute leukaemias. *Bleomycin* is used to treat lymphomas. Mucositis and skin pigmentation occur. Dose-related pulmonary fibrosis limits prolonged use.

Amyloidosis

Amyloidosis is characterized by the tissue deposition of fibrillar proteins that stain with Congo red. Excess κ and λ light chains, associated with abnormal plasma cell proliferation, can form AL-type amyloid. In reactive (secondary or AA-type) amyloidosis, amyloid A protein is deposited, usually after many years of an inflammatory response induced by chronic infection or rheumatic disease. Amyloid A is a 76-amino-acid polypeptide fragment of an acute-phase protein termed serum amyloid A.

Although any organ can be involved, proteinuria is the most common presenting feature. Other sites commonly involved are the gastrointestinal tract, heart and liver.

In long-term dialysis, the patient's β_2-microglobulin is deposited as amyloid in musculoskeletal tissue and the carpal tunnel. In Alzheimer's disease and Down syndrome amyloid plaques are found in the cerebral cortex.

Drug Overdoses

Self-administered drug poisoning accounts for 10% of all acute medical admissions to hospital. Accidental poisoning is common in children and drugs are best kept in child-proof containers out of their reach. In adults the common drugs taken are: the tricyclic antidepressants (e.g. amitriptyline, nortriptyline, protriptyline), the benzodiazepines (e.g. diazepam, nitrazepam, chlordiazepoxide), household substances (e.g. bleach, detergents), paracetamol, co-proxamol and aspirin. Barbiturates are now less commonly abused. The weed-killer paraquat and insecticides (e.g. organophosphates) are occasionally taken accidentally. Carbon monoxide poisoning from domestic gas no longer occurs in areas where North Sea gas is used and carbon monoxide poisoning is usually now a result of incomplete combustion from blocked flues and car exhausts.

Clinical presentation (Table 19.1)

Most patients who take overdoses are still conscious when seen and will usually state which tablets they have taken and/or bring the bottle. If unconscious, the other causes of coma must be considered even if a bottle is found in the pockets. It is well worth searching for a diabetic (to exclude hypoglycaemia) or steroid card, or a hospital outpatient card. Relatives or friends may know whether the patient is currently under treatment. Patients often take more than one drug and very often alcohol in addition.

Management

1 Maintain the airways and ventilation.
2 Absorption and removal of drugs.
3 General care of the unconscious patient—nursing, physiotherapy, fluid balance maintenance of renal function and treatment of shock.
4 Psychiatric assessment.
5 Poisons centres.

Ventilation

After ensuring that the airway is clear the patient should be admitted to hospital. It may be necessary to insert an endotracheal tube and give oxygen. Artificial ventilation is rarely necessary but spontaneous ventilation should be assessed regularly and the decision to ventilate decided on the basis of blood gas measurements.

NB Severe respiratory depression from morphine or dextropropoxyphene is reversed with naloxone.

Absorption and removal of drugs

Gastric lavage is of doubtful value if performed more than 1 h after ingestion. Activated charcoal can bind poisons in the stomach reducing their absorption.

Alkaline diuresis and dialysis. Salicylates in severe overdose may be removed by alkaline diuresis, and also by peritoneal dialysis or haemodialysis: amitriptyline, diazepam, nitrazepam and paracetamol cannot. The alkalinity is more important than the quantity of urine and a normal urine output is adequate for effect (1.5–2 l/24 h) as long as the patient is well hydrated. The decision to use these techniques depends upon the patient's general condition, particularly if this is deteriorating. It is useful to know the initial blood level of salicylate because an initially high level in a deteriorating patient is an indication for diuresis or dialysis. Contraindications are renal failure, shock and heart failure. The value

COMMON DRUG OVERDOSE

Drug	Clinical features	Notes	Diuresis or dialysis	Specific antidotes
Opioids	Depressed consciousness, respiratory depression, pinpoint pupils	CPR may be needed		Naloxone 1–2 mg repeat as necessary
Cocaine	Confusion, aggression, hallucination, seizures, CVA, MI, delirium,	Diazepam sedation β-Blocker for arrhythmias CPR		
+ 'crack'	+ thermal injury to respiratory tract + pneumothorax, pneumomediastinitis, hyperthermia			
Aspirin	Hyperventilation, visual disturbance, tinnitus, nausea, vomiting, acidosis	May be well on admission and later very ill Bicarbonate intravenously for severe acidosis	Alkaline diuresis successful Start if initial blood level over 2.8 mmol/l (500 mg/l) or if condition deteriorates	Nil
Barbiturates	Drowsiness and coma, hypotension, hypoventilation, red wheals on pressure points of limbs, wide dilated pupils, absent reflexes	Most patients require supportive therapy only. Ventilation rarely required	Rarely required	Nil
Amfetamines (and 'E')	Hyperalertness, Arrhythmias, dilated pupils, hyperthermia, hyponatraemia, hyperkalaemia, rhabdomyolysis, cardiac arrest	Fluid replacement, dantrolene if core $T° > 39°C$		
Digoxin	Nausea and vomiting arrhythmias	Common if potassium levels are reduced (diuretic therapy)	Not indicated	Fab digoxin-specific antibody fragments
Benzodiazepines	Drowsiness to coma	Rarely fatal and very rarely requires ventilation (potentiated by alcohol)	No value	Flumazenil
Phenothiazines (e.g. chlorpromazine)	Hypotension, hypothermia, arrhythmias and dystonic movements; respiratory and cerebral depression	May require: 1 Diazepam for fits 2 Antiarrhythmics 3 Orphenadrine for dystonia	No value	Nil

Table 19.1 Clinical features of common drug overdose.

continued on p. 316

COMMON DRUG OVERDOSE

Drug	Clinical features	Notes	Diuresis or dialysis	Specific antidotes
β-Blockers	Bradycardia and shock	Glucagon for severe reduced blood pressure 10 mg intravenous infusion 3 mg/h	No value	
Lithium	Nausea, vomiting, muscle tremor, rigidity and twitching with or without nystagmus and dysarthria. Apathy proceeding to coma		Forced diuresis or haemodialysis if concentration is 5 mmol/l acutely	Nil
Tricyclic antidepressants	Dry mouth, convulsions, arrhythmias, fits, respiratory depression, coma, dilated pupils	1 Diazepam for hyperexcitability 2 Physostigmine to block anticholinergic effects	No value	Nil
Paracetamol	Hepatotoxicity is usually apparent at 48 h (LFTs + INR)	Monitor liver function for up to 2 weeks if INR initially abnormal		N-acetylcysteine intravenously
Paraquat	Respiratory failure 10–14 days later	Oral Fuller's earth, followed by oral $MgSO_4$	Haemodialysis early (about 6 h) if more than minimal quantities	
Iron	Nausea and vomiting, agitation, liver damage	Usually seen in children Chelate gastric iron with desferrioxamine solution for gastric lavage. Chelate absorbed iron with desferrioxamine intramuscularly	No value	Desferrioxamine
Methanol and ethylene glycol	Blurred vision, acidosis	Gastric lavage with 3% HCO_3^- and give ethanol to block methanol acetaldehyde	With heavier intoxication	Ethanol

CPR, Cardiopulmonary resuscitation; CVA, cardiovascular accident; INR, international normalized ratio; LFTs, liver function tests; MI, myocardial infarction.

Table 19.1 (continued)

of these techniques for other specific poisons may be obtained by contacting specialist poisons centres.

In paracetamol overdose, the use of oral methionine or intravenous N-acetylcysteine is determined by the initial blood level and the time after ingestion using standard charts that are available for reference (usually pinned to casualty department notice boards).

Care of the unconscious patient and shock
Expert nursing is essential and aimed at care of the airway and prevention of chest infection and bed sores. Fluid intake and output and assessment of renal function may be critical, particularly if the patient is hypotensive. This is commonly seen with barbiturate and phenothiazine poisoning. Most young patients will maintain good renal function at a systolic blood pressure of 80 mmHg and sometimes less. In the elderly or if there is doubt about renal perfusion, monitor the central venous pressure to detect hypovolaemia (maintain at 2–5 cm of water) and continuously monitor the urine output.

Chest infections caused by inhalation or recumbency should be treated energetically with physiotherapy and antibiotics.

Psychiatric assessment
When the patient has recovered a careful assessment is required with the object of aiding the acute problem and preventing further attempts. About 10% of patients who take overdoses seriously intend suicide and 10–20% take a further overdose. It is useful to interview family and friends about the immediate background and their willingness to help in care after discharge. The patient may admit to planning a future suicidal attempt and a lack of plans for the future may be evidence of depression. The patient should be asked about:
• previous depression and suicide attempts;
• personal instability with a history of many jobs and different personal relationships;
• evidence of schizophrenic personality and schizophrenic thoughts;
• family history of depression, schizophrenia, alcohol abuse; and
• social history, especially living alone.
NB:
• Both aspirin poisoning and hypoglycaemia produce sweating.
• Both aspirin poisoning and diabetic ketoacidosis produce confusion, hyperventilation and glycosuria.
• Most patients with drug overdose rarely require more than active supportive therapy.
• Keep drugs away from children and in childproof containers.

Specialist centres
If in doubt, or the poison is unusual, specialist poisons centres provide advice and maintain a central database.

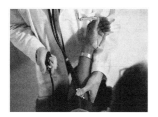

Imported and Infectious Diseases

Within the community virus infections of the upper respiratory and gastrointestinal tract are the most common, followed by common virus infections usually of children such as measles, rubella, chickenpox and mumps, and the venereal diseases. Infections seen more frequently in hospitals usually relate easily to a single body system and are dealt with there (pneumonia, p. 239; endocarditis, p. 284; gastroenteritis, p. 44; hepatitis, p. 207; pyelonephritis, p. 188; and meningitis, p. 106; and Table 8.2, p. 107).

Less frequent, but in diagnostic and management terms more difficult, are the imported diseases, septicaemia, pyrexia of unknown origin and infections of the immunosuppressed. The common infections, likely organisms and antibiotics of choice are shown in Table 20.1.

Imported diseases

The common diseases of travellers (Table 20.2) returning to temperate climates are malaria, acute gastroenteritis including typhoid, infectious hepatitis and worm infestation. Diarrhoea in returning travellers requires investigation for worms and parasites (especially *Giardia* and amoeba) but usually no organism is found and the symptoms settle spontaneously or with simple therapy. Other diseases common in the tropics but rarely seen in returning travellers include tuberculosis, schistosomiasis, hydatid disease, poliomyelitis, tetanus, cholera, leprosy and trypanosomiasis.

Malaria

Malaria is a disease of the subtropics and where the anopheline mosquito is found. Transmission is via the mosquito, which carries infected blood from infected to uninfected humans. The mosquito lives chiefly between latitude 15° north and south and not more than 1500 m (5000 feet) above sea level.

Clinical features

The patient presents with fever and rigors usually within 4 weeks of returning from or travelling through a malarial zone. Occasionally, symptoms may not develop for 12 months or more. The patient has usually failed to take antimalarials regularly, not slept under mosquito nets or failed to continue prophylaxis for 6 weeks after returning. The fever may be tertian (a 3-day pattern with fever peaking every other day (*Plasmodium vivax* and *P. ovale*)), quartan (a 4-day pattern with fever peaking every third day), or subtertian (a nonspecific febrile pattern; *P. falciparum*). Diagnosis depends upon clinical awareness and then seeing the parasite in a blood film. The species of parasite may be differentiated by an experienced observer. In the UK, *P. falciparum* and *P. vivax* are most frequently seen in travellers from Africa and Asia. Malignant tertian malaria refers to *P. falciparum* which, very occasionally, produces high levels of parasitaemia (only *P. falciparum* gives red blood cell parasitaemia of > 1–2%), serious complications of cerebral malaria or acute haemolysis and renal failure (blackwater fever).

Prophylaxis

Prophylaxis is by a combination of mosquito control, sleeping under mosquito nets and specific prevention with proguanil (Paludrine) 200 mg/day, with chloroquine 300 mg twice

INFECTIONS AND ANTIBIOTICS

Infection	Likely organism	Antibacterial of choice (adult doses while awaiting microbiology)
Ear, nose and throat*†		
Sore throat	Viral	Nil
	Haemolytic streptococcus (*Streptococcus pyogenes*)	Pencillin V or erythromycin 250 mg q.d.s. if allergic to penicillin
Sinusitis	*Streptococcus pneumoniae* (pneumococcus) *Haemophilus influenzae*	Amoxicillin or trimethoprim
Otitis media	As above plus haemolytic streptococcus *Haemophilus influenzae* in under 5s	Amoxicillin under 5 years old
Acute epiglottitis	*Haemophilus influenzae*	Maintain airway plus cefotaxime or chloramphenicol
Urinary tract		
Acute cystitis	*Escherichia coli* (85%)	Trimethoprim; or amoxicillin, or
Acute pyelonephritis	*Proteus vulgaris* (5%)	cephalosporin
Bone and soft tissue‡		
Cellulitis	Haemolytic streptococcus *Staphylococcus aureus*	Flucloxacillin and penicillin
Drip sites	*Staphylococcus aureus*	
Erysipelas	Haemolytic streptococcus	Penicillin (by injection initially if severe)
Osteomyelitis	*Staphylococcus aureus* *Haemophilus influenzae* in under 5s	Clindamycin alone or flucloxacin + fusidic acid. If *Haemophillus influenzae* give amoxycillin
Gastrointestinal infections§		
Acute gastroenteritis	Viral	Nil
	Campylobacter	Erythromycin or ciprofloxacin
Dysentery	Bacillary (*Shigella* species)	Ciprofloxacin or trimethoprim
	Amoebic—*Entamoeba histolytica*	Metronidazole
Typhoid	*Salmonella typhi*	Ciprofloxacin or cefotaxime or chloramphenicol
Salmonella food poisoning	*Salmonella* species (> 1000)	Nil (usually) unless invasive when ciprofloxacin or trimethoprim are used
Pseudomembranous colitis	*Clostridium difficile*	Metronidazole or vancomycin
Acute cholangitis	*Escherichia coli*	Gentamicin or cefotaxime (one-third of biliary coliform-resistant to ampicillin/amoxicillin)
Chest infections—in hospital practice Gram-stain of sputum may identify the organism		
Acute bronchitis	Viral	Nil
Acute on chronic bronchitis	Bacterial (*H. influenzae*) (*Streptococcus pneumoniae*)	Amoxicillin or tetracycline or erythromycin

INFECTIONS AND ANTIBIOTICS

Infection	Likely organism	Antibacterial of choice (adult doses while awaiting microbiology)
Bronchopneumonia (off the streets)	S. pneumoniae Mycoplasma pneumoniae Legionella pneumoniae (rare H. influenzae 5% psittacosis)	Erythromycin 500 mg b.d. plus amoxicillin 500 mg–1 g q.d.s.
In very unwell or immunosuppressed	Consider Coliforms Klebsiella Staphylococci during influenza epidemics Pneumocystis in AIDS	Erythromycin plus third-generation cephalosporin (cefotaxime, cefoxitime) Pentamidine by inhalation Septrin by mouth or i.v.
Meningitis (adult)–most are viral (90%) Viral Herpes simplex Bacterial Pneumococcal	Streptococcus pneumoniae	Acyclovir Cefotaxime. Substitute penicillin if sensitive
Meningococcal	Neisseria meningitidis	Penicillin or cefotaxime
Haemophilus (more common in children)	Haemophilus influenzae	Cefotaxime (chloramphenicol is an alternative)

*Recurrent infection or 'odd' organisms, e.g. Klebsiella, Pseudomonas, suggest an underlying abnormality such as stone or tumour and further investigation is required. It is rarely possible to clear infection if there is an indwelling catheter (only treat if systematically ill). It is best to remove it if possible and, if not, try instilling an antiseptic, e.g. chlorhexidine 0.2%. Antibiotic use encourages the development of resistant organisms.
†Persistent bacteriuria is difficult to eradicate but patients can be kept relatively symptom-free with regular daily ampicillin 500 mg or nitrofurantoin 100 mg nocte or trimethoprim 100 mg nocte.
‡Treatment of osteomyelitis may be started by injection for 5–7 days depending upon response and may need to continue for about 6 weeks.
§Patients with mild gastroenteritis without systemic illness or suspected systemic infection and who are excreting Shigella or Salmonella (including S. typhi) do not require antibiotics. The major problem is usually dehydration which may lead to deep venous thrombosis and pulmonary embolism in adults. Children need fluid and electrolyte replacement. Dioralyte sachets or electrosol tablets (which contain no dextrose) dissolved in water are satisfactory except in severe depletion.

Table 20.1 Common infections and antibiotics of first choice. NB Most hospitals have local policies.

weekly. For regions known to have chloro-quine-resistant malaria, Maloprim (pyrimetha-mine with dapsone) and mefloquine are used. Prophylaxis should be continued for 6 weeks after returning home.

NB Before advising travellers, check whether they are entering a malarial zone, and seek advice from the nearest centre for tropical diseases about the current recommended prophylaxis because drug resistance, particularly of P. falciparum malaria, is continually changing.

Treatment

See Table 20.3.

DISEASES OF THE RETURNING TRAVELLER

Common	Malaria
	Typhoid
	Diarrhoea often viral as pathogens rarely found but consider:
	Giardia lamblia and worms
	Amoebic colitis ⎫ which must be distinguished from
	Salmonella and ⎬ ulcerative colitis and Crohn disease
	Shigella infection ⎭
	Tropical sprue
	Infectious hepatitis
Rare	Tuberculosis—usually not acute and more likely in Asian immigrants
	Amoebic liver abscess
	Hydatid liver cyst
Exceedingly rare	Rabies
	Cholera
	Exotic viruses
	Lassa fever
	Marburg
	Ebola

Table 20.2 Infections imported by returning travellers.

Acute attacks

Patients with malaria should be given oral quinine. Intravenous quinine is potentially dangerous because it may produce cardiac asystole but is used in those who are vomiting or too ill to take oral therapy. Exchange transfusion may be required in very ill patients with high parasitaemia—consider levels above 10%. Some require full intensive care, including treatment of cerebral oedema, renal and liver failure and shock. Hypoglycaemia from a combination of liver failure and quinine-induced insulin secretion is easily overlooked; pulmonary oedema from fluid overload is common in those treated for shock.

After treatment of the acute attack, falciparum malaria is cleared with Fansidar or tetracycline, and vivax malaria with primaquine (check the glucose-6-phosphate dehydrogenase status first).

Typhoid

Clinical features

Symptoms begin with malaise, headache, dry cough and vague abdominal pain, up to 21 days after returning from a typhoid area. Travellers to any area with poor sanitation are at risk and typhoid occasionally occurs in non-travellers. In the first week fever is marked with dry cough and constipation which are typical features. In the second week, the fever persists, the abdomen distends, diarrhoea may or may not occur and rose spots develop as crops of pale pink macules on the sides of the abdomen. Delirium and death (10%) may occur in untreated cases. NB Symptoms of dry cough, constipation and fever should be sufficient to alert the clinician, particularly in returning holiday-makers.

Investigation

Leukopenia and neutropenia may or may not be present. Blood culture is mandatory if typhoid is suspected and culture of urine and stool should also be performed.

Treatment

Salmonella typhi responds to ciprofloxacin. Trimethoprim is also effective.
NB
• It is unnecessary to give antibiotics to patients who are clinically well, but from whom *S. typhi* is grown from the stools. If these

ANTIMALARIAL DRUGS

Drug	Important side-effects	Comments
Chloroquine	GI upset, headache, retinal damage and cataracts, rarely myelotoxicity, psychosis. Contraindicated in epilepsy.* Reduce dose in renal failure	Resistance is widespread, but confined to *Plasmodium falciparum*. Not active against dormant hepatic forms (hypnozoites) of *P. vivax* and *P. ovale*
Proguanil	GI upset, rarely mouth ulcers. Reduce dose in renal failure	Prophylaxis only
Quinine	Tinnitus, hypoglycaemia, headaches, flushing, GI upset, rash, myelotoxicity	Agent of choice for treatment of chloroquine-resistant or severe *Plasmodium falciparum* malaria
Fansidar (pyrimethamine and sulfadoxine)	Skin rash, myelotoxicity	For eradication of *Plasmodium falciparum* infection
Maloprim (pyrimethamine and dapsone)	Skin rash, myelotoxicity	Prophylaxis only
Halofantrine	Contraindicated in pregnancy. GI upset, pruritus, transient elevation of serum transaminases, cardiotoxicity	Treatment of uncomplicated *Plasmodium falciparum* infection
Primaquine	GI upset, haemolysis, particularly in G6PD deficiency	Eradication of dormant hepatic forms (hypnozoites) of *Plasmodium vivax* and *P. ovale*
Mefloquine	Contraindicated in first trimester, breast-feeding, neurological disease, epilepsy* (including family history), liver disease, concurrent β-blocker therapy. Causes neuropsychiatric effects and GI upset. Avoid pregnancy for 3 months after stopping treatment. Treatment duration should not exceed 1 year	Prophylaxis and treatment of chloroquine-resistant. *Plasmodium falciparum* malaria

*Doxycycline is an alternative in epileptic patients.
GI, Gastrointestinal; G6PD, glucose-6-phosphate dehydrogenase.

Table 20.3 Antimalarial drugs. (Reproduced with permission from Wilks, Farrington & Rubenstein, *The Infectious Diseases Manual*, Blackwell Science, 1995.)

patients are given antibiotics, they are more likely to become chronic excretors of resistant *S. typhi* (antibiotic-induced resistance).
• Typhoid must be reported to the public health authorities.
• Excretors of *S. typhi* are not allowed to work in the food industry.

Dysentery

Bacillary dysentery

Bacillary dysentery is caused by the genus *Shigella. S. sonnei* is the most common and occurs in outbreaks in children's homes. It produces the most serious clinical form of the disease, including septicaemia.

It is transmitted by faecal contamination of food and water and 2–4 days after ingestion produces acute diarrhoea, sometimes accompanied by abdominal colic, vomiting and tenesmus. If severe, there is rectal blood, mucus and pus.

Asymptomatic carriage can occur.

The disease is prevented by good sanitation, clean water supplies and good personal hygiene.

Infected patients should be isolated and rehydrated. Antibiotics (ciprofloxacin or trimethoprim) are required if the patient is septicaemic.

The public health service must be informed and patients and close contacts should not handle food until the stool cultures are negative.

Shigella dysentery can be confused with *Salmonella* food poisoning, amoebic and ulcerative colitis (p. 220).

Amoebic dysentery

This is an infection of the colon by the protozoon *Entamoeba histolytica*. In the acute dysenteric form, the illness begins suddenly with fever, abdominal pain, nausea, vomiting and diarrhoea containing mucus and blood. More commonly, amoebic colitis presents less acutely with intermittent diarrhoea with or without abdominal pain, mucus and blood.

The major complications are hepatic abscesses and pericolic amoebomas which can be confused with colonic carcinoma. The diagnosis is made by finding trophozoites or cysts in fresh faeces, rectal mucus or rectal biopsy and supported by a positive complement fixation test.

Metronidazole is the treatment of choice for all invasive forms of amoebiasis, but abscesses may have to be drained if they do not resolve on drug therapy. Diloxanide is used to eradicate chronic amoebic cysts.

Cyst excretors should not handle food, and the contacts should be screened. Acute amoebiasis can be confused with bacillary dysentery, *Salmonella* food poisoning and ulcerative colitis, and chronic infection with *Giardia lamblia*, tropical sprue, ulcerative colitis and diverticular disease (p. 228).

Giardiasis

G. lamblia is a flagellate protozoon which infects the small intestinal wall but not the blood. Viable cysts are ingested with contaminated food and may be excreted asymptomatically, or produce diarrhoea and steatorrhoea.

The diagnosis is confirmed by the presence of trophozoites or cysts in stools or duodenal aspirates.

Tinidazole and metronidazole are the drugs of choice.

Pyrexia of unknown origin

There are many definitions of pyrexia of unknown origin. In practice, the difficulty arises when the cause is unidentified after the clear clinical possibilities have been excluded, and a basic set of tests performed. It is usually a hospital problem. A broad-spectrum antibiotic has usually been given. The causes are listed in Table 20.4.

Special points in the history
• Exposure to infection (meals away from home, febrile illness in household contacts, unpasturized milk or cheese, undercooked eggs and poultry).
• Occupation, especially if a doctor or nurse (factitious fever). Farmer, veterinary surgeon, sewer worker, forester (for *Brucella*, *Leptospira*, anthrax, cat-bite fever, Lyme disease).
• Drug history, e.g. antibiotics, methyldopa, hydralazine, phenytoin, including non-prescribed preparations.
• Travel (malaria, amoebiasis) and sexual history.
• Pets, including dogs, cats and birds.

Special points in examination
NB Repeat regularly, e.g. on alternate days, if the fever persists.
• *Cardiovascular*. Murmurs, especially if changing, suggest infective endocarditis. Tender temporal arteries. Dressler syndrome.
• *Respiratory*. Crackles (crepitations or rales) for early pneumonia (e.g. Legionnaires dis-

MNEMONIC—*IMAGINE*		
Infections	*Bacterial.* Bacillary endocarditis and septicaemia (including culture-negative)	
	*Collections of pus	
	Subphrenic	
	Intrahepatic	
	Perirenal	
	Pelvic	
	Pleura	
	Bone (osteomyelitis)	
	Viral/rickettsial	
	(including hepatitis B)	
	Protozoal	
	Malaria, amoeba, spirochaetes	
	Specific	
	Tuberculosis* (all sites), typhoid, *Brucella*, Lyme disease (*Borrelia burgdorferi*)	
Malignancy	Kidney and liver (primary and secondary)	
	Pancreas, micrometastases, lymphoma (Hodgkin and non-Hodgkin), leukaemia	
Autoimmune	*Systemic lupus erythematosus, polyarteritis nodosa, systemic vasculitis	
diseases	Chronic active hepatitis	
	Rheumatoid disease, Still disease (including adult Still disease, p. 134)	
Granulomas	Sarcoid	
	Crohn disease	
Iatrogenic	Drug fever	
Nurses and	Factitious fever	
doctors and all		
paramedicals		
Etcetera	Consult exhaustive lists in big books, but remember that the cause is more often a rare manifestation of a common disease than a common manifestation of a rare disease	

*Denotes a more likely cause of pyrexia of unknown origin—all are treatable and potentially curable.

Table 20.4 Mnemonic list (*imagine*).

ease). Sinuses. Consider recurrent pulmonary thromboembolic disease.
• *Abdomen.* Palpable liver, gall bladder or spleen (with or without tenderness).
• *Musculoskeletal.* Muscle stiffness and tenderness of collagen diseases, e.g. polymyalgia rheumatica.
• *Skin rashes* (drugs, rose spots of typhoid). Splinter haemorrhages. Osler's nodes.
• *Lymphatic.* Glands (all group).
• *Check all orifices*: mouth (teeth for apical abscesses), ears, perineum (anus and genitourinary tract).

Basic screening tests already performed (check)
Most will need to be repeated until a diagnosis has been achieved.

• *Haemoglobin.* If anaemia is present and considerable, it is usually relevant. If iron-deficient and there is no overt blood loss, exclude gut malignancy.
• *White blood cell* (WBC) count. Neutrophilia is associated with pyogenic infection and neoplasia, and neutropenia with viral infection. Lymphocytosis may suggest tubercle. Leukaemia and infectious mononucleosis are usually associated with abnormal peripheral counts and cell types (remember direct tests for infectious mononucleosis). Eosinophilia may suggest parasites or polyarteritis nodosa.
• *Erythrocyte sedimentation rate.* If over 100 mm/h, check for myeloma, polymyalgia rheumatica, and secondaries from carcinoma in bone or liver (see also p. 300).
• *Mid-stream urine.* Haematuria, possibly

microscopic, occurs with bacterial endocarditis, renal carcinoma, polyarteritis nodosa and leptospirosis. WBCs in infection. Early morning urine for acid-fast bacillus (AFB). NB Glycosuria suggests infection somewhere.

• *Chest X-ray.* Carcinoma (primary or secondary) in lungs, and bone metastases. Miliary shadowing in miliary tuberculosis and sarcoid. Hilar nodes in tuberculosis, lymphoma, sarcoid and carcinoma.

• *Sputum* for microorganisms, including AFB.

• *Liver function tests* (LFTs) for secondary or primary malignancy, abscess, biliary disease, hepatitis (p. 39).

• *Infectious mononucleosis* screening test, e.g. Monospot.

• *Blood culture* ($\times$ 3).

Further tests commonly required as determined by clinical leads

• Agglutination enzyme-linked immunosorbent assay (ELISA) tests for *Salmonella*, *Brucella* and *Coxiella*.

• Viral, mycoplasma and human immunodeficiency virus (HIV) antibody titres immediately and 2 weeks later.

• Antistreptolysin O titre and rheumatoid factors.

• Autoimmune screen (etc.).

• Ultrasound or computed tomographic (CT) scan of abdomen for liver abscesses, and for secondaries, for renal tumours and abscesses, and for splenic enlargement, and of the pelvis for pelvic lesions.

• Echocardiography for vegetations.

• CT scanning of chest for lymphadenopathy and infection.

Invasive procedures as indicated

• Temporal artery biopsy.

• Liver needle biopsy (tuberculosis, granulomas, neoplasm).

• Muscle biopsy.

Go back again and again to take a new history, to re-examine the relevant areas, and to repeat selected investigations, especially those which might have been performed too early, i.e. before they could have become abnormal.

Other imported pathogens: nematodes, schistosomes

The worms listed in Table 20.5 are found worldwide and not uncommonly in travellers who live rough or enter areas of poor sanitation.

COMMON WORMS

Worm	Major clinical features	Treatment
Threadworm	Anal itch	Piperazine
(*Enterobius vermicularis*)	Worm on stool	Thiabendazole (treat all household members to prevent reinfection)
Roundworm	Worm on stool	Piperazine
(*Ascaris lumbricoides*)		
Hookworm	Nil. If severe infection,	Bephenium (Alcopar)
(*Necator americanus*:	iron-deficient anaemia;	Pyrantel
Ancylostoma duodenale)	malnutrition in children	Tetrachloroethylene
	Eggs or worms in stools	
Schistosoma	Fever and eosinophilia	
1 *S. mansoni* (spur on side)	Initially diarrhoea	
2 *S. haematobium* (spur on tail)	Haematuria	Praziquantel (for both)

Table 20.5 Worms commonly found in areas of poor sanitation.

Septicaemia (bacteraemia)

Traditionally this is classified as Gram-positive, Gram-negative or unknown. In practice, bacteraemia occurs most often postoperatively. Less commonly, patients are admitted from home with suspected bacteraemia, often without an obvious source or site of infection (Table 20.6).

Postoperative bacteraemia

The clinical features are of fever, often swinging and with rigors, and later hypotension and oliguria. The major differential diagnosis of postoperative shock is pulmonary embolism.

Management

General measures include good nursing care and fluid and electrolyte balance, and in severe cases intensive therapy, including treatment of shock and renal failure.

Special measures

A wound abscess is often the site of infection and obvious pus must be drained. This may result in a rapid fall in temperature and obviate the need for antibiotics.

The choice of antibiotic depends upon the organism grown from the wound or blood. If the patient's condition demands that treatment must be started before microbiological cultures are available, the type of operation allows a best guess at the likely organism. The choice of antibiotic depends in turn upon the likely organism and local knowledge of antibiotic sensitivities (see Table 20.1, p. 320).

The key management points are:

1 Drain pus.
2 Antibiotics (see Table 20.1 for guidelines for appropriate choice).
3 Expert nursing care.
4 Fluid balance and monitor renal function.

If the patient is shocked:

5 Treat hypovolaemia with plasma or equivalent.
6 Intensive care monitoring of:
   (a) renal function and fluid balance
   (b) right atrial pressure
   (c) left atrial pressure (pulmonary artery flow catheter).
7 Inotropes—dopamine to increase pumping efficiency for hypotension and increased renal

---

SEPTICAEMIA—THERAPY

Postoperative
1 Drain pus
2 Expert supportive or intensive care:
   • Fluids
   • Electrolytes
   • Urine output and renal failure
   • Shock
   • DIC
3 Treat infection with antibiotics

Operation site	Likely organism	Antibiotics of choice ('blind therapy' while awaiting cultures)
Gastrointestinal	Coliforms and anaerobes	Gentamicin, metronidazole plus ampicillin (ampicillin plus gentamicin for *Streptococcus faecalis*)
Hepatobiliary	Coliforms and *Streptococcus faecalis*	Gentamicin or cefotaxime
Urinary	Coliforms	Quinolone or cefotaxime
Gynaecological	Staphylococci (skin) and anaerobes (vagina)	Flucloxacillin and metronidazole (Augmentin for minor infection)
Cardiothoracic/CNS	Staphylococci (skin)	Flucloxacillin

SEPTICAEMIA—THERAPY

Off the streets (differential diagnosis influenza, or malaria in travellers)

1 Observe for site of infection:
  - Throat
  - Leg ulcer
  - Wound
  - History of urinary or chest infection
  - Rash—drugs, virus, staphylococcus/streptococcus
  - Hidden infection—ear, nose and throat, teeth, pelvis, liver, kidney

2 Urgent investigation:
  - White blood cells
  - Chest X-ray
  - Urine examination and culture
  - Blood cultures (± stool)
  - Ultrasound of liver and kidney for abscesses

3 Management:
  - Drain pus if present
  - General expert supportive or intensive care
  - Antibiotic therapy

Skin	Staphylococci (± toxic shock syndrome) β-Haemolytic streptococcus	Flucloxacillin (vancomycin if MRSA suspected)
Gynaecological (vaginitis, abortion)	*Escherichia coli* anaerobes *Streptococcus faecalis, Clostridium, Staphylococcus, Streptococcus* (coliforms and *Streptococcus faecalis*)	Penicillin and gentamicin and metronidazole (anaerobes)
Nil obvious	Probably *Staphylococcus* or *Streptococcus*	Cefotaxime plus metronidazole
	Abscess:	
	Liver (*Streptococcus milleri*, amoebae)	Drain plus penicillin Drain plus metronidazole
	Biliary (*Escherichia coli* and *Streptococcus faecalis*)	Gentamicin plus ampicillin
	Renal (*Escherichia coli* and *Streptococcus faecalis*)	Cefalosporin or quinolone

NB *Shocked patients*:
- Monitor right atrial pressure (+ 8–10 cm H_2O) and maintain circulating volume.
- Monitor left atrial pressure (pulmonary artery flow catheter).
- Inotropes (dopamine, dobutamine).
- Monitor urine output and renal function—dialysis may be required.
- Treat DIC.

NB Antibiotic choice:
- Always seek expert microbiological advice as choice and dosage alters with changing character of organisms.
- Use intravenous therapy initially to guarantee adequate blood levels.

CNS, Central nervous system; DIC, disseminated intravascular coagulation; MRSA, methicillin-resistant *Staphylococcus aureus*.

Table 20.6 Septicaemia: guidelines to initial therapy. Check with local hospital policy.

blood flow. Dopamine will also cause arteriole relaxation to reduce afterload if systemic vascular resistance is high.

8 Treat disseminated intravascular coagulation (DIC) by replacing deficient blood factors as measured. The presence of DIC indicates a poor prognosis, and the best means of treatment remains uncertain. Endotoxin triggers both extrinsic and intrinsic coagulation systems leading to consumption of coagulation factors and in turn to the widespread bleeding of DIC. NB Steroids are not of proven value in septicaemic shock unless there is associated adrenal damage (short Synacthen test).

Human immunodeficiency virus infection

HIV-1 and HIV-2 are members of the Lentivirus family of retroviruses. The virus preferentially infects CD4+ helper T lymphocytes, leading to a decline in CD4 cell counts with impaired cell-mediated immunity. Eventually, the immune system becomes clinically compromised and the patient develops the infectious, neurological and neoplastic complications characteristic of acquired immunodeficiency syndrome (AIDS).

HIV-2 shares 45% sequence homology with HIV-1, and is found mainly in West Africa. It is less pathogenic *in vitro*, and transmission rates appear to be lower.

Viral transmission is through sexual contact (homo- and heterosexual) or blood-borne (intravenous drug abuse or transfusion of blood or blood products). Blood for transfusion must be routinely screened. Approximately 20% of children born to HIV-positive mothers are infected, some through breast-feeding.

Clinical features

Half of cases develop a febrile illness with malaise, headache, pharyngitis, lymphadeno-pathy and maculopapular rash 2–4 weeks after infection. Antibody tests for HIV become positive 2–6 weeks after this illness. Patients then remain free from serious illness for a number of years. They may then develop symptoms

of malaise, fever, weight loss with features of mild immunodeficiency (e.g. oral *Candida*, cutaneous herpes zoster or herpes simplex) or immune dysfunction (immune thrombocytopenia, drug allergies). There may be generalized lymphadenopathy.

Progression to AIDS is defined in the UK by the development of one of the AIDS-defining illnesses listed in Table 20.7. In the USA, a CD4 count $< 200/mm^3$ is diagnostic of AIDS. The rate of progression to AIDS varies considerably—maintenance of normal CD4 counts and low levels of viral RNA in plasma are markers of slower progression.

Opportunistic infections

These remain the most frequent complications of HIV infection.

Candidiasis

Oral *Candida albicans* infection is common, presenting with typical white plaques or mucosal erythema or candidiasis. Topical treatments (nystatin or amphotericin lozenges) may be effective, but oesophageal or genital candidiasis are indications for systemic therapy with fluconazole.

Pneumocystis carinii pneumonia

Exposure is common in the general population, but clinical disease only occurs in severe immunodeficiency. Up to 85% of AIDS patients develop *Pneumocystis carinii* pneumonia (PCP), 60% at presentation. Cough and progressive dyspnoea are accompanied by fever, cyanosis, tachycardia, tachypnoea and confusion. Auscultation of the chest may be normal.

Chest X-ray is normal early in the disease, but widespread, diffuse interstitial shadowing develops. Twenty per cent of cases have atypical features of lobar consolidation, upper zone shadowing or hilar lymphadenopathy. Pneumothorax is a recognized complication. Patients are usually hypoxic.

Diagnosis depends on identification of the organism by microscopy in sputum, bronchoalveolar lavage or transbronchial biopsy, although treatment is often commenced on clinical grounds.

AIDS-INDICATOR DISEASES

AIDS-indicator disease	Comments and qualifications
Bacterial infections, recurrent or multiple	In a child less than 13 years
Candidiasis	Affecting oesophagus, trachea, bronchus or lungs
Cervical carcinoma	Invasive
Coccidioidomycosis	Disseminated or extrapulmonary
Cryptococcosis	Extrapulmonary
Cryptosporidiosis	With diarrhoea for more than 1 month
Cytomegalovirus disease	Onset after age 1 month, not confined to liver, spleen and lymph nodes
Cytomegalovirus retinitis	
Encephalopathy (dementia) caused by HIV	HIV infection and disabling cognitive and/or motor dysfunction, or milestone loss in a child, with no other causes by CSF examination, brain imaging or postmortem
Herpes simplex	Ulcers for longer than 1 month or bronchitis, pneumonitis or oesophagitis
Histoplasmosis	Disseminated or extrapulmonary
Isosporiasis	With diarrhoea for more than 1 month
Kaposi's sarcoma	
Lymphoid interstitial pneumonia and/or pulmonary lymphoid hyperplasia	In a child less than 13 years
Lymphoma	Burkitt's or immunoblastic or primary in brain
Mycobacteriosis	Disseminated, extrapulmonary or pulmonary
Pneumocystis carinii pneumonia	
Progressive multifocal leukoencephalopathy	
Recurrent non-typhoidal Salmonella bacteraemia	
Recurrent pneumonia	Two episodes within 12 months
Toxoplasmosis of brain	Onset after age 1 month
Wasting syndrome resulting from HIV	Weight loss (over 10% of baseline) with no other cause, and 30 days or more of either diarrhoea or weakness with fever

Table 20.7 AIDS-indicator diseases. (Reproduced with permission from Wilks, Farrington & Rubenstein, *The Infectious Diseases Manual*, Blackwell Science, 2002.)

Treatment is high-dose co-trimoxazole (100 mg/kg/day sulfamethoxazole and 20 mg/kg/day trimethoprim) in divided doses orally or intravenously for 21 days. Adverse reactions are common, and intravenous pentamidine 4 mg/kg/day is an alternative. High-dose oxygen and mechanical ventilation may be required in severe disease. Steroids improve survival in patients with hypoxia ($Pa_{O_2} < 9.3$ kPa).

Prophylaxis is continued with co-trimoxazole 960 mg/day three times per week, or monthly inhaled pentamidine.

Mycobacterial infections

Mycobacterium tuberculosis infection may occur as a result of reactivation or primary infection at any stage of HIV infection. Pulmonary presentation may be with typical apical cavitation and fibrosis, or more generalized lung infiltrates. Extrapulmonary tuberculosis (lymph nodes, bone, bone marrow, genitourinary tract, liver, spleen, skin, peritoneum, central nervous system) occurs in 50% of patients. Standard treatment regimens (e.g. isoniazid with pyridoxine, rifampicin, pyrazinamide and

TRIALS BOX 20.1

The **Canadian HIV Trials Network Protocol 010 Study Group** compared rifabutin, ethambutol and clarithromycin (three-drug group) with rifampicin, ethambutol, clofazimine and ciprofloxacin (four-drug group) in 229 patients with AIDS and *Mycobacterium avium*-complex bacteraemia. The three-drug regimen led to more frequent and more rapid resolution, with better survival rates. *N Engl J Med* 1996; **335**: 377–383.

Pierce *et al.* compared clarithromycin with placebo as prophylaxis against *M. avium*-complex infection in 333 patients with advanced AIDS. Clarithromycin was well-tolerated, prevented *M. avium*-complex infection, and reduced mortality. *N Engl J Med* 1996; **335**: 381–391.

The **California Collaborative Treatment Group** compared prophylaxis with weekly azithromycin, daily rifabutin, or both in 693 HIV-infected patients with CD4 counts < 100/mm^3. Combination therapy was most effective but poorly tolerated. Weekly azithromycin was more effective than daily rifabutin, and infrequently selected for resistant isolates. *N Engl J Med* 1996; **335**: 392–398.

Perriens *et al.* assessed whether, among patients with human immunodeficiency virus (HIV) infection and primary tuberculosis in Zaire, treatment should be extended from 6 to 12 months. They concluded that extending treatment from 6 to 12 months reduces the rate of relapse but does not improve survival, and that a 6-month programme of partly intermittent antituberculous treatment may be an acceptable alternative when resources are limited. *N Engl J Med* 1995; **332**: 779–784.

ethambutol) are used, although the duration is usually prolonged (see Trials Box 20.1). Multidrug-resistant tuberculosis is a particular problem in the USA.

Disseminated *Mycobacterium avium* complex infection is one of the most common systemic bacterial infection in HIV-infected adults. It causes fever, night sweats, weight loss, abdominal pain and diarrhoea, and is associated with shortened survival. Clarithromycin monotherapy is effective treatment, but relapses associated with bacterial resistance are common. Combination treatment with rifabutin, ethambutol and clarithromycin may improve long-term survival. A number of studies have highlighted the advantages of prophylaxis.

Cytomegalovirus
Cytomegalovirus (CMV) retinitis occurs in 10% of AIDS patients, usually presenting as unilateral visual loss. Asymptomatic lesions may be detected as fluffy white areas of necrosis and haemorrhage on fundoscopy. Untreated progression to bilateral blindness occurs. Initial treatment is with intravenous ganciclovir. Maintenance therapy with oral or intravenous ganciclovir is continued, although ultimately progression occurs.

CMV encephalitis presents with cognitive loss, motor and behavioural abnormalities. It can be difficult to distinguish from other causes of AIDS dementia complex (direct effect of HIV infection, herpes simplex encephalitis, *Toxoplasma gondii*), although diagnosis can be established by brain biopsy. Response to ganciclovir is limited.

Cryptococcal infection
Cryptococcus neoformans is a capsulate yeast, widely present in bird droppings. Infection occurs by inhalation. Meningitis is the most common manifestation in AIDS, although pneumonia and skin sepsis also occur.

Presentation of cryptococcal meningitis is usually non-specific, with prolonged fever, headache, malaise, nausea and vomiting. Diagnosis is confirmed by identification of capsulate yeasts or cryptococcal antigen in cerebrospinal fluid. Treatment is with intravenous amphotericin followed by oral fluconazole, continued as life-long maintenance therapy.

Toxoplasma
Primary infection with the protozoan *Toxoplasma gondii* is usually acquired during childhood by eating infected cat faeces or

undercooked meat. An infectious mononucle-osis-type illness is followed by persistence of *Toxoplasma* cysts in the central nervous system and elsewhere. Vertical transmission from mother to child also occurs and causes fetal abnormalities, including central nervous system abnormalities.

Reactivation of *T. gondii* in AIDS usually manifests with neurological features, including fever, confusion, fits and focal neurological deficit. Choroidoretinitis may precede en-cephalitis. Patients are seropositive for *T. gondii* and cranial CT reveals multiple hypodense lesions. Treatment is with pyrimethamine and folinic acid (to reduce haematological toxic-ity of pyrimethamine) and sulfadiazine or clindamycin.

Diarrhoea
Abdominal pain, diarrhoea and weight loss are common, and usually indicate infection, although no specific pathogen is identified in 25–50% of cases. Bacterial pathogens such as *Salmonella*, *Shigella*, *Campylobacter jejuni*, *Giardia lamblia* and *Entamoeba histolytica* should be excluded by stool microscopy and culture. *Cryptosporidium parvum* usually causes a self-limiting illness in normal in-dividuals, but causes severe, prolonged diar-rhoea in AIDS patients who may also develop cholangitis and cholecystitis. It may respond to paromycin.

Herpes simplex
Recurrent oral, genital or perianal ulceration is common and usually responds to systemic (oral or intravenous) acyclovir. Herpes simplex encephalitis typically presents with headache, fever, confusion and temporal lobe abnormal-ities. Culture of cerebrospinal fluid is usually negative for herpes simplex. Diagnosis can be established by brain biopsy, but treatment with intravenous acyclovir is usually started on clinical grounds.

Herpes zoster
Cutaneous dissemination of typical herpes zoster (p. 296) can occur. Treatment is with intravenous acyclovir.

Progressive multifocal leukoencephalopathy
Progressive multifocal leukoencephalopathy (PML) is caused by reactivation of the Poly-omavirus JC which is a common asymptomatic infection in childhood. Two per cent of AIDS patients develop PML with development of multiple, progressive, neurological defects. CT scan shows multiple non-enhancing lesions. Brain biopsy may be required to exclude other treat-able lesions. There is no specific treatment for PML.

Malignancy
Kaposi's sarcoma, non-Hodgkin's lymphoma and cervical carcinoma are all AIDS-defining illnesses.

Kaposi's sarcoma occurs almost exclusively in homosexual males, suggesting that an addi-tional sexually transmitted agent is important. Palpable, violaceous cutaneous nodules occur most commonly on the head and neck. Lesions also occur in other organs, including lungs and gastrointestinal tract. Radiotherapy can cause regression of local disease.

Non-Hodgkin's lymphoma often presents with widespread extranodal disease. Differentiation of central nervous system lymphoma from *Toxoplasma gondii* infection can be difficult and require brain biopsy.

Cervical carcinoma, abnormal cervical cyto-logy and human papillomavirus infection are all more common in HIV-infected women, who should have cervical smears at least annually.

Primary treatment of HIV
The development of therapies for AIDS requires an understanding of how the HIV-1 virus integrates into the human genome, and how viral replication and viral gene expression are regulated.

The proviral genome of HIV-1 is 9–10 kb long, and has three main structural genes:
• The *gag* (group-specific antigen) gene encodes the core protein antigens of the virion (intact virus particle). These are formed as the cleaved products of a larger precursor protein.
• The *pol* (polymerase) gene encodes the viral reverse transcriptase, and also the IN protein required for integration of viral DNA into the host genome.

TRIALS BOX 20.2

The **Viral Activation Transfusion Study (VATS)** assessed the benefit of highly active anti-retroviral therapy (HAART) in 528 HIV-infected patients with cytomegalovirus (CMV) seropositivity or who were receiving a first red blood cell transfusion for anaemia. The data supported an independent reduction in mortality and opportunistic events attributable to HAART, even in patients with very advanced HIV disease. *Ann Intern Med* 2001; **135**: 17–26.

The **HIV Outpatient Study Investigators** studied morbidity and mortality among patients with advanced human immunodeficiency virus infection. Data was analysed on 1255 patients, each of whom had at least one CD4 cell count below 100 cells/mm^3. Mortality among the patients declined from 29.4 per 100 person-years in the first quarter of 1995 to 8.8 per 100 in the second quarter of 1997. The incidence of any of three major opportunistic infections (*Pneumocystis carinii* pneumonia, *Mycobacterium avium*-complex disease, and cytomegalovirus retinitis) declined from 21.9 per 100 person-years in 1994 to 3.7 per 100 person-years by mid-1997. The decline in morbidity and mortality as a result of AIDS was attributed to the use of more intensive antiretroviral therapies. *N Engl J Med* 1998; **338**: 853–860.

The **Multicenter AIDS Cohort Study Investigators** studied the effectiveness of potent antiretroviral therapy on time to AIDS and death in men with known HIV infection duration. In the calendar period when potent antiretroviral therapy was introduced, the time to development of AIDS and time to death were extended, and rate of CD4 cell count decline was arrested. *J Am Med Assoc* 1998; **280**: 1497–1503.

The **EuroSIDA Study Group** examined the change in mortality rates of HIV-1-infected patients across Europe during 1994–98, and assessed the extent to which changes can be explained by the use of new therapeutic regimens. The mortality rate from March to September 1995 was 23.3 deaths per 100 person-years of follow-up, and fell to 4.1 per 100 person-years of follow-up between September 1997 and March 1998. From March to September 1997 the death rate was 65.4 per 100 person-years of follow-up for those on no treatment, 7.5 per 100 person-years of follow-up for patients on dual therapy, and 3.4 per 100 person-years of follow-up for patients on triple-combination therapy. A large proportion of the reduction in mortality could be explained by new treatments or combinations of treatments. *Lancet* 1998; **352**: 1725–1730.

The first trial (**HIV-1 Vaccine Trial Group**) of an HIV-1 vaccine, called 'ALVAC-HIV', which uses a live recombinant canarypox vector to express envelope and core genes of HIV-1, has started in Africa. *Br Med J* 2002; **324**: 226–229.

• The *env* gene encodes the two envelope glycoproteins, which are cleaved from a larger precursor.

When the HIV virion binds to a CD4 molecule on the cell surface, a conformational change occurs in the envelope glycoprotein, and the virus enters the cell via fusion of lipid bilayers at the cell surface. The uncoated core of the virion then uses its viral reverse transcriptase to transcribe one of the two identical strands of positive-sense RNA into DNA. This DNA is duplicated by a host cell DNA polymerase, and migrates to the nucleus where it is integrated at a random site into the genome. Transcription of the integrated viral DNA is regulated by both host factors (such as the DNA-binding protein NFκB), and viral regulatory proteins such as the tat and rev proteins. Virally encoded proteins are processed and assembled in the cytoplasm, and then bud from the cell surface as new infectious virions.

Therapy for AIDS

Despite increased understanding of the molecular biology of HIV infection, therapies remain elusive and AIDS remains a progressive, fatal disease. Several sites in the viral life cycle have been targeted, and effective treatment requires combination therapy (see Trials Box 20.2).

Inhibition of reverse transcriptase. Zidovudine (AZT) was the first anti-HIV drug to be introduced. It is a nucleoside analogue, which bind preferentially to viral reverse transcriptase compared to human DNA polymerase. Other nucleoside reverse transcriptase inhibitors include didanosine (ddI), dideoxycytosine (ddC; zalcitabine), abacavir, lamivudine and stavudine. Efavirenz and nevirapine are non-nucleoside reverse transcriptase inhibitors.

Protease inhibitors. Ritonavir, indinavir, amprenavir, lopinavir, nelfinavir and saquinavir prevent viral maturation. Gastrointestinal side-effects are common (nausea, diarrhoea, abdominal pain, vomiting). Protease inhibitors are associated with lipodystrophy, and hyperlipidaemia, insulin resistance and hyperglycaemia.

Highly active antiretroviral therapy. Combination anti-retroviral therapy for HIV infection has revolutionized the treatment of HIV and AIDS. Such treatment, which usually includes two nucleoside reverse transcriptase inhibitors and at least one protease inhibitor or one non-nucleoside reverse transcriptase inhibitor is called highly active antiretroviral therapy (HAART). Cohort studies has shown that HAART reduces morbidity and mortality.

HIV vaccines

Emphasis is currently being placed on the development of vaccines against HIV. In addition to their importance in prevention, vaccines may also induce additional immunity to any immunity generated as a consequence of natural infection in patients.

A number of therapeutic trials using either modified whole virus particles or recombinant HIV proteins are currently in progress. The majority of current vaccines are based on the extracellular envelope protein gp120, or the envelope precursor protein gp160. One factor that may limit the success of these vaccines is the high variability of the envelope proteins between different strains of HIV.

Infectious mononucleosis

(glandular fever)

Infectious mononucleosis is a common disease of the young, usually transmitted by saliva, with an excellent prognosis, It is caused by the Epstein–Barr virus (a herpesvirus). Seroprevalence is > 90% in adults.

Clinical presentation

Malaise, fever, sore throat, muscle and joint aches. Examination reveals a tonsillar exudate and palatal petechiae with generalized lymphadenopathy and splenomegaly. A macular–papular rash is common, and more frequent if ampicillin is given for the sore throat. Mesenteric adenitis with appendicitis may occur.

Investigation

The disease is confirmed by a leucocytosis (10–50×10^9/l), with an absolute ($> 4 \times 10^9$/l) and relative ($> 50\%$ of total white cells) increase in mononuclear cells. Patients with infectious mononucleosis produce IgM antibodies that bind to and agglutinate red cells from other species.

Thrombocytopenia and abnormal liver function tests are common but rarely severe.

Complications

Tonsillar enlargement may be severe and prevent swallowing of saliva and even threaten airway obstruction. Rare complications include splenic rupture, autoimmune haemolytic anaemia, encephalitis, transverse myelitis, Bell's palsy and Guillain–Barré syndrome. Lethargy may last for several months.

Differential diagnosis

The disease may be confused with:
• acute tonsillitis;
• infections which produce a similar rash, e.g. measles, rubella;
• infections which produce similar malaise and lymphadenopathy, e.g. toxoplasmosis, brucellosis and tuberculosis;

SUMMARY OF BTS RECOMMENDATIONS

	Initial phase	Months	Continuation phase	Months
Respiratory and non-respiratory	I, R, P, (E)*	2	I, R	4
Meningitis/central nervous system	I, R, P, (E)*	2	I, R	10

I, isoniazid; R, rifampicin; P, pyrazinamide; E, ethambutol.
Liver function tests (LFTs) should be checked before starting therapy. Transient asymptomatic increases in serum transaminases are very common after starting treatment. Discontinuation is not indicated unless there are symptoms of hepatitis (anorexia, vomiting, hepatomegaly) or jaundice. It is not necessary to monitor LFTs except in patients known to have pre-existing liver disease. Steroids are used in life-threatening or widespread tuberculosis in an attempt to reduce acute inflammation and allow time for drugs to work. They are usually indicated for pericarditis, extensive pulmonary disease, moderate or severe meningitis, ureteric tuberculosis and pleural effusion.
*Ethambutol may be omitted in certain circumstances.

Table 20.8 British Thoracic Society (BTS) recommendations for treatment of tuberculosis. (For full recommendations see *Thorax* 1998; **53**: 536–548.)

- lymphomas and leukaemias;
- AIDS;
- drug hypersensitivity; and
- acute appendicitis.

NB Diphtheria should not be forgotten.

Treatment

Usually rest, aspirin gargles and anaesthetic lozenges for the sore throat are sufficient. If the tonsillar enlargement is great and swallowing is difficult or the airway threatened (anginose glandular fever—usually with severe general symptoms), a short course of steroids (prednisolone 40 mg/day for 5–10 days) rapidly reduces the symptoms.

Tuberculosis

Tuberculosis most commonly causes pulmonary disease (p. 247) but can affect any site, including the central nervous system (p. 109). In the UK it is a statutory requirement to notify all cases of tuberculosis, an this initiates contact tracing if appropriate. The Joint Tuberculosis Committee of the British Thoracic Society recommends a 6-month short course regimen (Table 20.8), with four drugs in the initial phase,

should be used for all forms of tuberculosis, except meningitis, in children and adults. The fourth drug (ethambutol) can be omitted in patients with a low risk of resistance to isoniazid. In the UK these are previously untreated HIV-negative white patients who are not known to have been in contact with drug-resistant organisms. Drug-resistant tuberculosis is increasing and it is vital to confirm bacteriological diagnosis and drug susceptibility whenever possible. Treatment of drug-resistant tuberculosis, and in particular multidrug-resistance, requires specialist expertise and close collaboration with *Mycobacterium* reference laboratories.

Chronic fatigue syndrome

A report of the joint working group of the Royal Colleges of Physicians, Psychiatrists and General Practitioners used this term to describe the syndrome characterized by a minimum of 6 months of severe physical and mental fatigue and fatigability, made worse by minor exertion. The term myalgic encephalomyelitis (ME) was first used in 1955 to describe an unexplained illness in the staff of the Royal

Free Hospital. Although ME has been linked to chronic fatigue syndrome, it describes a specific pathological process which is not found in these patients.

Apart from profound fatigue, there are no other features or physical signs that distinguish chronic fatigue syndrome. Associated psychiatric disorders, particularly anxiety and depression, are common. There is no convincing evidence that common viral infections are a risk factor for chronic fatigue syndrome, with the exception of the fatigue that follows less than 10% of Epstein–Barr virus infections.

Investigation

No laboratory tests can confirm the diagnosis. The following should be performed to exclude other causes of fatigue:
- full blood count, erythrocyte sedimentation rate;
- urea and electrolytes, liver function test, C-reactive protein;
- thyroid and adrenal function;
- creatine kinase;
- urinalysis for protein and sugar.

Management

A gradual planned increase in exercise is the main objective. Cognitive behaviour therapy helps achieve this in some patients. Antidepressants should be given if there is evidence of an associated depressive disorder.

TRIAL BOX 20.3

The **Centers for Disease Control** in Atlanta produced the CDC-1994 criteria for chronic fatigue syndrome (*Ann Intern Med* 1994; **121**: 953–959):

1 Clinically evaluated unexplained persistent or relapsing fatigue that is not:
- of new onset
- the result of ongoing exertion
- substantially alleviated by rest

and results in substantial reduction in previous levels of occupational, educational, social or personal activities.

2 With four or more of the following symptoms, concurrently present for ≥ 6 months:
- impaired memory or concentration
- sore throat
- tender cervical or axillary lymph nodes
- muscle pain
- multijoint pain
- new headaches
- unrefreshing sleep
- postexertion malaise.

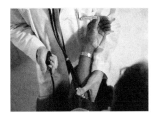

Appendices

Glossary of useful pharmacological terms

FIRST PASS METABOLISM

Metabolism of drugs after absorption from the gut lumen and before entry to the systemic circulation. This usually (but not exclusively) occurs in the liver. For example, glycerol trinitrate (GTN) given sublingually bypasses the liver.

PHARMACODYNAMICS

The study of the action of drugs at their sites of action, or 'the action of drugs on the body'.

PHARMACOGENETICS

The study of the different reactions to drugs based on hereditary differences, e.g. acetylation—'fast' and 'slow' of isoniazid and hydralazine.

PHARMACOKINETICS

The study of drug absorption, distribution, metabolism and excretion, or 'the action of the body on drugs' (Fig. 21.1).

RECEPTORS

Molecules with which drugs interact to produce pharmacological effects. The following terms describe this interaction:
• *Affinity*—a measure of how avidly the drug binds to its receptor.
• *Agonist*—a molecule that interacts with a receptor to produce a response.
• *Antagonist*—a molecule that binds to a receptor but does not activate it. They block the action of agonists.
• *Competitive antagonists* bind reversibly to the receptor—high doses of agonist can overcome the effect.

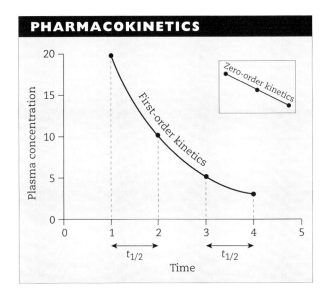

Fig. 21.1 Pharmacokinetics ($t_{1/2}$ = half life).

• *Irreversible antagonists* cannot be overcome by increasing concentrations of agonist.
• *Partial agonists* do not elicit the same response as full agonists, and antagonize the effect of full agonists.

THERAPEUTIC RATIO

The *toxic therapeutic ratio* is better termed the non-toxic therapeutic range. It is the plasma concentration range sufficient to produce a desired effect but below the toxic dose. The greater the ratio (e.g. penicillin when enormous doses are required to cause toxicity), the better.

TRIALS

Phase I

Small studies in normal volunteers to determine the effective dose range and to detect and monitor side-effects and toxicity.

Phase II

Studies on patients which include dose-ranging studies and small clinical trials.

Phase III

Clinical trials comparing the drug with other agents or placebo.

HALF-LIFE ($T_{1/2}$)

The time for the plasma concentration of a drug to fall by half.

ZERO-ORDER KINETICS

The rate of fall of plasma concentration is independent of concentration (e.g. ethanol).

FIRST-ORDER KINETICS

The rate of fall of plasma concentration is related to the concentration, i.e. the more present, the faster the fall in plasma concentration (most drugs).

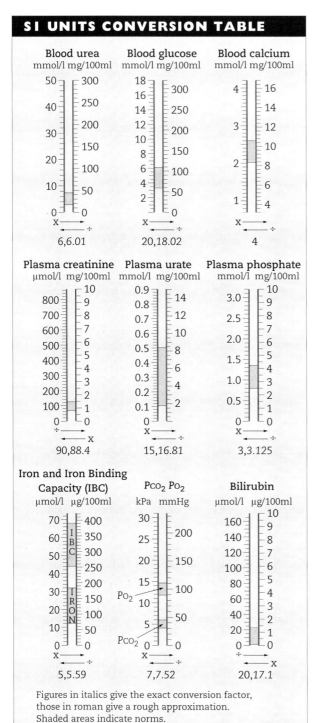

SI UNITS CONVERSION TABLE

Figures in italics give the exact conversion factor,
those in roman give a rough approximation.
Shaded areas indicate norms.

Fig. 21.2 SI units conversion table.

Index